WHAT REVIEWERS ARE SAYING ABOUT

Could It Be My Thyroid?

The American Association of Clinical Endocrinologists website:
"Simply put, this is one of the best, if not THE best patient source for Thyroid Information ..."

Kenneth D. Burman, M.D., in *Trends in Endocrinology and Metabolism:*
"Each chapter is informative, well written, and easy to read and digest ... the book is highly recommended for those who want to understand thyroid disease and its potential treatment."

Robert P. Uller, M.D., in *Thyroid,* the journal of the American Thyroid Association:
"This book is clearly written for the patient ... The book's tables and pictures contain excellent summaries ... All in all, I would advise a patient with a thyroid problem to read *Could It Be My Thyroid?*

Elizabeth E. Puscheck, M.D., in *Fertility News,* a publication of the American Society for Reproductive Medicine:
"One of the more attractive aspects of this book is the section talking about famous people who have thyroid disease ... Famous people can be role models for others affected with thyroid disease and can re-enforce the concept that thyroid disease is common, treatable, and not incapacitating."

Joanne Swenson, RN, MSN, in the Endocrine Nurses Society Newsletter:
"The book is extremely thorough and all aspects of thyroid disease are addressed."

Mary Shomon of The Mining Company (Internet)
"The book features more useful illustrations that I've typically found in other thyroid books, and definitely more photographs, and various tables and charts with summary information. These charts, graphics and tables help make the information more understandable.

"The book is current, and is written in simple, understandable language that does not complicate the issues for those of us without medical degrees."

COULD IT BE MY THYROID?

SHELDON RUBENFELD, M.D.

with a Foreword by President George H.W. Bush

M. Evans and Company, Inc.
New York

M. Evans and Company, Inc.
216 East 49th Street
New York, NY 10017

First M. Evans Edition

ISBN 1-59077-038-2

Library of Congress Cataloging-in-Publication Data

Rubenfeld, Sheldon.
Could it be my thyroid? / Sheldon Rubenfeld, with a foreword by George H. W. Bush.—1st M. Evans ed.
p. cm.
Includes index.
1. Thyroid gland—Popular works. 2. Thyroid gland—Diseases—Popular works. I. Title.
RC655.R83 2004
616.4'4—dc22 2003021280

Editing and Layout by Kathy Kobos

Photography by Bruce Bennett and Mary Urech Stallings

Text Illustrations by Thomas Nash

Printed in the United States of America

This book is dedicated to
Linda, Jesse, and Sarah Rubenfeld.
It could not have been written
without their loving support.

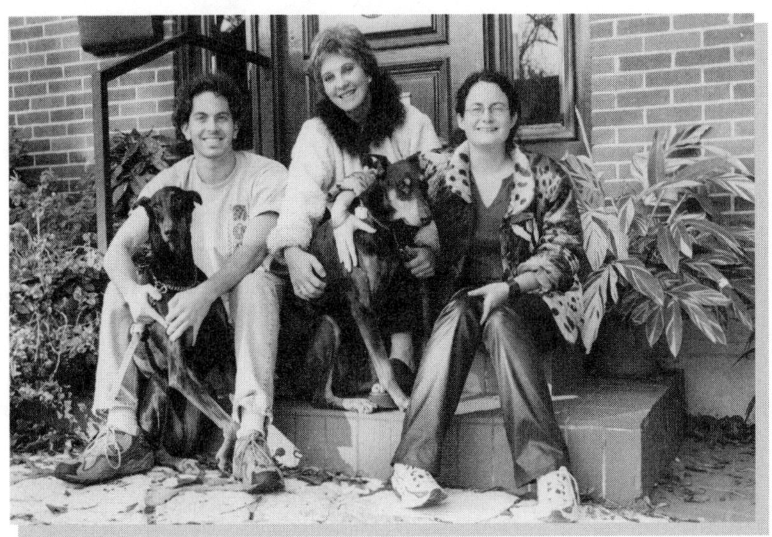

CONTENTS

FOREWORD

Barbara and I are among the more than twenty million Americans who have been affected by thyroid disease. Fortunately, our condition, Graves' disease, was diagnosed early and treated promptly, and now we continue to live full and productive lives.

As the result of the national media scrutiny our disease attracted, many Americans contacted Barbara and me for more information about thyroid disease. We learned that there are millions of Americans who are unaware that thyroid disease is the source of their symptoms. Diagnostic tests and effective treatment are readily available if you know where to turn. It is for this reason that accurate information and public education about thyroid disease is critical.

Could It Be My Thyroid? is an ideal source of information for people living with thyroid disease. It is an up-to-date, comprehensive source of thyroid facts written just for lay people. Within the covers of this book, you will find illustrations, photographs, and tables included with the text to help you understand more clearly what is, and is not, thyroid disease. You can find answers to questions you think of after you leave your doctor's office. And while reading the true-life stories of other thyroid patients and how they have dealt with thyroid disease, you may recognize similarities in your situation or that of a friend or family member.

Dr. Rubenfeld's book contains information that is empowering. If you have, or someone you know has, thyroid disease, Barbara and I encourage you to read this book and to tell others about it.

George H. W. Bush
41st President of the United States

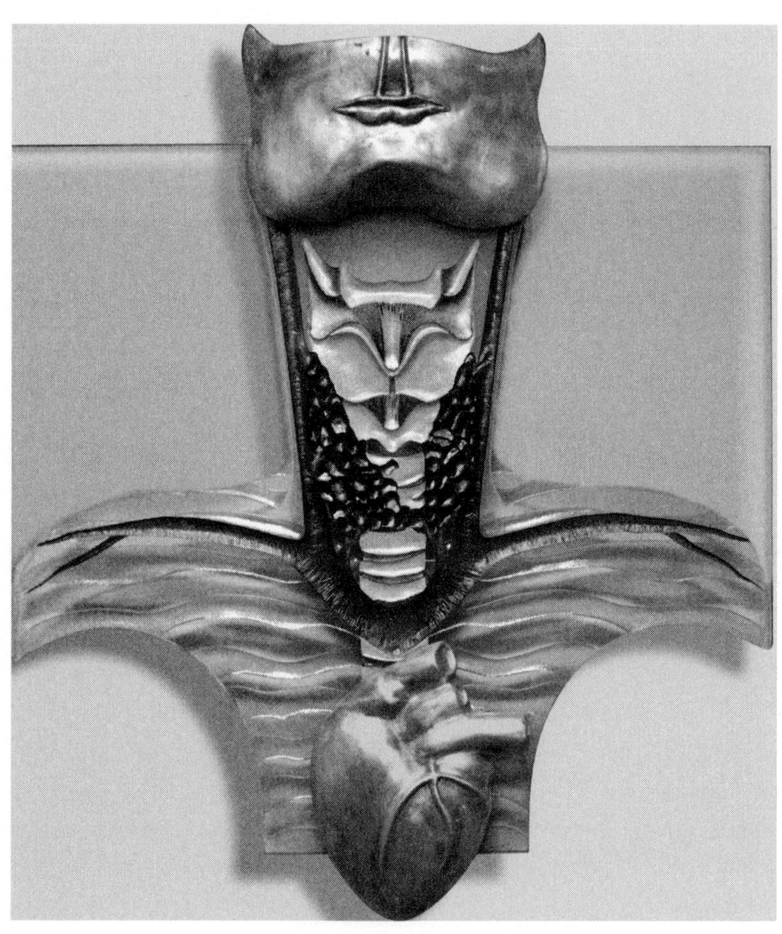

La Tiroide Roja by Patricia Baez

PREFACE

Over the years, I have been asked the same question again and again by patients—"Could it be my thyroid?" Either a friend, a relative, or their doctors have suggested that their fatigue, change in weight, depression, menstrual difficulties, or hair loss is due to a thyroid problem. In some cases, patients recognize in themselves certain signs and symptoms they have seen in their mothers, aunts, sisters, grandmothers, or friends with thyroid disease and wonder if they, too, are suffering from thyroid disorders.

Thyroid disease is very common. Unfortunately, so is misinformation about the thyroid gland from the media and well-intentioned friends and relatives. Misinformation creates fear, anxiety, and doubts about thyroid disease and its treatment. Even though well-informed physicians can provide answers to patients' questions, they may not have either the time or the inclination to do so during an office visit. Patients also often think of questions after they leave a doctor's office. For these reasons, patients need a book that they can refer to as questions arise.

Many symptoms of thyroid dysfunction are also associated with other diseases, leading many people with thyroid disease to believe they are suffering from something else. Patients with known thyroid disease who develop new symptoms may wonder if these symptoms are also related to thyroid dysfunction. On the other hand, many people without thyroid disease believe they have it because they know thyroid patients with the same complaints. I hope that the information provided in this book, together with a physician's guidance, will clarify what is, and is not, thyroid disease.

I have written *Could It Be My Thyroid?* as a reference book for lay people. Every attempt has been made to describe the thyroid gland and thyroid disease in a comprehensive and easily understood fashion. "Translating" medical terminology into everyday language is always a challenge; it is even more so when trying to explain the complexities of the thyroid gland. Some sections, especially Chapter 4, "How Is Thyroid Disease Diagnosed?", may appear complicated and difficult to read. If this should happen, readers may choose to read other sections first, particularly the ones that apply to them.

Since 80 to 85% of thyroid disease occurs in women, a patient is referred to as "she" throughout the book. Similarly, a doctor is referred to as "he" since the majority of practicing doctors are men.

My experience has taught me that most people initially read only the chapter of the book that relates to their own problem. Therefore, each chapter has been written to stand alone. Those patients who read this book from cover to cover may benefit from the built-in repetition of new terms and concepts. I believe the repetition of unfamiliar and complex material will reinforce an understanding of thyroid disease.

To further help readers recognize, understand, and relate to thyroid disease, I have included "Patient Profiles." At the end of most chapters, readers will discover patient stories based on interviews with forty thyroid patients. These patients describe their personal experiences in their own words and offer a unique insight into the impact of thyroid disease on their lives. Some of the patients have had common problems that many readers may relate to, while others have had uncommon experiences that are fascinating.

Each story has more than one point to make about the diagnosis, treatment, or nature of thyroid disease. Any given story could have been placed in one or more chapters. Therefore, it is my hope that you will read all of the "Patient Profiles," since each of these stories is so intriguing and informative—and they put a human face on the technical details of the diagnosis and treatment of thyroid disease.

You will find detailed information that

- describes recent medical developments
- responds to patients' questions about the disease
- counters *mis*information found on the Internet
- recognizes heightened awareness of thyroid disease

Many patients with thyroid disease will pick up this book, read a section, and immediately recognize their own illness. They may be reassured that their symptoms are not unique and that they will get better. After learning more about thyroid disease, readers may suggest to a friend or relative the possibility that they, too, may have a thyroid problem. Some thyroid diseases run in families, and it is likely that a thyroid patient will have a relative with some type of thyroid dysfunction.

I hope that you will share what you have learned from this book with your friends and family. People who have thyroid disease, and people who think they may have thyroid disease, need accurate information. I have written this book to provide answers to questions, to calm fears about thyroid disease and its treatment, and to help patients comply with recommended therapies. Now let us begin to answer the question, "Could it be my thyroid?"

ACKNOWLEDGMENTS

I am grateful to all my thyroid patients who have taught me so much over the years. Their personal observations and insights have given life and meaning to my study of thyroid disease—it has been a privilege and a pleasure to care for them. I especially appreciate those patients who have allowed me to include their stories and pictures in this edition. They have been more than generous in sharing their personal experiences.

I also wish to thank Kathy Kobos of The Kobos Group for her unflagging energy and tireless devotion to this project. She interviewed the patients for the "Patient Profiles," edited the manuscript, designed the layout, and supervised various aspects of the production of the book. Her compassion and sensitivity are evident throughout this book.

A special thank you goes to Phyllis Applebaum, Susan Cashman, Linda Rubenfeld, and Sarah Rubenfeld, who volunteered their time to proofread the manuscript; to Kate Wilson, who offered technical and design advice; to Albert Throckmorton, who corrected my grammatical excesses and omissions; and to Tony Sakkis of Evras Communications, who fine-tuned the final manuscript. I am also indebted to Bruce Bennett and Mary Urech Stallings, whose beautiful photographs enhance the text; to Thomas Nash, whose attractive and precise illustrations clarify difficult concepts; and to Patricia Baez of Elemento Magico who designed the magnificent glass and sculpted pewter creation, "La Tiroide Roja," which hangs in my waiting room and is pictured on page x.

I gratefully acknowledge the contributions of my professional colleagues who reviewed the manuscript. Drs. Mario Maldonado and Victor Silverman graciously reviewed all chapters. Drs. Leonard Wartofsky, Martin I. Surks, Jerald C. Nelson, Charles Soparkar, David G. Orloff, Sam Weber, Ron Moses, and Tom Wheeler kindly reviewed individual chapters. Drs. John Kirkland, Michael Kazim, James Patrinely, Warren Moore, Lynn Hoffman, John Dallas, and Satish Jhingran offered helpful advice regarding their areas of expertise. Dr. Patrinely also contributed photographs of patients' eyes, Dr. Soparkar invited Debbie to contribute

"Debbie's Story," and Dr. Wheeler conceived the sketches of follicular and papillary cancers in Chapters 9, 10, and 11. Pharmacists Shara Zatopec and Kenneth Hughes clarified issues in Chapter 6 related to prescribing levothyroxine. Dr. Usha Joseph contributed the thyroid image seen in Figures 2.4 and 8.3. Dr. Proctor Harvey, a master teacher of cardiology, introduced me to the concept of the "five-finger rule."

Thank you to Dr. Brian Poteet for educating me about thyroid diseases in dogs and cats. And thank you to my nurse, Julie Petru, for introducing me to Dr. Poteet after her cat became hyperthyroid.

In 1979, I first visited the offices of Dr. Joel Hamburger. I thank him for encouraging my interest in thyroidology and for demonstrating how valuable a book like this could be for thyroid patients.

This book would not be in your hands right now without the persistence of my agent, Sheree Bykofsky, and her able assistants, Janet Rosen and Megan Buckley, as well as my editor, P. J. Dempsey, and her able assistant Matt Harper. Thank you very much.

I began my Endocrinology Fellowship at Baylor College of Medicine in 1976, a time when the current president of the Oregon Health Sciences University, Peter O. Kohler, M.D., was chairman of Baylor's Endocrinology Division. Thank you, Pete, for your early and frequent encouragement and support of my choice of a career in thyroidology.

Finally, I wish to thank the celebrities who kindly donated their photographs and statements. Their success stories offer encouragement and inspiration to the more than twenty million Americans with thyroid disease.

Sheldon Rubenfeld
Houston, Texas

COMMONLY USED ABBREVIATIONS

CAT scan – computerized axial tomography

ENT – ear, nose, and throat doctor

I^{131} – radioactive iodine

MRI – magnetic resonance imaging

ob-gyn – obstetrician-gynecologist

PET scan – positron emission tomography

PTU – propylthiouracil

T_3 – triiodothyronine

T_4 – thyroxine or levothyroxine

TSH – thyroid-stimulating hormone

UNITS OF MEASUREMENT

mm – millimeter

cm – centimeter

mcg – microgram

mg – milligram

mU/L – milliunits per liter

pg/mL – picograms per milliliter

ng/mL – nanograms per milliliter

ng/dL – nanograms per deciliter

CHAPTER 1

WHAT IS THE THYROID GLAND?

The thyroid gland is an endocrine gland located in the neck. Its functions are production, storage, and secretion of two thyroid hormones—thyroxine (T_4) and triiodothyronine (T_3). Hormones are chemicals that travel through the blood to every part of the body; thyroid hormones regulate the body's use of energy.

Endocrine glands secrete (release) hormones into the bloodstream. Examples of endocrine glands, in addition to the thyroid gland, are the pituitary gland, parathyroid glands, adrenal glands, ovaries, testes, and those parts of the pancreas that make insulin. Endocrine glands are not to be confused with either sweat glands or with "swollen glands"—a term that people sometimes use to describe swelling of lymph nodes. Doctors who care for patients with disorders of the endocrine glands are called endocrinologists.

The word "thyroid" is derived from the Greek *thyreoeides*, which means shield-shaped. Dr. Thomas Wharton gave the thyroid gland its name in 1656 because of its proximity to the thyroid cartilage, which is shaped like a shield. The thyroid cartilage, commonly called the "Adam's apple," is more prominent in men than in women.

Thyroid diseases may be viewed as disorders of structure and disorders of function. Since disorders of structure and function frequently overlap, and since patients may have more than one thyroid problem, this distinction is somewhat artificial; nonetheless, it will simplify understanding what is, and is not, thyroid disease.

A

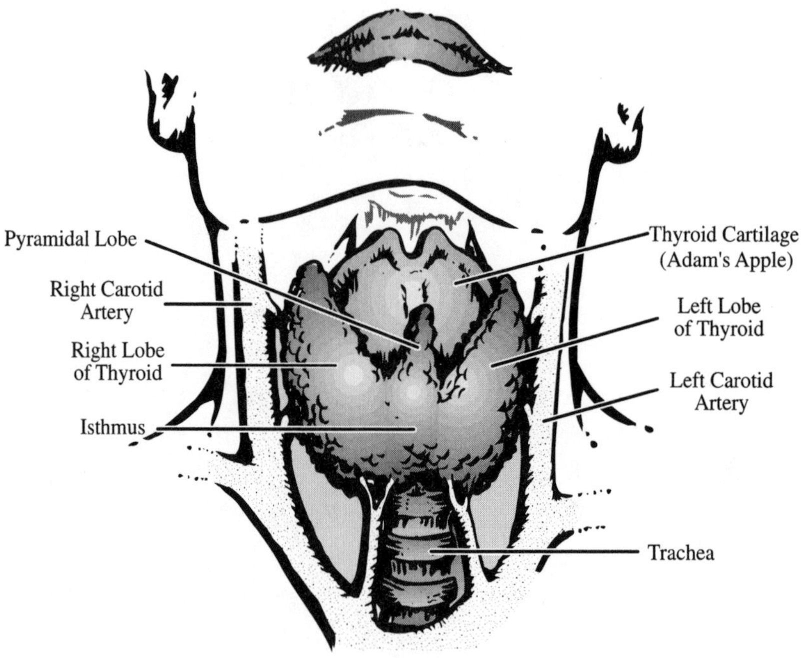

B

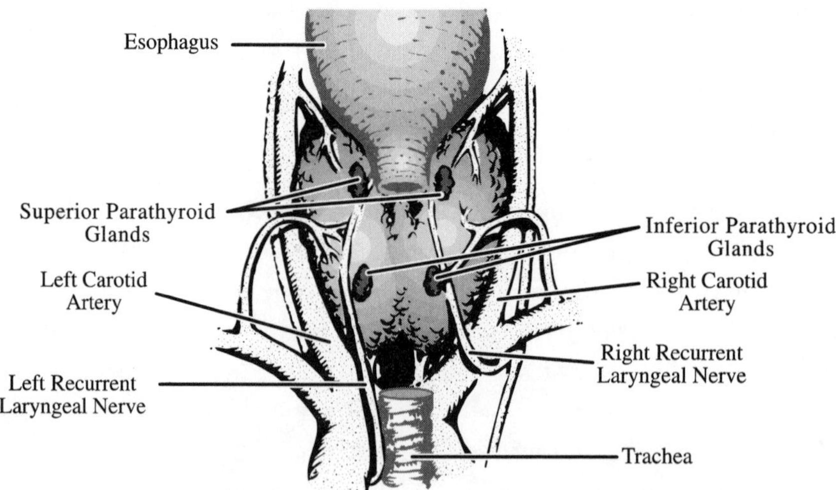

Figure 1.1. The thyroid gland, not drawn to scale. (A) Front view of neck and thyroid gland. (B) Rear view.

Thyroid Structure

The normal thyroid gland, which is shaped like a butterfly, has two lobes connected by an isthmus, and, occasionally, a small pyramidal lobe rising upward from the isthmus. The thyroid gland's relation to other structures in the neck is shown in Figure 1.1. Located in the lower part of the neck, in front of the windpipe (trachea), the thyroid gland moves with swallowing and is often visible, especially when it becomes enlarged. Understandably, the thyroid gland is more easily seen in people with long, thin necks than in people with short, thick necks. Ordinarily, the thyroid gland weighs less than an ounce and has the consistency of muscle. Frequently, the right lobe of the thyroid gland is slightly larger than the left lobe.

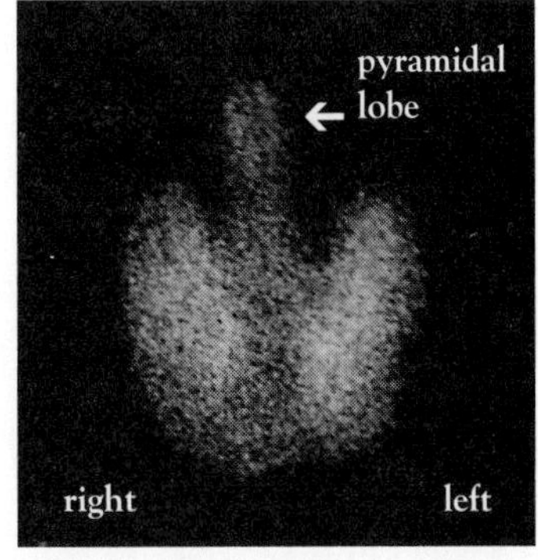

Figure 1.2. Thyroid image of patient with overactive thyroid. Note the large pyramidal lobe.

The parathyroid glands are located close to the thyroid gland. Usually four parathyroid glands are found on the back of the thyroid gland (see Figure 1.1.B). Typically, one parathyroid gland is at the top and one is at the bottom of each lobe of the thyroid gland. The parathyroid glands make parathyroid hormone, which is responsible for maintaining normal calcium levels in the blood. If the parathyroid glands are damaged during thyroid surgery, patients may suffer from hypocalcemia (low calcium).

When viewed under the microscope, the thyroid gland is composed of distinct units called follicles (see Figure 1.3). These are spherical structures lined by follicular cells that make thyroid hormone. In the center of each sphere is a gelatinous material called colloid, which stores thyroid

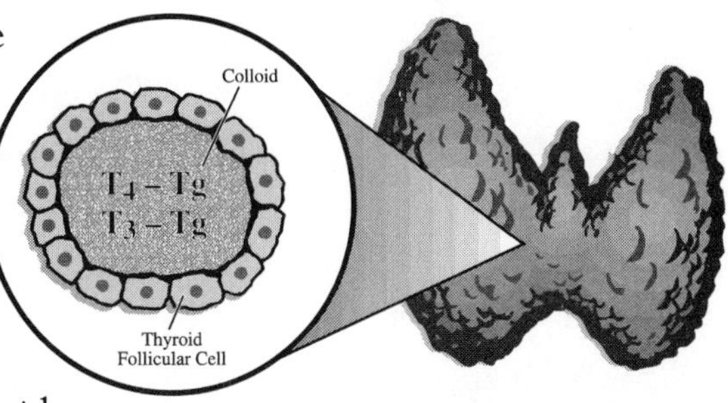

Figure 1.3. Close-up of thyroid follicle.

hormones attached to thyroglobulin (Tg), a protein in which thyroid hormones are made. Malignant tumors arising from follicular cells are called either differentiated (papillary and follicular) or undifferentiated (anaplastic) thyroid cancer (see Chapter 11).

C cells (parafollicular cells) are located in the thyroid gland, next to follicular cells. C cells produce calcitonin, a hormone whose function is unknown. Tumors may arise from C cells and produce too much calcitonin; these tumors are called medullary thyroid cancers.

The majority of thyroid structural abnormalities are either goiters or nodules. The word "goiter" is derived from the Latin *guttur*, meaning throat. A goiter is any enlargement of the thyroid gland. The enlargement may occur uniformly throughout the thyroid gland or may affect one lobe more than the other. Goiters may be caused by an inflammation of the thyroid gland, degeneration of growths within the thyroid gland leading to cyst formation, or a functional disorder of the thyroid gland. Goiters are not commonly cancerous.

A thyroid nodule is a lump in the thyroid gland. If a patient has a solitary thyroid nodule, there is up to a 10% chance that it will be cancerous. Generally speaking, patients with multiple nodules are less likely to have thyroid cancer.

Congenital Abnormalities

People are sometimes born with structural abnormalities of the thyroid gland (congenital anomalies). Approximately one out of every 4,000 infants is born with hypothyroidism (too little thyroid hormone); many times it is caused by thyroid agenesis, the absence of any thyroid gland. On rare occasions, one lobe, typically the left, may fail to develop. When only half of the thyroid develops, it is called hemiagenesis (see "Rhonda's Story" on pages 31–34 and "Kitty's Story" on pages 121–122).

During fetal development, the normal thyroid gland begins to form at the back of the tongue. As development progresses, it moves to its proper location just below the Adam's apple. Occasionally, it does not migrate far enough, in which case thyroid tissue may appear at the base of the tongue (lingual thyroid) or in any place between the base of the tongue and the normal location of the thyroid gland (see "Janet's Story" on pages 9–10). Sometimes the thyroid gland migrates too far and goes into the chest, behind the breastbone (sternum), in which case it may form a substernal goiter. Thyroid tissue may also deviate from its usual path and appear in other places in the neck (aberrant thyroid).

The thyroglossal duct, the connection between the thyroid gland and the tongue, normally disappears after it migrates downward. Sometimes the thyroglossal duct does not disappear completely, and it may appear as a thyroglossal duct cyst, a cystic structure between the tongue and the normal thyroid gland. A thyroglossal duct cyst can be identified by its upward movement when a patient sticks out her tongue. It may become infected and may need to be removed (see "Ralph's Story" on pages 10–12).

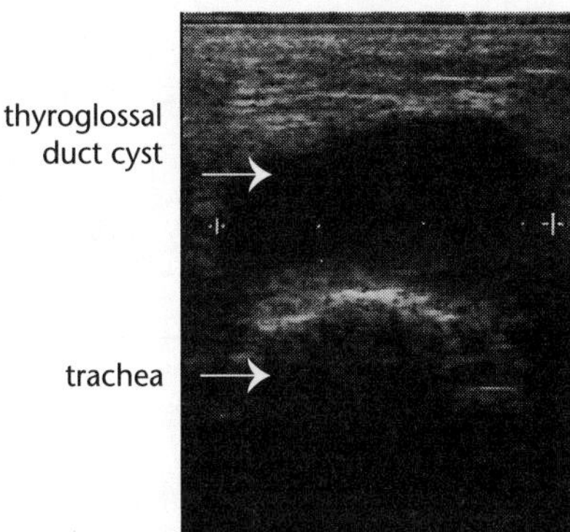

Figure 1.4. Ultrasound of thyroglossal duct cyst (transverse view).

When patients have developmental structural abnormalities, such as lingual thyroid, hemiagenesis, or aberrant thyroid, they may also have functional abnormalities. The abnormal thyroid tissue may enlarge (hypertrophy) and still not be able to produce enough thyroid hormone, resulting in hypothyroidism.

Environmental Factors

Environmental factors can influence the structure of the thyroid gland. For example, insufficient iodine in the diet can cause a goiter. Worldwide, iodine deficiency is the most common cause of thyroid structural abnormalities. An estimated 1.6 billion people living in 130 countries are at risk for iodine deficiency disorders. Approximately 655 million people have goiters from iodine deficiency. In many areas outside the United States, entire populations suffer from enlargement of the thyroid gland due to iodine deficiency (endemic goiter).

Ionizing radiation from nuclear accidents (such as that at Chernobyl), from treatment of cancers such as Hodgkin's disease, or from treatment of a large thymus at birth can cause thyroid nodules. Certain foods, such as cabbage, contain compounds that can block production of thyroid hormone (goitrogens). When eaten in excess, especially in iodine-deficient areas, these foods can cause thyroid enlargement. Medications, such as lithium and amiodarone, can also induce enlargement of the thyroid in susceptible individuals.

Thyroid Function

The functions of the thyroid gland are production, storage, and secretion of thyroid hormones—thyroxine (T_4) and triiodothyronine (T_3). One of the main components of thyroid hormones is iodine. Thyroxine is called T_4 because it contains four atoms of iodine; triiodothyronine is called T_3 because it contains three atoms of iodine.

The thyroid gland, when working properly, maintains a normal balance of these hormones. When patients have normal thyroid function, they are euthyroid. Patients with too little thyroid hormone are hypothyroid; patients with too much thyroid hormone are hyperthyroid.

Thyrotropin (thyroid-stimulating hormone, or TSH), is produced in the pituitary gland and controls production of thyroid hormones in the thyroid gland. TSH is controlled by both thyrotropin-releasing hormone (TRH) from a part of the brain called the hypothalamus and by thyroid hormones in the blood (see Figure 1.5).

TSH circulating in the blood is captured by thyrotropin receptors on thyroid cells, which, in turn, stimulate the thyroid cells to make thyroid hormones. A receptor is a specific site on a cell that selectively captures its corresponding hormone—the hormone fits in the receptor like a key in an ignition switch. When the TSH receptors on the thyroid follicular cells capture TSH, they combine to stimulate, or "ignite," thyroid hormone production.

Once manufactured by thyroid follicular cells, thyroid hormones remain attached to a chemical called thyroglobulin and are stored in the gelatinous colloid located within the thyroid follicle (see Figure 1.3).

The Feedback Mechanism

The pituitary gland controls the thyroid gland much like a thermostat controls an air conditioner (see Figure 1.5). When thyroid hormone production goes down, the pituitary gland (thermostat) senses it and secretes additional TSH. The additional TSH stimulates the thyroid gland (air conditioner) to bring production of thyroid hormone back to normal. When thyroid hormone production increases, TSH production decreases, and thyroid hormone production is reduced to normal. This feedback mechanism maintains the proper level of thyroid hormones in the blood.

Additional information concerning regulation of thyroid hormone stimulation is relayed to the pituitary gland from the hypothalamus via thyrotropin-releasing hormone. Less is known about the influence of thyrotropin-releasing hormone on pituitary and thyroid function than about

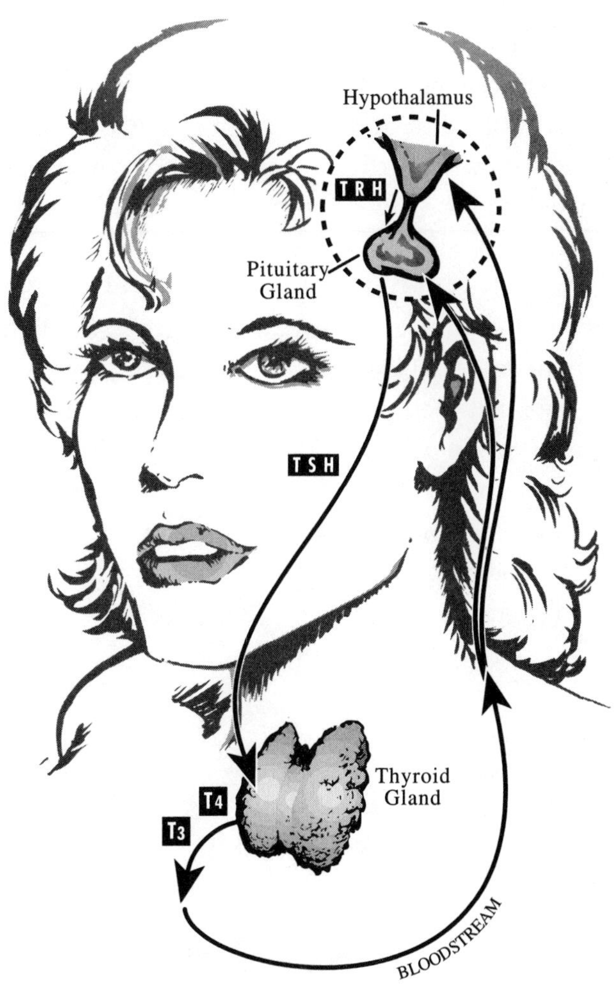

Figure 1.5. Feedback mechanism: hypothalamus, pituitary gland, and thyroid gland.

the influence of TSH on thyroid function.

Although it rarely happens, when the pituitary gland is not working properly (for example, if it forms a tumor), the pituitary's ability to make TSH could be affected. An even rarer condition, known as resistance to thyroid hormone (RTH), may arise if the pituitary's feedback mechanism is defective (see "Bob's Story" on pages 12–14).

Thyroid Hormone-Binding Proteins

Under the influence of TSH stimulation, the appropriate amounts of thyroid hormones are released into the bloodstream. More than 99% of thyroid hormones in the blood are bound to thyroid hormone-binding proteins. Therefore, only 0.03% of T_4 and 0.3% of T_3 are "free" (unbound) in the bloodstream to affect human function and well-being. Abnormalities in these thyroid hormone-binding proteins may have an effect on thyroid hormone function and a profound effect on certain thyroid function test results.

Estrogens, such as those found in birth control pills and in medications given to menopausal women, affect thyroid hormone-binding proteins and, therefore, will alter certain thyroid function test results. If doctors are aware that their patients are taking estrogens, they can take that factor into account when interpreting test results.

Measurements of free T_4 and free T_3 have always been preferred over calculations of free thyroid hormones that rely on indirect estimates of thyroid hormone-binding proteins. Advances in thyroid function testing have now made free T_4 and free T_3 measurements technically and economically feasible (see Chapter 4).

Congenital Abnormalities

As early as the tenth to twelfth week of pregnancy, the fetus develops a recognizable thyroid gland and some thyroid function. Production of thyroid hormones within the thyroid gland requires several enzymes (helpers) to facilitate chemical reactions. Deficiencies of these enzymes can cause enlargement of the thyroid gland and hypothyroidism in the fetus and the newborn. Because these enzymes are not easily measured, their deficiency is most often presumed, rather than proven.

Environmental Factors

Environmental factors can influence thyroid function just as they can alter thyroid structure. Approximately 1.6 billion people worldwide are at risk for iodine deficiency disorders, which include hypothyroidism, mental retardation, reproductive problems, and a wide range of neurological and physical disorders. Iodine deficiency is the leading cause of preventable mental retardation and brain damage in the world. The International Council for the Control of Iodine Deficiency Disorders estimates that iodine deficiency disorders account for varying degrees of mental deficiency in more than 43 million people. Of this number, approximately eleven million are cretins (congenitally hypothyroid patients with severe mental retardation and short stature).

Radiation can cause hypothyroidism by damaging thyroid cells. The resulting hypothyroidism may not become apparent for years, or even decades, after exposure to the radiation. Iodine excess from x-ray dyes and medications containing iodine can also cause thyroid dysfunction. Finally, a variety of medications, such as lithium and amiodarone, can cause changes in thyroid function.

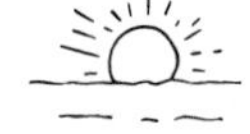

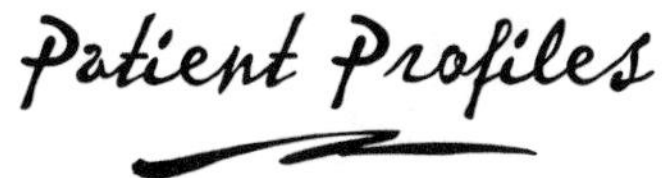

JANET'S STORY

In 1983, while she was in law school, Janet visited her ear, nose, and throat doctor (ENT) because of a persistent sore throat.

> My ENT prescribed antibiotics, but my throat still hurt. While I was on vacation visiting my parents, I saw an ENT there who said he thought my thyroid was at the back of my throat. When I came home from vacation, I went to see another ENT who confirmed that I did indeed have a lingual thyroid. He referred

> me to [an endocrinologist].

Janet recalled that the doctor who performed her tonsillectomy when she was three years old had told her mother "something" about a lingual thyroid. However, since she had had no problems with it, she had forgotten about it until this episode of sore throats.

To confirm her diagnosis, Janet's ENT ordered a CAT scan and esophagram, which revealed a long, flat, broad-based sublingual thyroid projecting into her throat. He also performed a biopsy, which confirmed that the mass at the base of her tongue was a noncancerous lingual thyroid. Later on, Janet consulted an endocrinologist who diagnosed mild hypothyroidism and prescribed levothyroxine.

> I never really had any problems with it other than the sore throats in 1983. I've been taking [levothyroxine] since then. Somewhere between 1992 and 1995, I had to increase the dosage twice. I get tired sometimes, but I really don't sleep a lot. I don't think it has anything to do with my thyroid.

Lingual thyroids are not always apparent at birth. Although Janet's congenital thyroid abnormality did not cause her difficulty, other congenital defects, such as neonatal hypothyroidism, can cause irreversible damage if not detected at birth. Fortunately, neonatal screening programs have markedly reduced the consequences of congenital hypothyroidism.■

RALPH'S STORY

One morning in 1993, thirty-eight-year-old Ralph woke up and saw an unexpected sight in the mirror.

> I knew I had a problem. My throat was so swollen I had no chin. It was huge! Supposedly, I had mumps three times in a row when I was in the second grade. So my first thought was that it was mumps again. I went to my allergist who sent me to an ENT. He said he thought it might be my thyroid and sent me to [an

> endocrinologist]. I took antibiotics, and, within a week-and-a-half, the swelling went down.

During the physical examination, his endocrinologist felt an oval mass measuring 5 by 7 cm (centimeters) in the middle of Ralph's neck, just above the usual location of the thyroid gland. An ultrasound revealed a predominantly cystic mass above a large thyroid gland. Ralph's laboratory results showed that he had thyroid antibodies (indicative of Hashimoto's thyroiditis), low normal thyroid function test results, a high white blood cell count, and an elevated sedimentation rate (indicative of inflammation or infection). The physical examination, ultrasound, and laboratory tests were consistent with a diagnosis of an infected thyroglossal duct cyst.

> In testing me, [my endocrinologist] found out that I had Hashimoto's thyroiditis. He sent me to [a different ENT] who said he needed to take [my thyroglossal duct cyst] out now; it could swell again.

When Ralph visited this ENT, his thyroglossal duct cyst was half the size it had been when he first saw his endocrinologist.

> I put off surgery for a month, but it became swollen again, and I had to have emergency surgery to incise and drain it. Six weeks later, I had my thyroglossal duct cyst removed. Normally, [people] have them removed between the time they are seven and ten. A recurring sinus infection finally had infected my [thyroglossal duct] cyst.

Four months following Ralph's first visit, his endocrinologist felt a goiter and prescribed levothyroxine. Even though Ralph was euthyroid, the medication was prescribed in order to avoid further enlargement of his goiter and symptoms of hypothyroidism from progression of his Hashimoto's thyroiditis.

Some congenital thyroid abnormalities, like Ralph's thyroglossal duct cyst, may not become apparent for years or decades. The presentation of a congenital thyroid abnormality later in life may be confusing and dramatic, but, fortunately, it is usually easy to treat once properly diagnosed.■

BOB'S STORY

Fifty-seven-year-old Bob has always led an active lifestyle. In high school, he was a state-ranked champion sprinter. He worked in the oil fields and served in the military. After leaving military service, he became a state trooper and enjoyed weight lifting.

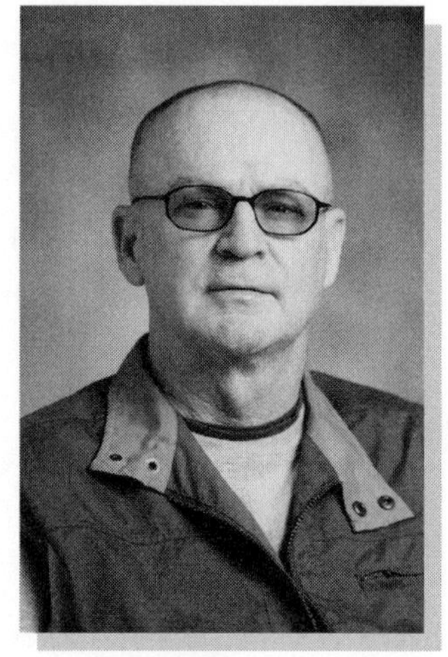

> There were times I didn't feel quite right, but I just worked through any symptoms I might have. I've always been hyper in general and had a hard time in high school with my schoolwork. I was always keyed up. Sometimes I think maybe it had to be my thyroid back then, but who knows? It's just no telling.
>
> When I was lifting weights, I realized my legs felt kind of weak, but I kept on trying. It's just not my nature to quit. I believe in mind over matter. Then I started feeling almost paranoid and was keyed up all the time. It was just unbelievable turmoil. I thought I should have it checked out, and my wife agreed I should get some help.
>
> I went to an endocrinologist, and he ran some tests and told me I had hyperthyroidism. He recommended radioactive iodine, and so I had it. Years later I found out it wasn't hyperthyroidism after all—I had been misdiagnosed.
>
> I went to [another endocrinologist] who found out I

> had thyroid hormone resistance. It was about seventeen or twenty years ago. He noticed that I had strange lab work. I had high TSH levels and still do.

Bob's TSH was quite elevated, as were his T_4 and T_3. After ruling out a pituitary tumor, it became evident that he had a very rare disorder—resistance to thyroid hormone. His endocrinologist referred him to a physician at the National Institutes of Health (NIH) who was a world renowned expert in the study of resistance to thyroid hormone.

> I went up to NIH twice; my whole family went up there, too. While I was there, they found out I had an aortic aneurysm and a bad heart valve. I had open-heart surgery later, but I could've died if I hadn't gone up there for the research study.
>
> [The doctor at NIH] said I had peripheral resistance to thyroid [hormone] and that it was almost absolute that it would affect 50% of the family. My brother doesn't have it, but one of my daughters does. She was about eight years old when we went for the research study and is twenty-eight now.
>
> As far as anyone else in the family, I had an aunt with a goiter, but back then people just didn't know about the thyroid. I take Cytomel—5 micrograms twice a day. I've been taking it for years. At one time, I took both [levothyroxine] and Cytomel, but that didn't seem to work any better.

Although resistance to thyroid hormone is not usually treated with thyroid hormone, Bob's situation presented one of those occasions when treatment with T_3 might be indicated.

> My TSH fluctuates quite a bit; it's always high. But I have no real symptoms. I do things even if I'm feeling weak or tired. I mentally make myself do it. I just keep going through the pain; I do what I got to do. I try to

> stay physical. I do stretching and walking. I walk three miles a day, three times a week.

Resistance to thyroid hormone continues to intrigue researchers, even as the genetic defects in families with this disorder are discovered. Hopefully, when patients with this and other rare conditions are identified, they will be as willing as Bob to work with medical scientists.■

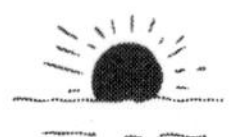

Chapter 2

WHAT IS AND IS NOT THYROID DISEASE?

A disease may be considered a condition in which some part of the body—in this case, the thyroid gland—does not work properly. Thyroid dysfunction can affect every organ in the body and can cause many symptoms of varying severity. In addition, nonthyroidal illnesses are often confused with thyroid disease. This chapter will explain what is, and is not, thyroid disease.

Before turning to that explanation, a word must be said about the nature of suffering, as opposed to the nature of disease. Suffering is an individual's perception of personal experience with a disease and its treatment. For example, some patients may suffer after successful treatment of their thyroid disorder because they continue to have symptoms, which they are convinced are caused by thyroid disease. These patients may suffer not only because they continue to have symptoms but because they also feel misunderstood. Therefore, compassionate physicians will continue working with their patients to identify and explain the true causes of these ongoing symptoms. If patients are open to the possibility that their symptoms are not caused by thyroid disease, then they can begin to find relief of their suffering.

What Is Thyroid Disease

Thyroid disease is common; in fact, it affects more than twenty million Americans. Unfortunately, more than thirteen million Americans have a thyroid condition and are unaware of it. Women are much more likely than men are to have thyroid disease. For reasons that are unclear,

The Prevalence of Thyroid Disease in the United States

THE DISORDER	WHO IT AFFECTS
hypothyroidism	6 – 7 million adults 1 out of 10 women over 65 1 out of every 4,000 newborns
subclinical hypothyroidism	7 – 9% of adult women 3% of adult men
hyperthyroidism	2.5 million people
Hashimoto's thyroiditis	5% of the adult population
postpartum thyroiditis	5 – 9% of women after delivery
thyroid nodules	4 – 7% of the adult population
goiter	5% of the adult population
thyroid cancer	17,000 people per year 1,300 deaths per year

approximately 80% of all thyroid disease occurs in women. The ancients thought the thyroid gland was larger in women than in men to make their necks more beautiful. Regardless of the reasons, women in particular should be aware of the signs and symptoms of thyroid disease as well as the impact it can have on their well-being.

Accurately diagnosing thyroid disease may be complicated since abnormal thyroid function test results are common and many diseases with similar symptoms masquerade as thyroid disease. It is easy to confuse other diseases and abnormal thyroid function test results with actual thyroid disease.

Overall, thyroid diseases may be viewed as disorders of structure and disorders of function. Since disorders of function and structure frequently overlap, and since patients may have more than one thyroid

Women and Thyroid Disease

The following diseases occur more frequently in women than in men:

thyroid nodules	4 times more
Hashimoto's thyroiditis	at least 5 times more
Graves' disease	5 to 10 times more
thyroid cancer	2 to 3 times more
subacute thyroiditis	3 to 6 times more
postpartum thyroiditis	exclusively in women

problem, this distinction is somewhat artificial; nonetheless, it will simplify understanding what is, and is not, thyroid disease.

Functional Diseases

Functional diseases are those involving either too much thyroid hormone (hyperthyroidism) or too little thyroid hormone (hypothyroidism), as opposed to a normal amount of thyroid hormone (euthyroidism). Functional disorders may be permanent or temporary. For example, in certain types of thyroiditis, patients may be hyperthyroid for months and then become hypothyroid for months before returning to the euthyroid state.

Functional diseases may be so mild that they do not cause obvious symptoms. If there are no obvious symptoms and if only the thyroid-stimulating hormone (TSH) level is abnormal, the resulting disease is called subclinical. Asymptomatic patients with elevated TSH and normal thyroid hormone levels have subclinical hypothyroidism, or mild thyroid failure. Asymptomatic patients with low TSH and normal thyroid hormone levels have subclinical hyperthyroidism, or mild hyperthyroidism.

In addition, there are abnormalities in thyroid function test results that may masquerade as thyroid disease. At least two-thirds of all patients hospitalized with nonthyroidal illnesses will have striking abnormalities of their thyroid function test results. This misleading occurrence is so common that it has been given its own name—nonthyroidal illness syndrome (NTIS) or euthyroid sick syndrome (ESS). In these circumstances, it is not the patient's thyroid function that is abnormal; it is the patient's thyroid function *test results* that are abnormal (see "Maiko's Story" on pages 36–40).

Structural Diseases

A person may develop structural disease of the thyroid gland or may be born with a structural defect. Acquired structural diseases of the thyroid gland may be classified as diffuse enlargement of the thyroid gland (goiter) and lumps in the thyroid gland (thyroid nodules). In this book, "goiter" will mean any enlargement of the thyroid gland.

If the enlargement is generalized, relatively symmetrical, and free of nodules, it is referred to as a diffuse goiter. On the other hand, an enlarged thyroid gland that has multiple growths or nodules is called a multinodular goiter. A multinodular goiter should be distinguished from a thyroid gland with only one thyroid nodule, the solitary thyroid nodule, because, in general, solitary thyroid nodules are more commonly cancerous than those nodules found in multinodular goiters. However, a dominant nodule within a multinodular goiter may have the same malignant potential as a solitary thyroid nodule. Diffuse goiters are

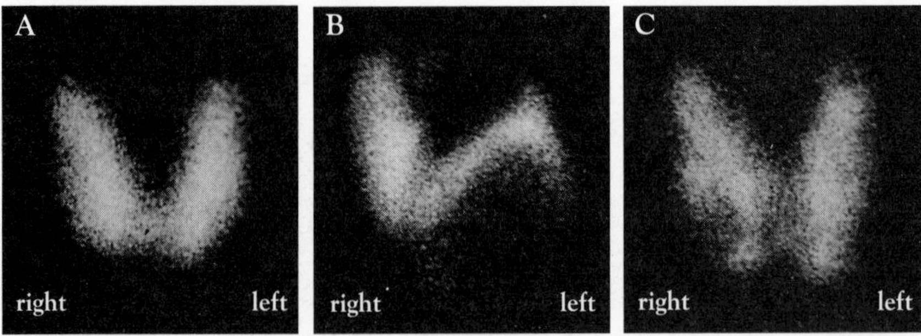

Figure 2.1. Images of thyroid glands. (A) Normal thyroid gland with uniform white appearance. (B) Thyroid nodule, dark area in lower left lobe. (C) Multiple thyroid nodules, dark areas scattered throughout both lobes.

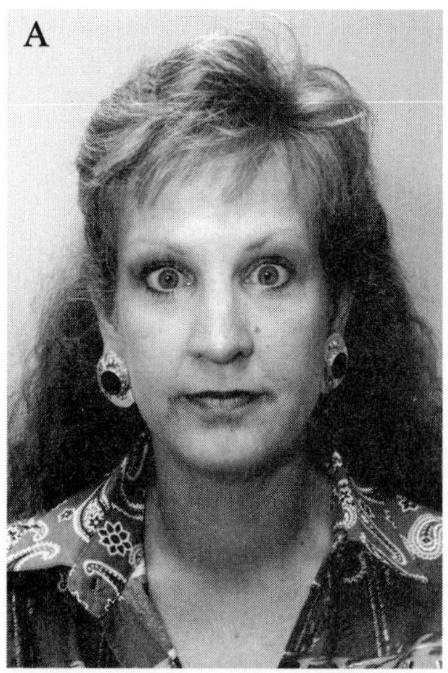

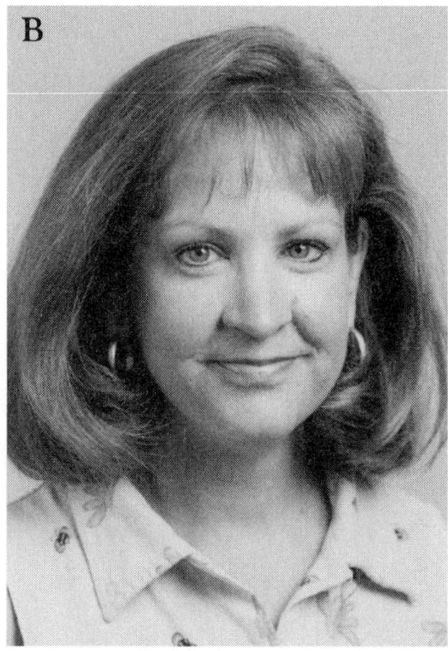

Figure 2.2. Before and after pictures of hyperthyroid patient with a goiter. (A) Note the stare and the fullness in the lower portion of the neck. (B) Note the same areas after successful treatment.

seldom cancerous (see Chapter 9).

The presence of a diffuse goiter, a multinodular goiter, or a solitary thyroid nodule does not indicate whether the patient is hyperthyroid, hypothyroid, or euthyroid. In other words, it is possible to have many combinations of thyroid structural abnormalities and thyroid function (see "Rhonda's Story" on pages 31–34). For example, a toxic multinodular goiter (TMNG) is a goiter with multiple lumps (structural disease) that causes hyperthyroidism (functional disease).

Factors Affecting Thyroid Function and Structure

Several additional factors may influence thyroid function and structure. These modifying factors include:

- autoimmunity
- iodine deficiency
- radiation

- food and drugs
- congenital abnormalities
- fetal factors
- inflammatory processes
- smoking

Autoimmunity

Autoimmunity refers to development of antibodies against one's own body. Ordinarily, antibodies protect against outside invaders, such as bacteria or viruses. However, sometimes the body produces antibodies against its own tissue. Two thyroid disorders, Hashimoto's thyroiditis and Graves' disease, are classic examples of autoimmune disease.

In Hashimoto's thyroiditis, the most common cause of hypothyroidism in the United States, the body develops antibodies to certain elements within the thyroid gland. Graves' disease, the most common cause of hyperthyroidism in the United States, is thought to be caused by antibodies to the thyroid gland, eyes, and, possibly, skin. In a most remarkable fashion, the antibodies formed against the thyroid gland duplicate the function of thyroid-stimulating hormone and stimulate the thyroid to produce too much thyroid hormone.

Even though Hashimoto's thyroiditis causes hypothyroidism and Graves' disease causes hyperthyroidism, each can also cause a goiter. The presence of a goiter does not indicate whether a patient is hypothyroid, hyperthyroid, or euthyroid.

Iodine Deficiency

Iodine deficiency is the leading cause of thyroid disease worldwide, and it is the most common cause of preventable mental retardation and brain damage in the world. Iodine deficiency disorders (IDD) include goiter, hypothyroidism, cretinism (severe mental retardation and short stature), reproductive problems, and a wide range of neurological and physical disorders.

Since iodine has been added to table salt, milk, bread, and other foods, it is very uncommon, if not unheard of, to see thyroid disease as a result of iodine deficiency in developed countries such as the United

The World Health Organization's Recommended Minimum Daily Iodine Intake	
90 mcg	children up to 5 years old
120 mcg	children 6 to 12 years old
150 mcg	adults
200 mcg	pregnant and lactating women

States. Indeed, the average iodine intake in the United States is 300 to 500 mcg (micrograms), compared to a recommended minimum daily requirement of 150 mcg in nonpregnant adults. Nonetheless, iodine deficiency remains a large public health problem in at least 130 of the world's 191 countries.

The risk of iodine deficiency disorders is increased in geographic regions where there is little iodine in the soil. Therefore, crops grown in that soil and animals grazing on the affected land do not yield enough iodine for the people who eat the produce and meats from that region. These soil conditions are most likely to occur in high mountainous areas, in regions with frequent flooding, and in countries far inland. Some of these areas are called "goiter belts" since so many of the people living there eventually develop goiters.

At one time, people dismissed goiters caused by iodine deficiency as merely cosmetic problems. Now iodine deficiency disorders are recognized as major medical problems that can present a threat to the social and economic development of many countries. Therefore, in 1990, the United Nations World Summit for Children issued a mandate to eradicate iodine deficiency disorders by the year 2000. The International Council for the Control of Iodine Deficiency Disorders (ICCIDD), an international, nonprofit, nongovernmental organization with a multidisciplinary network of experts from eighty-two countries, worked with the United Nations to achieve this goal through salt iodination programs. Through these collaborative efforts, the number of countries with salt iodination programs has increased from forty-six to ninety-three.

Iodized salt is the preferred way to add iodine to the diet and eliminate iodine deficiency disorders. There are several reasons that iodizing salt is the ideal method of thyroid disease prevention: salt is universally and regularly consumed; it is inexpensive; the technology to iodize salt is simple; and it is very effective. A teaspoon of iodine is all that a person requires during a lifetime. However, because the body cannot store iodine for long periods, very small amounts are required on a regular basis.

Radiation

Thyroid dysfunction may also occur as a result of exposure to radiation. Years ago, some children were treated with radiation for conditions such as tonsillitis, acne, ringworm, or an enlarged thymus. It is now known that goiters, thyroid nodules, thyroid cancers, and hypothyroidism may result from radiation treatments. Some patients may be unsure whether they had radiation treatments when they were very young. The answers to several questions could suggest whether they had such procedures.

- ***Were parents and medical personnel asked to leave the room during treatment?*** Parents and nonessential medical personnel were asked to leave the room when radiation was used. Nonpatients were not asked to leave the room when children were treated with purple ultraviolet or "UV" light, which does not use radiation and, therefore, does not cause thyroid dysfunction.

- ***Was the treating physician a dermatologist, and was the treatment for the scarring form of acne?*** If the answer is yes, it is likely that radiation was used.

- ***Were rods placed in the nose to shrink the tonsils and adenoids?*** Radiation-tipped rods were sometimes inserted for this purpose. Fortunately, only a very small amount of radiation reached the thyroid gland with this type of treatment.

Patients treated with radiation for cancers, such as Hodgkin's disease, may also develop thyroid problems, particularly hypothyroidism. The dosage of radiation used to treat patients with Hodgkin's disease is much larger than that given to children with acne, tonsillitis, or ringworm. Although one might think that these larger doses of radiation would be more harmful to the thyroid gland than smaller doses would be, this is not the case. Smaller doses appear to stimulate development and growth of thyroid nodules and cancers, whereas larger doses tend to destroy the thyroid gland and cause hypothyroidism.

Radiation from the 1986 nuclear accident in Chernobyl caused thyroid disease, particularly thyroid cancer in children. Nuclear tests conducted by a variety of countries in the 1950s probably caused an increased incidence of thyroid disease in people exposed to the fallout. Similarly, people living near nuclear materials production plants may have an increased incidence of thyroid disease. On the other hand, people who live near incident-free nuclear power plants do not have an increased incidence of thyroid disease.

A different disorder, radiation-induced thyroiditis, may occur as the result of high dosages of external-beam radiation used to treat cancers; it may also result from large doses of radioactive iodine given for a variety of thyroid disorders. The course of this disease is similar to other disruptive forms of thyroiditis (see Chapter 8).

Finally, radiation to the head, for either a benign or malignant brain tumor, can damage the pituitary gland so that it does not produce enough TSH to stimulate the thyroid gland. When hypothyroidism results from a failure of the pituitary gland, it is called secondary hypothyroidism.

Food and Drugs

Food alters the absorption of prescribed thyroid hormone. Medicines, especially those containing iron and calcium, can also interfere with the absorption of thyroid hormone. Therefore, thyroid hormone should be taken with water on an empty stomach one or more hours before taking any other medicines. Other drugs, such as amiodarone, lithium, and interferon alpha, can induce, alter, or profoundly affect thyroid disease and its treatment.

Too much iodine will aggravate many thyroid disorders, including

Hashimoto's thyroiditis and multinodular goiter, as well as interfere with tests and treatments using radioactive iodine. Supplements containing thyroid hormones will also aggravate thyroid disorders and interfere with tests and treatments. Unfortunately, over-the-counter iodine and thyroid supplements are readily available on the Internet, in health food stores, and in some grocery and drug stores. Many well-intentioned patients erroneously assume that supplementing their diets with these products will help them. However, many products will actually harm them by causing or worsening thyroid dysfunction, as well as interfering with tests and treatments.

If patients search the Internet for information about thyroid disease, they are likely to see advertisements and links to sites selling natural products for thyroid dysfunction, weight loss, or energy. Very few sites list the ingredients or the amounts of the ingredients in these products. Therefore, patients cannot actually know what they are taking, and neither can their physicians.

Similarly, products from health food stores may not be adequately labeled. The labels on a variety of supplements contain terms such as "thyroid" or "thyro," leading some consumers to assume the products contain thyroid hormone. A closer look will show that few of these supplements actually list thyroid tissue as an ingredient. If they do, they usually do not state the source or the amount of the thyroid hormone in the products. Typically, iodine from kelp is among the ingredients listed on the labels of these products. The recommendations stated on some labels may range from 450 to 600 mcg of iodine daily, well above the minimum 150 mcg of iodine recommended by the World Health Organization for nonpregnant adults. Since the average daily intake of iodine in the United States is already 300 to 500 mcg, supplementing the typical American diet with iodine is unnecessary and potentially harmful.

Some x-ray dyes contain large amounts of iodine. These dyes can sometimes cause thyroid function test result abnormalities and, uncommonly, symptomatic thyroid dysfunction. CAT scans, arteriograms, intravenous pyelograms (IVPs), heart catheterizations, and myelograms are x-ray procedures that typically use injectable dyes with iodine. On the other hand, the injectable dyes used for MRIs do not contain iodine and, therefore, do not affect thyroid function. Finally, iodine is also found in certain medications (see Chapter 4). In most cases, iodine-free substitutes are available.

Congenital Abnormalities

Congenital abnormalities are those present at birth. Examples include absence of the thyroid gland (agenesis), development of only half of the thyroid (hemiagenesis), and an abnormal location of the thyroid. The thyroid gland may be located at the back of the tongue (lingual thyroid) or behind the breastbone (substernal thyroid). Stories of patients with congenital thyroid abnormalities can be found in the following "Patient Profiles": "Janet's Story" on pages 9–10; "Ralph's Story" on pages 10–12; "Rhonda's Story" on pages 31–34; and "Kitty's Story" on pages 121–122.

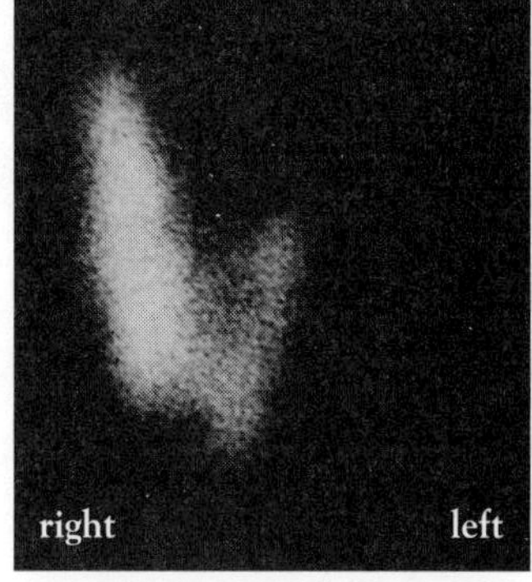

Figure 2.3. Image of hemiagenesis of thyroid gland: right lobe and isthmus are present; left lobe is absent.

Any one of these developmental abnormalities may be associated with functional disease of the thyroid. For example, congenital absence of the thyroid gland will result in hypothyroidism. Congenital hypothyroidism—whether from agenesis, enzyme deficiencies, or other causes—occurs in one in 4,000 births. Therefore, all newborns in the United States, Canada, Israel, Japan, Australia, New Zealand, and most countries in Europe are screened for congenital hypothyroidism.

Fetal Factors

A pregnant woman's thyroid hormone levels may have an impact on the health of her unborn child. A recent study described the impact of maternal hypothyroidism during pregnancy on childhood intellectual performance. Results indicated that the average IQ of children born to inadequately treated hypothyroid mothers may be four points lower than the average IQ of children born to mothers without hypothyroidism. The average IQ of children born to untreated hypothyroid mothers was seven points lower than the average IQ of children born to mothers without hypothyroidism. In addition, the frequency of children born with IQs below 85 increased when their mothers received no treatment for their hypothyroidism. The results of this study underscore the importance of maintaining adequate thyroid hormone levels in expectant mothers.

Neonatal hyperthyroidism may occur in an infant born to a mother who has Graves' disease. The antibodies that stimulate the mother's thyroid gland to produce excessive amounts of thyroid hormone can cross the placenta and also stimulate the fetus' thyroid gland. This condition resolves once the thyroid-stimulating antibodies are metabolized by the infant. Neonatal hyperthyroidism occurs in approximately one of every 100 births to women with Graves' disease.

Inflammatory Thyroid Diseases

Thyroiditis, or inflammation of the thyroid gland, may result from viral infection (subacute thyroiditis) or bacterial infection (acute suppurative thyroiditis). In addition to infection, radiation and antibodies can also cause inflammation of the thyroid gland, as discussed in Chapter 8.

Smoking

Findings of a recent study indicate that people who smoke are three times more likely to develop thyroid disease, especially autoimmune thyroid diseases such as Hashimoto's thyroiditis and Graves' disease. Smokers who have Graves' disease are at a greater risk than nonsmokers for developing Graves' eye disease.

Smoking can also worsen subclinical hypothyroidism. For example, one study of women with subclinical hypothyroidism found that those who smoked two or more cigarettes per day had higher TSH levels and higher cholesterol levels than those who did not smoke. The more a woman smoked, the higher her TSH and low-density lipoprotein (LDL, the "bad" cholesterol).

Summary of What Is Thyroid Disease

Thyroid disease is very common and may occur at any age. The thyroid gland may be larger than normal, smaller than normal, diffusely enlarged, irregular, lumpy and bumpy, symmetrical or asymmetrical, and may be associated with either hyperthyroidism, hypothyroidism, or euthyroidism in various sequences and combinations. Since the course of thyroid disease can be so varied, new symptoms could cause a thyroid patient to wonder, "Could it be my thyroid?" Additionally, a person without thyroid disease may develop similar symptoms and ask, "Could it be my thyroid?" In answering this question, it is helpful to understand what is *not* thyroid disease.

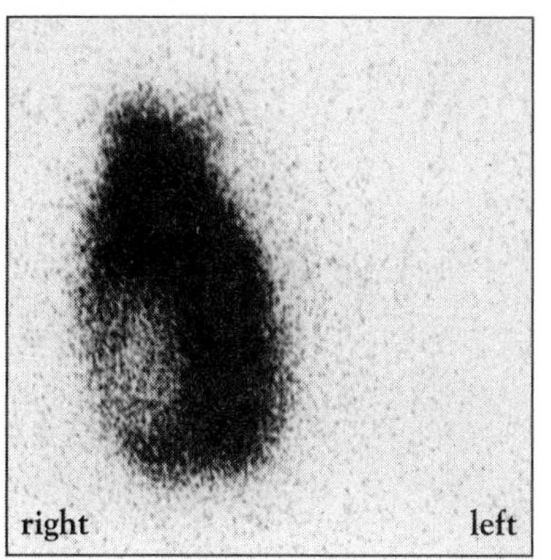

Figure 2.4. Thyroid image of a patient with multiple thyroid diseases: congenital hemiagenesis with absence of left lobe and isthmus; thyroid cancer (light area) in right lobe; Hashimoto's thyroiditis was also found at surgery. The patient was euthyroid prior to surgery, hypothyroid after surgery, and temporarily hyperthyroid after levothyroxine treatment.

What Is Not Thyroid Disease

Many myths and misconceptions have arisen about the thyroid gland. It is difficult to understand genuine thyroid dysfunction without first addressing and dispelling these myths and misconceptions.

Obesity

Many people think that hypothyroidism causes obesity; this is not true. Hypothyroidism may make it more difficult to lose weight, and hypothyroid patients may gain a few pounds; however, massive obesity is never caused by hypothyroidism. Furthermore, some patients have the misconception that taking thyroid hormone will make them gain weight or prevent them from losing weight. This is also untrue.

On the other hand, some patients believe that taking thyroid hormone will help them lose weight. Indeed, thyroid hormone can cause weight loss but only if taken in excess. People with normal thyroid function who take excessive amounts of thyroid hormone to lose weight become hyperthyroid. Much of the weight lost in hyperthyroid patients is muscle mass, not fat. In addition to losing weight, these patients risk becoming weak, losing their hair, developing irregular heartbeats, and experiencing other unpleasant symptoms.

Trying to lose weight may be very frustrating. People spend millions of dollars every year in search of a miraculous formula for weight loss. Thus far, there is no quick, effortless, and safe solution for losing weight. The safest, most effective way to lose weight and to keep it off is to reduce caloric intake, eat well-balanced meals, and exercise regularly (see "Kathy's Story" on pages 34–36).

Fatigue

Fatigue is one of the most common patient complaints. It is true that both hypothyroidism and hyperthyroidism can cause fatigue. However, the most common causes of fatigue are lack of sleep, overwork, stress, depression, and anemia. Euthyroid patients experiencing prolonged fatigue should consult a physician and have a thorough physical examination to search for the cause.

Infertility and Menstrual Dysfunction

Although hypothyroidism and hyperthyroidism may alter a woman's menstrual cycles and cause infertility, they are not common causes of these problems. Prior to the development of sensitive and accurate thyroid function tests, many women with reproductive disorders were treated with thyroid hormone. Some became pregnant during treatment—either because they actually had thyroid disease or because the underlying problem resolved spontaneously. Although a woman with a history of infertility or menstrual problems should be *tested* for thyroid disease, she should be *treated* only if the test results indicate the presence of thyroid disease. A patient with normal thyroid function should not be treated with thyroid hormone for menstrual dysfunction or infertility.

Attention Deficit Disorder

An association has been found between attention deficit disorder (ADD) and a very uncommon thyroid disease called resistance to thyroid hormone (RTH). Publication of this connection led to a flurry of thyroid function testing in children and adults with attention deficit disorder. It is important to understand that very few people with attention deficit disorder have resistance to thyroid hormone.

Osteoporosis

A good deal of misunderstanding exists about osteoporosis (thinning of the bones) and treatment with thyroid hormone. Treatment of thyroid dysfunction with the proper amount of thyroid hormone will not cause osteoporosis. Initial scientific studies found treatment with *too much* thyroid hormone caused osteoporosis, but subsequent studies disputed these findings. The important point to remember is that taking the proper amount of prescribed thyroid hormone will not cause osteoporosis.

Abnormal Thyroid Function Test Results

Abnormal thyroid function test results do not always indicate thyroid disease. For example, estrogen may cause abnormalities in certain thyroid function test results without causing thyroid disease. Many pregnant women, women taking birth control pills, and postmenopausal women taking estrogen will have some abnormal thyroid function test results—although the results are perfectly normal for women taking estrogens.

Depression

Symptoms of depression are among the most common reasons that patients consult physicians. These symptoms are similar to the symptoms of thyroid disease, especially hypothyroidism. For example, fatigue, sleeping excessively, inability to concentrate, apathy, and poor memory may occur in both disorders.

Both depression and hypothyroidism are common, especially in women. Depression may also be seen more often in patients with thyroid dysfunction than in euthyroid patients. Therefore, it is not unusual for patients to have both hypothyroidism and depression.

Hypothyroidism may aggravate symptoms of depression, but it does not ordinarily cause depression. To determine whether patients have depression or hypothyroidism, physicians may ask their patients to make the distinction between feeling sad and feeling tired. Similarly, they may ask their patients to make the distinction between losing interest in the activities of daily living and not having the energy to do them.

The proper diagnosis of both depression and hypothyroidism is important because both disorders are treatable, but the treatments for each illness are entirely different. Some confusion may arise when patients with normal thyroid function test results and depression are treated with thyroid hormone as well as antidepressants. The reason for adding thyroid hormone in this situation is that it may increase the effectiveness of certain antidepressants.

Even when test results indicate normal thyroid function, some patients are reluctant to consider that they could be suffering from depression. Misconceptions and the social stigma attached to the diagnosis of depression may make it a difficult diagnosis to accept. Nonetheless, if patients with thyroid dysfunction are also depressed, they will not get well without treatment of both their depression and their thyroid dysfunction.

Patient Profiles

RHONDA'S STORY

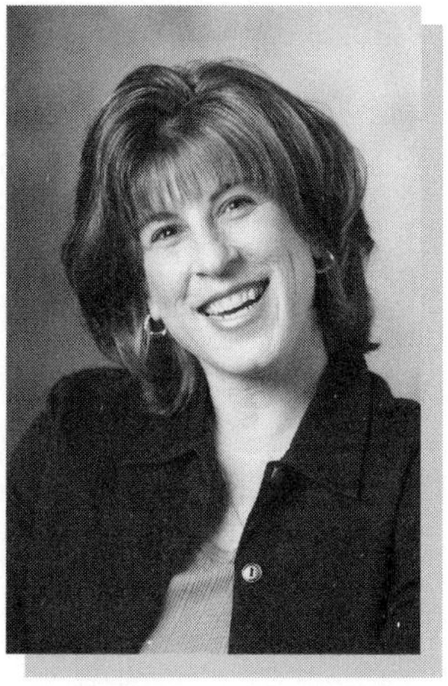

Rhonda is no stranger to thyroid disease. She first learned about thyroid disease when she was a teenager. Her mother had Hashimoto's thyroiditis and developed a large goiter, which was surgically removed. Years later, when Rhonda gave birth to a daughter, routine neonatal tests indicated that her daughter did not have enough thyroid hormone. Further investigation revealed that her daughter had congenital hypothyroidism and a lingual thyroid, thyroid tissue located at the back of the tongue.

> We saw a pediatric endocrinologist who started my daughter on thyroid pills when she was three weeks old. At first, I had to crush the pills, put it in applesauce, and shove it down her. When she was eighteen months old, she started chewing the pills herself. She was tested constantly. Her lingual thyroid shrank a little, and it put out some [thyroid hormone]. Fortunately, her lingual thyroid did not cause her to develop a speech impediment. I'm real proud of her; she's nineteen years old now and graduated with honors.

Rhonda's past experience dealing with her family's thyroid disease prepared her for what lay ahead. In October of 1988, she noticed a lump on her neck and made an appointment with an endocrinologist.

> He more or less dismissed the knot, saying that it was probably just my Adam's apple. But he did do some tests—an iodine uptake and an imaging scan. Then

he suggested that I take levothyroxine to shrink the nodule.

I was not pleased with this doctor so I went to [another endocrinologist]. He did a needle biopsy and told me that there was a remote possibility the knot was cancerous, so I was prepared and not upset. I didn't think for one minute that my life was threatened. I had such trust in him.

Rhonda's new endocrinologist examined her and reviewed her old and new studies. He told her that she had thyroid hemiagenesis, Hashimoto's thyroiditis, and thyroid cancer. In February 1989, a surgeon removed her only thyroid lobe and the malignant thyroid nodule.

I was in the hospital four or five days. The worst part was the drainage tube they left in my neck, but I wasn't in any real pain. I had had three C-sections, and this was nothing! I was not hoarse and didn't need calcium, but they checked it frequently.

About six to eight weeks after the surgery, I returned to the hospital for my first radioactive iodine treatment. The whole experience was weird, just weird. The people at the hospital that came into my room had on this strange get-up like a space suit. They unscrewed the cap on this thick cement thing, stuck a straw in it, and said drink it. Then they ran a Geiger counter over me. No one could come to see me. No one came into my room. They put my food on paper plates and left it at the door.

So I just talked on the phone and rested. It was sort of like a mini-vacation. I drank lots of water and ate sour candy to stimulate my salivary glands. The glands did get clogged up on one side, and they had to flush them out several weeks after the treatment. But I didn't have any more problems with them after that. After about

> a day-and-a-half in the hospital, they let me go home.
>
> I had three children under the age of eight. I called their pediatrician, and he said to stay several feet away from them and not to kiss them for about ten days. I also wore a surgical mask so that I wouldn't sneeze or accidentally spit on them.
>
> By the time I went in for the first radioactive iodine treatment, I was really tired. I couldn't take any thyroid medication until after the treatment. I started taking [levothyroxine], but it took at least six weeks for it to build up. So I was tired for twelve weeks!

Rhonda had a whole body scan nine months later to see if there was any residual thyroid tissue or cancer. In order to prepare for the scan, she had to stop taking all thyroid hormones two weeks before the scan was scheduled. When this scan showed residual tissue, Rhonda checked into the hospital for another radioactive iodine treatment.

> This was the first time I got a little worried because someone said that this treatment had to do it—they couldn't give me any more [radioactive iodine]. It wasn't so weird this time in the hospital. I knew what to expect. I took lemon drops with me and sucked on them and drank water all the time. I was really bored. I even went into the bathroom, turned out all the lights, and looked to see if I glowed. I was really disappointed that I didn't! When I went home, I stayed away from the kids again, but I wasn't as freaked out about it.
>
> Being off the [levothyroxine] pills was awful! I was so tired. I wasn't employed, but I was an active school volunteer. I decided to keep going instead of lying around the house feeling sorry for myself.

Rhonda's determination to stay active was rewarded when she won the Volunteer of the Year Award at the school her children attended. Her whole body scan the following year was clear (negative).

> I finally got back to my old self. It's been twelve years, and I don't think about it any more. I never really thought of myself as a cancer survivor. I'm not worried about myself because I trust my doctor completely.

Rhonda returns to her endocrinologist annually and takes her levothyroxine as prescribed. Despite having congenital, autoimmune, and malignant thyroid disease, she continues to do well.■

KATHY'S STORY

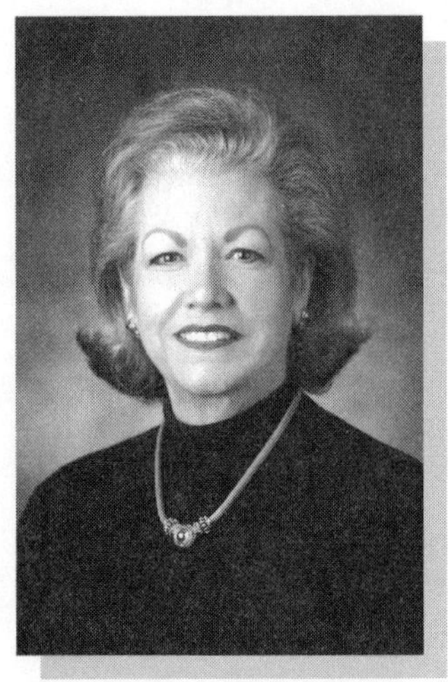

Kathy is a fifty-three-year-old wife, mother, editor, and layout designer. As the editor of this book, she has a unique perspective on thyroid disease, especially her own.

> I would love to blame my thyroid gland for my long-standing weight problem. It would certainly simplify my life. But I was overweight long before I was diagnosed with Hashimoto's thyroiditis and hypothyroidism, and I was overweight long after I began taking levothyroxine to correct my thyroid problem.
>
> Approximately ten years ago, I did what many other people do—I tried to blame the symptoms of hypothyroidism that I experienced on all the wrong things. When I started feeling tired, I thought it was because of the long hours I was working. When my skin became dry and itchy, I dismissed it because it was cold outside. But when my hair started falling out, that really got my attention!

My endocrinologist's office was one floor beneath my office. I hesitantly walked in and told him that I thought I had a thyroid problem. Lab results confirmed that I was hypothyroid. Within two months of taking levothyroxine, I felt much better, and my hair stopped falling out. I also lost the *one* pound I had gained.

For those people who think that you cannot lose weight if you are taking levothyroxine, I can cite at least one case when that was not true—my own! Eighteen months ago, after more than twenty years of being extremely overweight, I found out that I was diabetic and needed to take oral medication to control it. Visions of my mother's daily battle with diabetes and its side effects flashed before me. I did not want to go there.

I followed my doctor's advice and started seeing a diabetic educator/dietician. I made up my mind to change my lifestyle and to take control of my health. I followed the meal plan suggested by my dietician and also started something I never thought I would or could do—exercising. At first, I could only walk ten or fifteen minutes at a time. Huffing and puffing, I would get to the end of my block and think I was going to die. Everything hurt. My husband and son encouraged me to keep trying and would walk with me every day to ensure that I would go.

After six months, I lost fifty-seven pounds. To date, I have lost ninety pounds and plan on losing at least another ten. I no longer need to take medication to control my diabetes, and I'm the one dragging my family off the sofa to walk. I walk twenty to forty-five minutes a day, four to five days a week and feel like a new person, with energy to spare!

The solution to my weight problem did not come overnight or from an exotic, magic potion. In all honesty,

> I cannot say that losing weight has been easy, but it has been worth the effort and has become more natural every day. For all of you who think that a middle-aged, physically inactive, food-loving, hypothyroid person on levothyroxine can't lose weight, I'm here to tell you that this is one old dog who has learned a new trick…or two!

Kathy's story makes a clear distinction between what is and what is not thyroid disease. Unfortunately, treating hypothyroidism does not ordinarily result in significant weight loss without a commitment to eating less and exercising more.■

MAIKO'S STORY

Less than a year after he was married and moved to the United States from Brazil, twenty-eight-year-old Maiko and his wife recognized a change in his behavior and health.

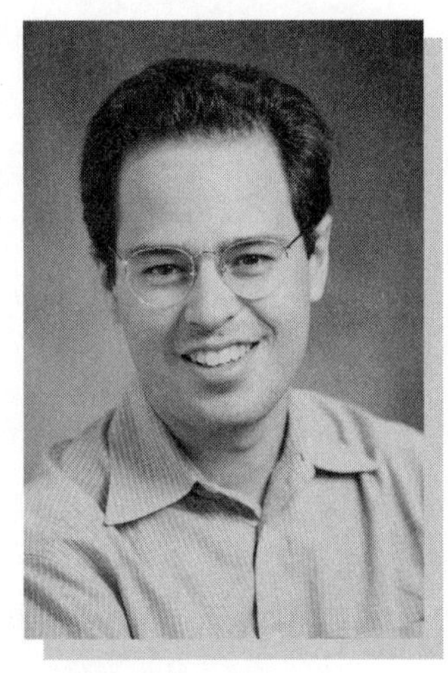

> After I was married, my wife noticed that I was more agitated. I had problems with my respiratory system and had difficulty breathing. I thought it was the pollen. It took a long time for me to recover from colds. I was sleeping less at night and waking up during the night full of energy, but my body was getting tired. I was sweating a lot at night.
>
> There were lots of changes in my life, and I thought they had caused more anxiety. But finally it got to the point I knew there was a problem.
>
> I went to a pulmonary doctor, who did all kinds of tests. All of them said I was okay. The doctor attributed my anxiety to life changes. But one morning I fainted

> when I woke up, and knew I had to do something.

During this time, Maiko and his wife visited his parents, who lived in New York. When he described what he was experiencing, his parents persuaded him to visit their physician.

> By this time, I was sleeping two hours a night. My parents' doctor discovered that I had high blood pressure, but we thought it was from the steroids I was taking for my respiratory problems.
>
> After returning home, I went to my [general practitioner], and he confirmed that I had high blood pressure. My blood work was unusual—it showed both hypothyroidism and hyperthyroidism. So I had scans and x-rays, but the doctor admitted he had no idea what was wrong with me. He said it might be my pituitary or thyroid and suggested I find a specialist, a good endocrinologist.

Because of his abnormal thyroid function test results, Maiko made an appointment with an endocrinologist who was recommended by a nurse he knew. The endocrinologist reviewed Maiko's previous blood tests, which revealed low total T_4, total T_3, and TSH, and a high T_3 resin uptake (T_3RU). After examining Maiko, the endocrinologist ordered tests for that day and the next day.

> I went home that night and woke up screaming. I started saying some strange things and really frightened my wife when I started running for no reason. She talked me down, and then she called my parents.

Maiko's parents arranged to fly in the next day, and his wife insisted they return to the endocrinologist. She hoped to speak to the nurse and doctor privately to describe Maiko's strange behavior:

> Maiko is a very good actor; he hid his emotions. When I asked if I could speak to the nurse outside, she

> explained that I had to talk in the presence of Maiko. But Maiko said I was exaggerating and nothing had happened. He said I was crazy!

Maiko vaguely remembered this period of time.

> I do recall saying, "I've lost my north," as in a compass; I felt as though I had lost my reference points. Then I got better as the day progressed.
>
> The amazing thing is that none of this affected me at work. I could function there. I got sweaty once in a meeting, but that was all. I was getting ready to start working in a new area, so this was happening at the perfect time.

That night, after his parents flew in, Maiko had another "episode." His family took him to a nearby emergency room early in the morning.

> They did a CAT scan and registered me as a mental patient. They said I was suffering from an anxiety disorder and that I needed a week of vacation.

The emergency room physician discharged Maiko that night. The next night his behavior became even more unmanageable.

> This time, my family took me to the emergency room of [a major medical center]. We waited eight hours to be treated. I was having hallucinations. I thought I was going to hell one moment and heaven the next. They were religious-type hallucinations.
>
> A psychiatrist came to evaluate me, but he said I was okay. He thought that maybe I had encephalitis, so they did a spinal tap. It was clear. My family asked the doctors to hospitalize me because they were quite concerned for my health.

> After that I went totally crazy, even during the day. I remember some of it. I called one of my friends and told him that my family had put me in jail. I was getting worse everyday. My wife and parents were really frightened. They took turns watching me. The doctors gave me Haldol to keep me calm. I would freeze in one position for two hours. It was very bizarre behavior! Throughout all of this, my wife remained very stable. My mother was quite emotional.
>
> I had lost thirty pounds; I weighed less than 100 pounds! When [my endocrinologist] came, he ordered a MRI. After a week, we had a diagnosis. I had a tumor on my right adrenal gland.

Tests confirmed that Maiko had a right adrenal gland tumor, which was producing excessive amounts of several hormones, including one that is not typically produced in the adrenal gland. This type of tumor is very rare—less than a dozen cases have been described in medical literature. The adrenal glands ordinarily make several hormones, including catecholamines and cortisol (steroids), which are necessary to sustain life. An adrenal tumor that makes excess catecholamines is called a pheochromocytoma. Incredibly, Maiko's pheochromocytoma was not only making catecholamines but also ACTH, a hormone that stimulates production of cortisol. ACTH was, in turn, stimulating excessive production of cortisol from both adrenal glands.

ACTH is usually produced in the pituitary gland, not in the adrenal glands. When a tumor makes a hormone that it does not normally make, production of the hormone is described as ectopic. Maiko had an ectopic ACTH-producing pheochromocytoma stimulating excessive cortisol production, which contributed, in part, to his abnormal thyroid function test results. His tumor was surgically removed.

> I went home ten days after surgery. I was feeling very good, but I felt impotent psychologically. I was indecisive. This lasted a few days. I started becoming more aware of my body and doing the right things.

> Suddenly, I became conscious that I was actually there. I could fully comprehend what had happened and what was happening now. Then I could make decisions. You could say I snapped into a more lucid state. It was the day I finally recovered—June 18. I felt like everything was back.

Following surgery, Maiko made a full recovery and his abnormal thyroid function test results quickly normalized. Remarkably, it was his abnormal thyroid function test results—caused by excessive steroids—that led him to the right doctor, an endocrinologist, for the wrong reasons. Maiko is now feeling well, on no medications, and working on a master's degree in business administration.■

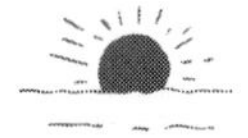

Chapter 3

WHO DIAGNOSES AND TREATS THYROID DISEASE?

The word "doctor" is derived from the Latin *docere*, which means "to teach." Doctors teach patients about their bodies, how best to care for them, and how to treat them when something goes wrong. Since doctors will be the most important individuals in determining whether patients have thyroid disease, patients should know as much as possible about their doctors.

How Doctors Are Trained after Medical School

After graduation from medical school, new doctors receive additional training called a residency. Hospitals and medical schools offer residencies in specific areas of study or specialties—such as internal medicine, obstetrics and gynecology, nuclear medicine, ophthalmology, pathology, and general surgery. Residencies last for a minimum of three years; the first year of residency is often called an internship. Following residency, doctors may take additional subspecialty training called a fellowship. For example, doctors who have completed three years of residency in internal medicine may then take an additional two or three years of fellowship training in endocrinology, cardiology, gastroenterology, rheumatology, or another subspecialty of internal medicine.

Once training is completed, physicians will either join the faculty of a medical school or go into private practice. Physicians who are employed by medical schools are said to be in academic medicine and are called full-time faculty members. Most of these physicians have training in research, and some may even have Ph.D.'s in areas related to medicine, such as biochemistry or cellular biology. They may have titles, such as instructor, assistant professor, associate professor, or professor. Physicians in private practice are not employed by medical schools, but they may volunteer to work with medical students, residents, or fellows. Doctors in private practice who teach are called voluntary faculty members and will have titles such as clinical instructor, clinical assistant professor, clinical associate professor, and clinical professor. Most physicians in private practice are not affiliated with any medical school at all.

Just like physicians, hospitals may or may not be affiliated with medical schools. If hospitals are affiliated with medical schools, they are called teaching hospitals. In addition to caring for patients, teaching hospitals may also conduct medical research and educate physicians. Generally speaking, teaching hospitals have a higher concentration of physicians with very specialized training.

Nearly all hospitals and most state medical boards require continuing medical education for physicians after they complete formal medical training. One way physicians can meet this requirement is by attending medical conferences offered by professional societies, such as the American Thyroid Association (ATA), the American Association of Clinical Endocrinologists (AACE), The Endocrine Society, and the American College of Physicians-American Society of Internal Medicine (ACP-ASIM). Members of some professional societies who meet certain additional requirements, such as publishing medical research, are recognized as fellows of that organization—such as Fellow of the American College of Endocrinology (F.A.C.E.) and Fellow of the American College of Physicians (F.A.C.P.).

How Doctors Are Licensed and Certified

Licenses

Each state licenses its own physicians after a thorough review of the applicants' credentials and experience. Medicine is one of the most heavily regulated, if not the most heavily regulated, of all the professions in the United States. State licensing boards keep a watchful eye on the physicians they license, and most states require annual renewal of physicians' licenses. In addition, hospitals usually require annual renewal of privileges by physicians. Physicians' credentials, experience, and continuing medical education may be reviewed. Hospital privileges and state licenses merely allow physicians to practice medicine, both in and out of a hospital. The licensing process and the granting of hospital privileges do not indicate how qualified physicians are in a particular area of medicine.

Board Certification

Physicians' qualifications and competence in a given area are certified by boards who give certifying examinations. For example, internists are permitted to take the certifying examination in internal medicine after three years of an internal medicine residency. If they pass this examination, they are board certified in internal medicine. Physicians who complete fellowships are eligible to take the certifying examination in their subspecialty to become board certified. Doctors who are qualified to take the examination, but have not yet taken or passed it, are said to be board eligible in a specialty or subspecialty.

In recent years, specialty boards have limited the period of certification, usually to ten years. At the end of that time, physicians must pass another examination to be recertified. Physicians who were certified before this policy change do not have to take the recertification examination.

How Doctors Practice Medicine

Solo and Group Practices

Doctors may practice as individuals, in which case they are in solo practices, or they may join together to form group practices. A group practice may include physicians in only one specialty, such as internal medicine, in which case the group is called a single specialty group. On the other hand, physicians with varying specialties (for example, internal medicine, surgery, psychiatry, pediatrics) may join together to form a multispecialty group.

Fee-for-Service vs. Managed Care

A great deal of change is occurring in the medical profession today. Traditional fee-for-service medicine is rapidly being replaced by managed care. At least 85% of all medical care is not paid directly by patients but by the so-called "third party," such as an insurance company or the federal government. This book is not the appropriate place to discuss the advantages and disadvantages of fee-for-service versus managed care, but certain broad principles should be borne in mind:

- Generally speaking, managed care is somewhat less expensive than fee-for-service medicine.
- Fee-for-service medicine offers an unlimited choice of physicians; some managed care companies provide incentives, if not outright limitations, regarding choice of physicians.

Patients must choose what is best for themselves and their families. However, the choice of medical insurance may have a tremendous impact on the type of medical care patients will receive.

Doctors Who Diagnose and Treat Thyroid Disease

Many doctors may be involved in the care of patients with thyroid problems. The following is a brief description of physicians with whom thyroid patients may have contact.

Thyroidologists

Thyroidologists are endocrinologists who see, almost exclusively, patients with thyroid disease. There are very few thyroidologists in the United States or worldwide. Almost all thyroidologists have completed fellowships in endocrinology; some have additional training in nuclear medicine. These physicians usually have done some research into the causes or treatment of thyroid disease and generally have accumulated experience with a large number of thyroid patients. Most thyroidologists belong to a professional organization called the American Thyroid Association.

Endocrinologists

Endocrinologists study the endocrine (hormone-secreting) glands of the body. These physicians specialize in the diagnosis and treatment of disorders of the endocrine glands. Examples of endocrine glands, in addition to the thyroid gland, are the pituitary gland, parathyroid glands, adrenal glands, ovaries, testes, and those parts of the pancreas that make insulin. After completing a residency in internal medicine, endocrinologists receive fellowship training in endocrinology, metabolism, and diabetes. There may be advantages for patients with thyroid disease who consult endocrinologists. According to the authors of a 1998 study in the *Journal of Clinical Endocrinology and Metabolism*, "Early referral of patients with suspected thyroid nodules to an endocrinologist results in significant savings in both cost and patient's time as well as increased precision of diagnosis."

Internists

Internists are physicians who specialize in the diagnosis and nonsurgical treatment of illnesses in adults. Endocrinology is one subspecialty of internal medicine, as are cardiology, gastroenterology, rheumatology, and oncology. People often assume that cancer specialists (oncologists) treat all patients with thyroid cancer. In fact, thyroidologists or endo-crinologists, in conjunction with surgeons and nuclear medicine physicians, treat most thyroid cancer patients.

Family Practitioners

Family practitioners are primary care physicians who treat both adults and children. They are considered generalists who have broad knowledge, as opposed to specialists or subspecialists who have in-depth knowledge about a given area.

Pediatricians/Pediatric Endocrinologists

Pediatricians are physicians who specialize in the treatment of diseases of children. Thyroid disease is much less common in children than in adults, but it definitely occurs. Children before the age of puberty who develop thyroid disease are usually treated by pediatricians. Many times these children are referred to pediatric endocrinologists.

Obstetricians and Gynecologists

Obstetricians and gynecologists (ob-gyns) specialize in the delivery of babies and the treatment of women with disorders of their reproductive systems. Ob-gyns deliver most babies born in the United States. For many women, they function as primary care physicians. Since thyroid disease occurs five times more frequently in women than in men, ob-gyns are often the first to suspect or diagnose thyroid disorders.

General Surgeons and Otorhinolaryngologists

There are two types of surgeons who operate on thyroid glands—general surgeons and otorhinolaryngologists (ear, nose, and throat physicians, or ENTs). Surgeons with a particular interest in thyroid surgery might join the American Thyroid Association and the American Association of Endocrine Surgeons.

Ophthalmologists

Ophthalmologists are surgeons who treat patients with diseases of the eye. Some ophthalmologists have accumulated additional expertise in treating Graves' eye disease and have formed professional organizations to share ideas, research, and experiences. The Orbit Society and the American Society of Ophthalmic, Plastic and Reconstructive Surgery are two such organizations.

Nuclear Medicine Physicians

Nuclear medicine physicians are specially trained in the use of radioactive materials for the diagnosis and treatment of diseases. A license to handle radioactive materials is granted by each state. Nuclear medicine physicians may see thyroid patients when they are having thyroid scans, receiving radioactive iodine for the treatment of hyperthyroidism, or receiving much larger doses of radioactive iodine for the treatment of thyroid cancer. Some endocrinologists are also licensed to handle selective radioactive materials, such as technetium and radioactive iodine.

Pathologists

Pathologists are experts in examining cells and tissue for disease (anatomic pathology) and in supervising laboratories where blood tests are performed (clinical laboratory medicine). The experience and expertise of pathologists are especially critical in interpreting thyroid biopsies and in assuring quality and accuracy of laboratory tests.

Radiologists

Radiologists are physicians who perform specialized imaging procedures, such as arteriograms or myelograms, and interpret x-rays, ultrasounds, and MRIs. Radiologists often discover thyroid nodules when imaging other parts of the neck, such as the carotid arteries or cervical spine.

Dermatologists

Dermatologists are experts in diseases of the skin. Thyroid patients with hair loss, vitiligo, changes in their nails, or Graves' dermatopathy may consult dermatologists.

Psychiatrists

Psychiatrists are physicians specializing in treatment of mental health disorders. Sometimes they are the first ones to suspect thyroid disease in patients with symptoms of depression or anxiety.

How to Find a Doctor Who Treats Thyroid Disease

Primary care physicians—who may be family practitioners, ob-gyns, pediatricians, internists, or endocrinologists—will most commonly be the doctors who first diagnose and treat thyroid disease. Depending upon the type of thyroid disease and the particular needs of each patient, one or more specialists may be required to treat certain thyroid disorders. It is important that patients be confident in, and comfortable with, their physicians. If they need to see a thyroid specialist, or if they want a second opinion about their thyroid condition, there are several avenues they may pursue.

If either patients or physicians believe that thyroid experts should be consulted, physicians are usually the best sources of referral. They generally know the doctors and the specific resources available in a given geographic area.

If patients wish to locate physicians on their own, the most important fact they should bear in mind is that *experience counts*. When inquiring into a doctor's qualifications, certain questions may be helpful to ask. For example:

- Is the doctor board certified?
- Does he belong to any professional organizations with a special interest in thyroid disease?
- How many patients with thyroid disease does he treat?
- How many years has he been treating thyroid patients?

If a surgeon is required, patients might also ask:

- How many thyroid surgeries does he perform a year?
- How many of his patients experience surgical complications, such as recurrent laryngeal nerve paralysis or permanent hypoparathyroidism ?

Patients seeking the names of physicians who treat thyroid disease also have other resources available to them. Several of these resources are listed in "Appendix A: Sources of Thyroid Information."

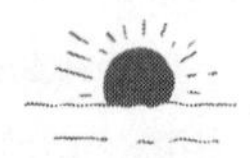

CHAPTER 4

HOW IS THYROID DISEASE DIAGNOSED?

Correctly diagnosing thyroid disorders is now easier than ever before; many advances have been made in tests and equipment over the last two decades. Nonetheless, the most important factors leading to a correct diagnosis remain the patient's medical history and physical examination. Most of the time, a doctor arrives at a correct diagnosis with information from the medical history and physical examination alone. A physician orders tests based upon conclusions drawn from the patient's medical history and physical examination in order to confirm a diagnosis and rule out other possibilities.

One way to understand how a physician diagnoses thyroid disease is to consider the "five-finger rule." Each finger of the hand represents one step taken by a physician to reach a diagnosis.

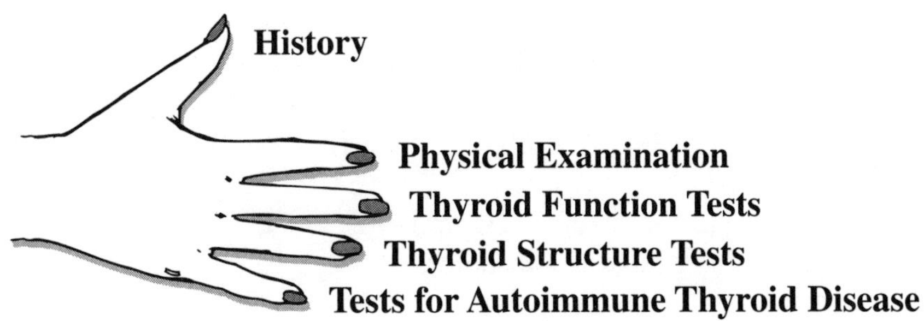

Figure 4.1. Five-finger rule.

As with the classification of thyroid diseases described in Chapter 2, there is much overlap between tests of thyroid function and tests of thyroid structure. Furthermore, not all patients will have all tests. For example, a patient will not ordinarily have a thyroid biopsy unless she has a thyroid nodule. Nonetheless, the five-finger rule may prove useful in understanding what is going on at the doctor's office.

The Medical History

A doctor begins a medical history with a general question, such as "How can I help you today?" or "What brings you to the doctor today?" In this way, a patient is encouraged to tell, in her own words, why she has come to see the doctor. Some responses may be brief and specific, such as "My doctor found a thyroid nodule, and I am here for a thyroid biopsy," or they may be nonspecific. In either case, a doctor should give a patient sufficient opportunity to describe the reason(s) for her visit.

A physician will then ask specific questions about the patient's complaints. Answers to these questions provide clues to the patient's illness. A patient may be asked about: medications affecting thyroid function, such as iodine, herbs, supplements, and lithium; radiation exposure; thyroid surgery; and family history of thyroid disease. A doctor may complete the medical history by asking questions about:

- past medical history including:
  - other medications
  - hospitalizations
  - surgeries
  - drug allergies

- social history including:
  - caffeine consumption
  - smoking habits
  - alcohol and drug use
  - marital status
  - pregnancies
  - children

sexual orientation
employment

- family history including:
  - the medical history of relatives
  - hereditary diseases

- review of systems including:
  - visual symptoms
  - menstrual history
  - breast discharge
  - cardiac history
  - sexual history
  - skin and hair changes
  - temperature intolerance
  - sleep disturbances
  - stress
  - psychiatric history

The Physical Examination

Most physical examinations begin with measurement of the patient's vital signs, including blood pressure, pulse rate, and, when indicated, respiratory rate and temperature. Weight and height should also be recorded since they serve as reference points for future examinations. The remainder of the physical examination depends, in part, on the type of physician being seen. For example, if a patient is seeing a gynecologist, her examination will almost certainly include a pelvic examination. On the other hand, if she has been referred to an endocrinologist to treat a thyroid disorder, then a pelvic examination is very unlikely.

Regardless of the type of physician seen, a physical examination includes a search for signs that indicate the presence, or absence, of thyroid dysfunction. A patient may be asked to hold out her hands to observe whether a tremor is present or to inspect the condition of her skin and nails. The physician may tap the inner elbows or ankles with a reflex hammer to determine the speed of reflexes. If hyperthyroidism is suspected, a great deal of attention may be paid to the eyes. To evaluate a patient's muscle strength, the physician may ask the patient to do deep-knee bends or other exercises.

A doctor may also examine other parts of the body, such as the lungs, heart, breasts, abdomen, and extremities. Some patients, both female and male, may be surprised when endocrinologists examine their breasts. By applying pressure to a woman's nipple, an endocrinologist can determine if there is a milky discharge (galactorrhea), a sign of hypothyroidism. Similarly, an endocrinologist may examine male breasts, looking for growth of glandular breast tissue (gynecomastia) sometimes found in hyperthyroid males.

Examination of the thyroid gland generally begins with a visual inspection. Enlargement of the thyroid gland is usually visible to the trained eye, and even to the untrained eye, if a person's neck is long and thin. Confirmation that the thyroid gland, and not something else, is enlarged may be obtained by asking the patient to swallow. The thyroid gland moves up and down with swallowing. A physician will sometimes give his patient a cup of water so that she can swallow

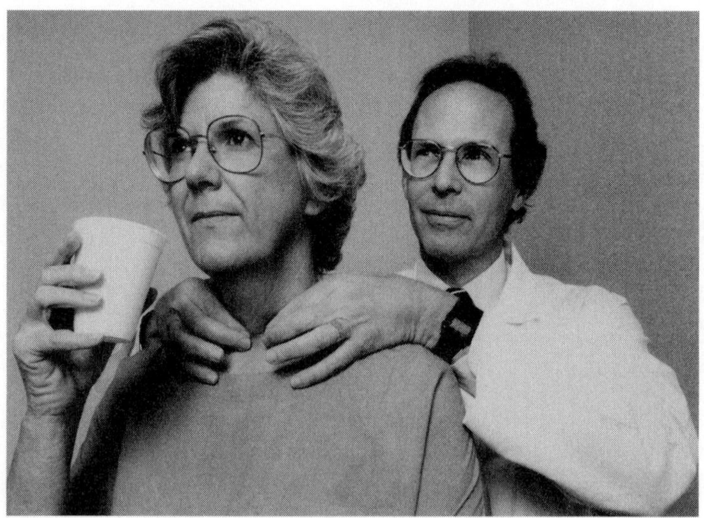

Figure 4.2. Physical examination of a patient's thyroid gland while she swallows water.

repetitively while the physician either observes or feels her thyroid gland. A doctor may examine the thyroid gland while standing in front of his patient or behind his patient. In this way, he can evaluate the size, texture, nodularity, and tenderness of the thyroid gland.

Incidentally, a patient can examine her own thyroid gland (see "Gail's Story" on pages 81–82). Figures 4.3 and 4.4 and the shaded information box on page 54 describe and illustrate how to perform this examination.

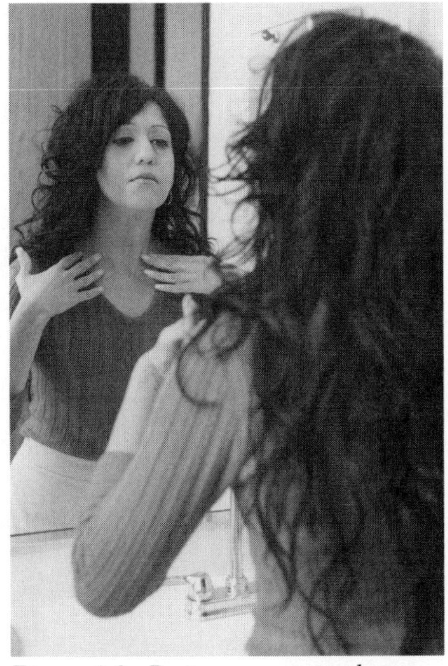

Figure 4.3. Patient examining her own thyroid gland.

Tests of Thyroid Function

Laboratories play a critical role in the evaluation of thyroid patients. Blood test results, which these laboratories provide, are essential in making the correct diagnosis. Laboratories are not equal in their ability to select the best test methodology and to perform tests accurately and precisely. One of the main functions of physicians is to ensure that the laboratories with which they work are of the highest quality.

TSH

The single most important test of thyroid function is the measurement of TSH (thyroid-stimulating hormone). The level of TSH (also called thyrotropin) indicates the pituitary gland's response to the amount of thyroid hormone in the blood.

A low TSH level suggests hyperthyroidism—too much thyroid hormone. On the other hand, an elevated TSH level suggests hypothyroidism—not enough thyroid hormone. Before reaching a conclusion

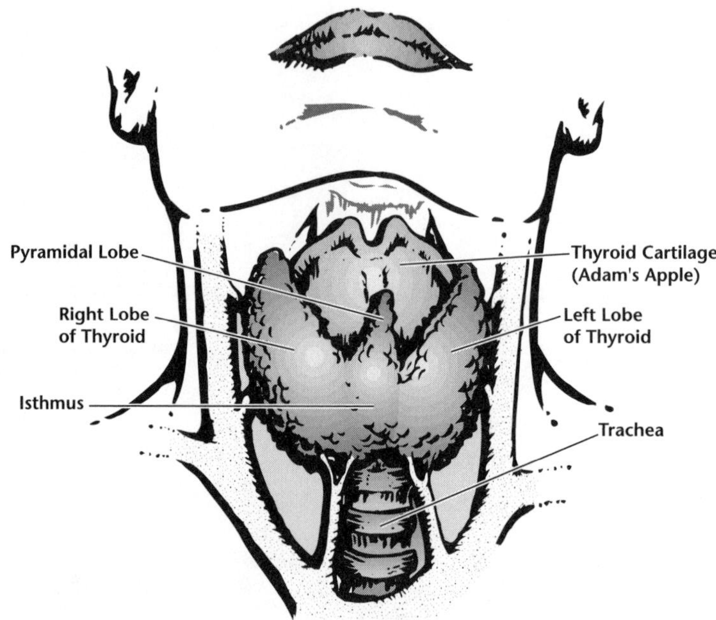

Figure 4.4. Front view of thyroid gland and neck, not drawn to scale.

Thyroid Self-Examination

You can actually examine your own thyroid gland if you can find your Adam's apple (thyroid cartilage). Begin by standing in front of a mirror with a cup of water. Then follow these steps:

- Locate your Adam's apple with your fingers.
- Drop down to the next tracheal ring of cartilage.
- Lift your head up and, while swallowing some water, look for the isthmus that lies over this ring of cartilage and for the thyroid gland that spreads out from the isthmus like a butterfly with its wings open.

Since the thyroid gland moves with swallowing, enlargement of your thyroid gland or lumps on your thyroid gland may become more apparent while swallowing.

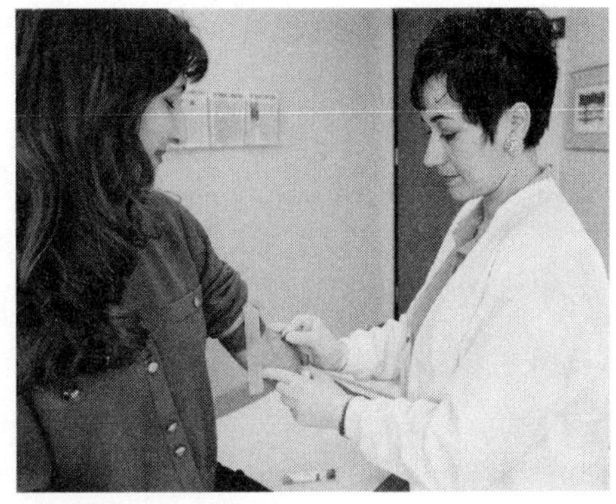

Figure 4.5. Nurse drawing blood for thyroid function tests.

about the correct diagnosis, the physician interprets a TSH result in light of each patient's circumstances. For example, even though low TSH most often means a patient is *hyper*thyroid, it may also indicate that the pituitary gland is unable to produce any TSH; this type of patient is actually *hypo*thyroid (see "Matilde's Story" on pages 119–120). Similarly, even though high TSH most often means a patient is hypothyroid, it may also indicate overproduction of TSH by the pituitary gland and hyperthyroidism (see "Seymour's Story" on pages 84–88).

The sensitivity of assays (tests) for TSH is continually increasing, and new superlatives are regularly applied to them. Terms that may be heard include sensitive, ultrasensitive, supersensitive, second generation, or third generation TSH test. Increased sensitivity of TSH tests translates into an increased ability to distinguish a low TSH from a normal TSH level.

TRH Test

Sometimes a single measurement of TSH does not give enough information about a patient's thyroid status. In this circumstance, a TRH (thyrotropin-releasing hormone) test may be performed. Thyrotropin-releasing hormone is secreted from the hypothalamus and stimulates TSH production and secretion from the pituitary gland. In the TRH test, a blood sample for TSH is drawn, and then thyrotropin-releasing hormone is injected intravenously. One or more blood samples for TSH are drawn at specified time intervals after the injection of thyrotropin-releasing hormone. The TRH test can be useful in several ways:

- to confirm the diagnosis of hyperthyroidism
- to confirm the adequacy of TSH suppression in thyroid cancer patients

- to confirm the diagnosis of pituitary or hypothalamic insufficiency
- to diagnose mild hypothyroidism

Free T_4 and Free T_3

The two active thyroid hormones in humans are thyroxine (T_4) and triiodothyronine (T_3). Most of the thyroid hormones in the blood are bound to three proteins: thyroxine-binding globulin (TBG), thyroxine-binding prealbumin (TBPA), and albumin. Unbound (free) T_4 and T_3 can be measured directly in tests called free T_4 and free T_3 assays. They are preferred over measurements of total (bound plus free) T_4 and T_3, since only free T_4 and free T_3 are available to affect human function and well-being.

Available methods for measuring free thyroid hormones differ in their speed and accuracy. For example, one test may be faster but not nearly as accurate as another test. There is frequently a trade-off between speed and accuracy, and doctors should be aware of what types of tests are being used to estimate free thyroid hormones. Equilibrium dialysis, a very specialized and time-consuming test, is considered the most accurate method (the "gold standard") for the measurement of free T_4 and free T_3.

In the diagnosis of hypothyroidism, measurement of free T_4 is more useful than measurement of free T_3. In many cases of hypothyroidism, free T_4 is low, while free T_3 is normal. In most cases of hyperthyroidism, both free T_4 and free T_3 are elevated. In some patients with hyperthyroidism—

Typical Results of
Preferred Thyroid Function Tests

Patient	TSH	Free T_4	FreeT_3
hypothyroid	high	low	not useful
hyperthyroid	low	high	high
with high estrogen level	normal	normal	normal

particularly those with toxic autonomously functioning thyroid nodules (TAFTN) or toxic multinodular goiters (TMNG)—the free T_3 may be elevated while the free T_4 is normal.

T_3 Resin Uptake (T_3RU), Total T_4, and Total T_3

Older thyroid function tests, such as the T_3 resin uptake (T_3RU), rely on indirect measurements of thyroid hormone-binding proteins. An estimate of free T_4 or free T_3 is then generated by combining the thyroid hormone-binding protein estimate with the result of a measurement of total (bound and free) thyroid hormone. For example, the free T_4 index (FTI) is calculated from the T_3RU and the total T_4. The free T_4 index (free thyroxine index) is only an estimate of free T_4.

Measurements of free thyroid hormones are preferred over estimates of free thyroid hormones, and, fortunately, these tests are now readily available. Test results from the T_3RU and total T_4 are altered by changes in thyroid hormone-binding proteins and can cause confusion. For example, estrogens increase thyroid hormone-binding proteins, and, therefore, the results of the T_3RU and total T_4 tests in patients with elevated estrogens are frequently out of the normal range. However, these "abnormal" test results are normal for people with elevated estrogens, such as pregnant women, women taking certain birth control pills, and menopausal women taking estrogen replacement. Using a direct measurement of free T_4 eliminates this confusion.

Patients with familial dysalbuminemic hyperthyroxinemia also have changes in thyroid hormone-binding proteins that alter total T_4

Typical Results of
Other Thyroid Function Tests

Patient	T_3RU	Total T_4	FTI	Total T_3
hypothyroid	low	low	low	not useful
hyperthyroid	high	high	high	high
with high estrogen level	low	high	normal	high

but not free T_4. Familial dysalbuminemic hyperthyroxinemia occurs most often in patients of Hispanic descent and is characterized by an abnormal albumin (a thyroid hormone-binding protein) that has a higher than normal binding capacity for T_4 but not T_3. Patients with familial dysalbuminemic hyperthyroxinemia may have high total T_4 levels, but they will have normal free T_4 levels.

The table on page 57 shows the typical results of these commonly used, but less desirable, indirect thyroid function tests in hyperthyroid and hypothyroid patients and in euthyroid patients taking estrogens. The table on page 56 shows the typical results of the preferred thyroid function tests in the same patients.

Radioactive Iodine Uptake

Since iodine is a key component of thyroid hormones, a test has been devised to see how the thyroid gland handles iodine. This test is called the radioactive iodine uptake (RAIU). The radioactive iodine uptake is performed by administering a specific amount of radioactive iodine orally to a patient. Six to twenty-four hours later, the amount of radioactive iodine in the thyroid gland is counted, usually by a gamma camera or a rectilinear scanner. The percentage of the administered radioactive iodine "taken up" by the thyroid gland is calculated and is called either a 6-hour radioactive iodine uptake or a 24-hour radioactive iodine uptake. A thyroid image (scan) is frequently made at the same time. The radioactive iodine uptake is most useful in diagnosing and treating patients with hyperthyroidism.

The radioactive iodine uptake may be misleading if patients have had other diagnostic tests using iodine within the preceding two to three months. For example, patients having CAT scans, myelograms, intravenous pyelograms (IVPs), or arteriograms may be given x-ray dyes that contain large amounts of iodine. The large amount of iodine given for the x-ray procedure dilutes the small amount of radioactive iodine given for the radioactive iodine uptake; therefore, interpreting the radioactive iodine uptake becomes difficult. Patients should postpone elective x-rays using iodinated dyes until after their radioactive iodine uptake is completed (see "Trina's Story" on pages 82–84).

Some patients are concerned about tests using radioactive iodine because they are allergic to iodine. The small amounts of iodine used in the diagnosis and treatment of thyroid diseases do not cause allergic reactions.

Pregnant women should never take radioactive iodine.

Although radioactive iodine used for diagnostic testing does not harm an adult, it may harm a fetus. Therefore, if a patient has any doubts about whether she is pregnant, any test or treatment using radioactive iodine should be delayed. The physician will ask about the possibility of pregnancy prior to performing any test involving radioactive materials. Breastfeeding women will need to temporarily discontinue nursing.

T_3 (Cytomel®) Suppression Test

Occasionally, a physician suspects that a thyroid nodule is functioning autonomously. When a thyroid nodule functions autonomously, it functions independently of the thyroid gland's normal control mechanisms. Ordinarily, TSH from the pituitary gland and thyroid hormone from the thyroid gland work as parts of a feedback mechanism, much like a thermostat and an air conditioner (see Figure 4.6 on page 60). When thyroid hormone production goes down, the pituitary gland (thermostat) senses it and secretes additional TSH. The additional TSH stimulates the thyroid gland (air conditioner) to bring production of thyroid hormone back to normal. When thyroid hormone production increases, TSH production decreases, and thyroid hormone production is reduced to normal. If a thyroid nodule fails to turn off its production of thyroid hormone despite suppression of TSH production, it is referred to as an autonomously functioning thyroid nodule (AFTN).

In the Cytomel suppression test, a radioactive iodine uptake is performed both before and after ten days of a high dose of Cytomel (the brand name of T_3). A thyroid nodule is functioning autonomously if the radioactive iodine uptake is not markedly reduced following ten days of Cytomel. This test is ordered infrequently, and it must be used carefully because excessive amounts of thyroid hormone can be harmful to some patients.

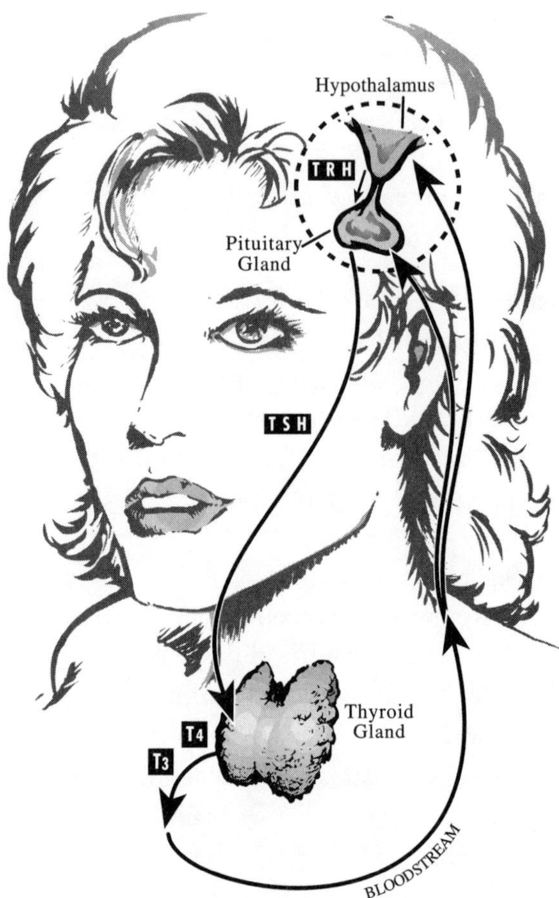

Figure 4.6. Feedback mechanism: hypothalamus, pituitary gland, and thyroid gland.

Factors that Can Affect Thyroid Test Results and Thyroid Patients

Many factors that affect thyroid function test results may or may not affect thyroid function. For example, estrogens will profoundly affect certain thyroid function test results, but will not affect thyroid function to any significant degree in people without thyroid disease. On the other hand, too much iodine will aggravate many thyroid disorders, including Hashimoto's thyroiditis and multinodular goiter, as well as interfere with tests and treatments using radioactive iodine. Supplements that contain thyroid hormones will also aggravate thyroid disorders and interfere with tests and treatments.

Unfortunately, over-the-counter iodine and thyroid supplements are readily available on the Internet, in health food stores, and in some grocery and drug stores. Many well-intentioned patients erroneously assume that supplementing their diets with natural products will help them. However, many products will actually harm them by causing or worsening thyroid dysfunction, as well as by interfering with tests and treatments.

If patients search the Internet for information on thyroid disease, they are likely to see advertisements and links to sites selling natural products for thyroid dysfunction, weight loss, or energy. Very few sites list the ingredients or the amounts of the ingredients in these products. Therefore, patients cannot actually know what they are taking, and neither can their physicians.

Similarly, products from health food stores may not be adequately labeled. The labels on a variety of supplements contain terms such as

Substances* Containing Iodine

amiodarone
- Cordarone®
- Pacerone®

iodoquinol
- Yodoxin®
- Vytone®

kelp

potassium iodide
- KI Syrup®
- Pediacof Syrup®
- Pima Syrup®
- SSKI® (Lugol's solution)

povidone-iodine douches
- Betadine® Medicated Douche
- Massengill® Medicated Douche

povidone-iodine topical ointments
- Betadine® Ointment

x-ray dyes
- CAT scans
- IVPs
- myelograms
- arteriograms

* *This list contains some, but not all, of the substances containing iodine that may affect thyroid patients.*

Other Substances* Affecting Thyroid Patients

5-fluorouracil (5-FU)
aluminum hydroxide
- Maalox®
- Mylanta®

amphetamines
- Adderal®

androgens
- Androderm®
- Androgel®
- Depo®-Testosterone
- Testoderm®

beta-blockers
- atenolol (Tenormin®)
- propranolol (Inderal®)

calcium
- Maalox®
- Os-Cal®
- Viactiv®

carbamazepine
- Tegretol®

cholestyramine
- Questran®
- Cholybar®

clofibrate
- Atromid-S®

colestipol hydrochloride
- Colestid®

danazol
- Danocrine®

estrogens
- birth control pills
- Premarin®

fiber
furosemide
- Lasix®

grapefruit juice
heparin
heroin
interferon alfa
- Rebetron®

iron
- Feosol®
- Fergon®
- prenatal vitamins

l-asparaginase
- Elspar®

lithium
- Duralith®
- Eskalith®
- Lithobid®

mefenamic acid
- Ponstel®

methadone
perphenazine
- Etrafon®
- Trilafon®

phenytoin
- Dilantin®

raloxifene **
- Evista®

rifampin
SSRI's
- Celexa®
- Paxil®
- Prozac®
- Zoloft®

salicylates
salsalate
- Disalcid®

slow-release niacin (nicotinic acid)
- Slo-Niacin®

soy products
steroids
- Decadron®
- Deltasone®

sucralfate
- Carafate®

tamoxifen
- Nolvadex®

thalidomide

** This list contains some, but not all, of the substances affecting thyroid patients and some, but not all, of the name brands of those substances.*

*** There is contradictory evidence about the effect of raloxifene on thyroid function test results.*

"thyroid" or "thyro," leading some consumers to assume the products contain thyroid hormone. A closer look will show that few of these supplements actually list thyroid tissue as an ingredient. If they do, they usually do not state the source or the amount of the thyroid hormone in the products. Typically, iodine from kelp is among the ingredients listed on the labels of these products. The recommendation stated on some labels may range from 450 to 600 mcg (micrograms) of iodine daily, well above the minimum 150 mcg of iodine recommended by the World Health Organization for nonpregnant adults. Since the average daily intake of iodine in the United States is already 300 to 500 mcg, supplementing the typical American diet with iodine is unnecessary and potentially harmful.

Iodine is also found in certain medications. In most cases, there are iodine-free substitutes available for medications containing iodine; however, sometimes an iodine-free substitute is not available. For example, some patients cannot discontinue amiodarone, a very effective iodine-rich medication for the control of dangerous heart rhythm disturbances (arrhythmias). Amiodarone can have a profound and unpredictable effect on thyroid test results and on thyroid function. Because of its high iodine content, amiodarone can cause abnormal thyroid function test results and, in a small number of patients, actual thyroid dysfunction (see "Jim's Story" on pages 88–90). Approximately 7% of patients taking this drug develop amiodarone-induced hypothyroidism (AIH), and approximately 5% develop one of two forms of hyperthyroidism known as Type I and Type II amiodarone-induced thyrotoxicosis (AIT). Amiodarone-induced hypothyroidism is discussed on page 102 in Chapter 5, and amiodarone-induced thyrotoxicosis is discussed on pages 198–199 in Chapter 7.

Finally, some x-ray dyes contain large amounts of iodine. Sometimes these dyes can cause thyroid function test result abnormalities and, uncommonly, symptomatic thyroid dysfunction. CAT scans, arteriograms, IVPs, heart catheterizations, and myelograms are x-ray procedures that typically use injectable dyes with iodine. On the other hand, the injectable dyes used for MRIs do not contain iodine and, therefore, do not affect thyroid function.

When thyroid function test results are altered by nonthyroidal illnesses, patients are said to have nonthyroidal illness syndrome (NTIS), which is also called euthyroid sick syndrome (ESS). Nonthyroidal illness syndrome is commonly seen in hospitalized patients and only occasionally in outpatients (see "Maiko's Story" on pages 36–40).

In patients taking prescribed thyroid hormone, there are additional factors that can affect thyroid function test results. For example, substances affecting thyroid hormone absorption, such as food and drugs, may lower thyroid hormone levels, although the resulting levels may still be in the normal range. These substances can alter more than just thyroid function test results. If they interfere with thyroid hormone absorption enough, they will cause euthyroid patients to become hypothyroid (see "Ken's Story" on page 145–147).

Pregnancy and Thyroid Function Tests

Confusion regarding thyroid function test results during pregnancy may arise because these results will vary depending on how far along women are in their pregnancies. Thyroid function test results, such as TSH and thyroid hormone (T_4 and T_3) levels, will fluctuate during normal pregnancies. These levels may go up and down and, yet, remain in the normal range for pregnant women. When pregnant women say that their hormones are bouncing all over the map, they are only scratching the surface of the problem. Below is a "simplified" description of some of the thyroid hormone changes during a normal pregnancy.

Several factors contribute to these fluctuations, including estrogens and human chorionic gonadotropin (hCG). Beginning in the early stages of pregnancy, estrogens cause an increase in thyroid hormone-binding proteins, which remain elevated until a few months after delivery. These increased thyroid hormone-binding proteins may cause a 10 to 15% decrease in free T_4 and T_3, even though they are usually within the normal range for pregnant women. Correspondingly, the TSH rises slightly between the first trimester and delivery.

During the first eight to fourteen weeks of pregnancy, hCG, a hormone produced by the placenta, rises significantly. If hCG rises sufficiently, it can mimic, to a mild degree, the function of TSH. Therefore, hCG can sometimes raise free T_4 and T_3 levels. Although the free T_4 and T_3 levels are still in the normal range, they may be sufficiently elevated to lower TSH levels during the first eight to fourteen weeks of pregnancy in up to 20% of pregnancies. These women have transient subclinical hyperthyroidism.

In a much smaller percentage of normal pregnancies, the effects of hCG can be so pronounced during this six-week period that free T_4 may be temporarily elevated out of the normal range for pregnant women. These laboratory findings (an elevated free T_4 and a low TSH) are sometimes referred to as gestational transient hyperthyroidism, gestational thyrotoxicosis, or gestational hyperthyroxinemia.

Tests That Evaluate Thyroid Structure

Thyroid Imaging or Scanning

A thyroid image, or thyroid scan, is a picture of the thyroid gland obtained after administering radioactive materials to a patient. The first instrument designed for this purpose was called a rectilinear scanner. This machine moves (scans) back and forth over the neck of the patient who remains stationary. A picture obtained using this device is called a thyroid scan and is life-size.

Today most thyroid imaging is done using a stationary gamma camera. It does not give a life-size picture of the thyroid gland, but it may be more sensitive than a rectilinear scanner for detecting minor abnormalities. The picture obtained from a gamma camera is called a thyroid image. The terms "image" and "scan" are frequently used interchangeably.

Different radioactive materials, or isotopes, are used to obtain images of the thyroid gland. Radioactive iodine is frequently used since both a picture and a radioactive iodine uptake can be obtained with only a single isotope. Various isotopes of radioactive iodine are available, but I^{123} is most commonly used for thyroid imaging. Although it is more expensive than I^{131} (the isotope used to treat hyperthyroidism and thyroid cancer), I^{123} delivers a much lower dose of radiation. Typically, a patient takes a dose of I^{123} orally, in the form of a liquid or a pill, in the morning and returns either in the afternoon or the next day. When she returns, both a thyroid image and a 6-hour or a 24-hour radioactive

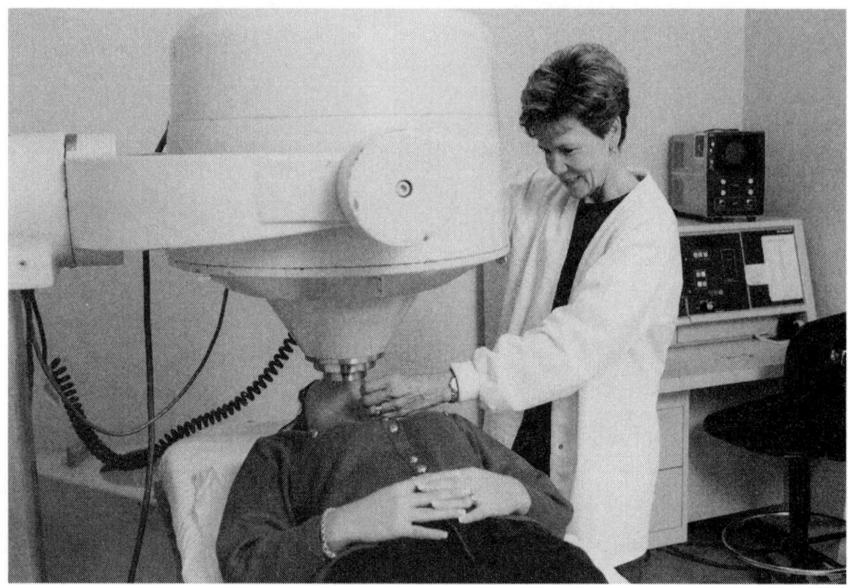

Figure 4.7. Nurse positioning patient for radioactive iodine uptake and thyroid image with gamma camera.

iodine uptake can be obtained.

Technetium is another isotope commonly used to obtain a thyroid image. Technetium is injected intravenously, and a thyroid image can be obtained as soon as twenty minutes later. Although this procedure is quick and involves less radiation than iodine, it has two disadvantages. First, a radioactive iodine uptake cannot be done with technetium. Second, technetium has given misleading results in a small number of patients with thyroid nodules. Technetium is taken up by the thyroid gland, but it is not used by the thyroid gland. Radioactive iodine is both taken up and used by the thyroid gland in the production of thyroid hormones. Therefore, technetium may sometimes suggest a nodule is over-functioning when, in fact, it is not.

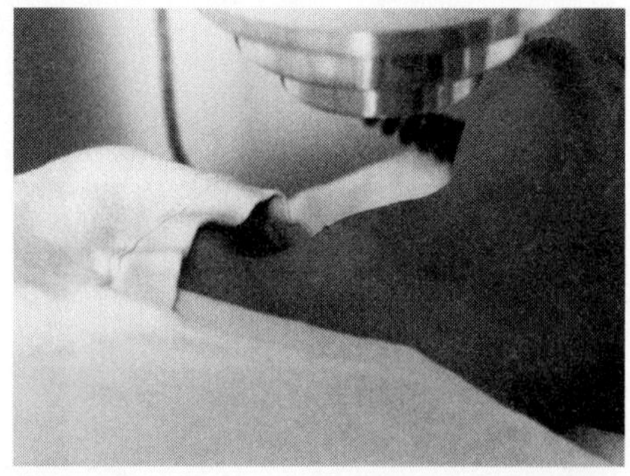

Figure 4.8. Patient with asymmetrical multinodular goiter under gamma camera for thyroid image.

Thyroid images or scans are most often performed to

evaluate thyroid nodules or to follow up on known thyroid cancers. Nodules are classified as hot, warm, or cold. These are relative terms that describe how much of the radioactive material is taken up by the nodule as compared to the surrounding thyroid tissue. A nodule that takes up more radioactive material than the surrounding thyroid tissue is said to be hot. Sometimes a nodule is so hot that it produces enough thyroid hormone to suppress the surrounding thyroid tissue. If this happens, the hot nodule will be the only thyroid tissue on the thyroid image. Hot nodules are almost never cancerous.

A nodule that takes up less radioactive material than the surrounding tissue is said to be a cold nodule. While most cold nodules are not malignant, almost all malignancies are cold on thyroid imaging. Examples of hot and cold nodules are shown in Figure 4.9. A nodule that is neither hot nor cold is called warm. While hot nodules are almost never malignant, warm nodules can be.

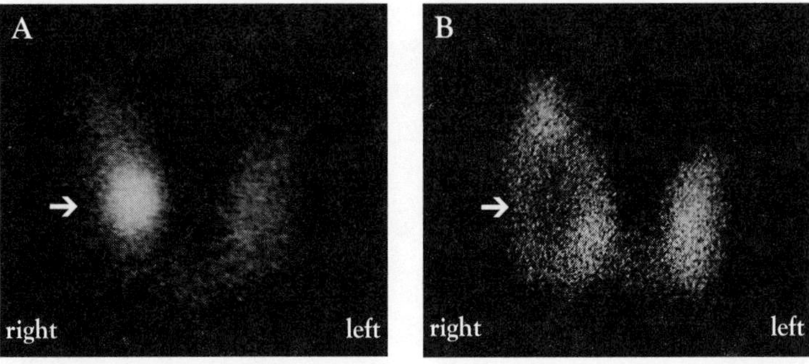

Figure 4.9. Thyroid images. (A) Hot nodule in right lobe. (B) Cold nodule in right lobe.

As mentioned earlier in this chapter, there is much overlap between tests of thyroid function and tests of thyroid structure. For example, thyroid scans not only demonstrate the presence of nodules (as well as other structural abnormalities), but they also indicate how the nodules are functioning.

In a patient with thyroid cancer, radioactive materials may be used to image not only the thyroid, but also other parts of the body to which cancerous thyroid cells may have spread. This scan is called a whole body scan. Most whole body scans are obtained forty-eight to seventy-two hours after administration of radioactive iodine. They are usually performed six weeks after removing a thyroid cancer and, if patients have been treated with radioactive iodine, eight to twelve months later.

Pregnant or breastfeeding women should not take radioactive materials.

Thyroid imaging, just like the radioactive iodine uptake, can be altered by certain other diagnostic tests done within the preceding six weeks. For example, a patient having a CAT scan, myelogram, IVP, or arteriogram may be given x-ray dyes that contain large amounts of iodine. The large amount of iodine given for the x-ray procedure dilutes the small amount of radioactive iodine given for the thyroid image. The amount of radioactive material taken up by the thyroid gland, therefore, may not be enough to produce a thyroid image. A patient should postpone elective x-rays using iodinated dyes until after her thyroid image is completed (see "Trina's Story" on pages 82–84). Injectable dyes may also be used in MRIs; however, the dyes used for MRIs do not ordinarily contain iodine and, therefore, do not affect thyroid function.

Thyroid Ultrasound

When sound waves are bounced off a structure, a picture can be obtained safely and painlessly. Thyroid ultrasound is particularly helpful in older patients and in patients with short, thick necks whose thyroid glands are difficult to feel.

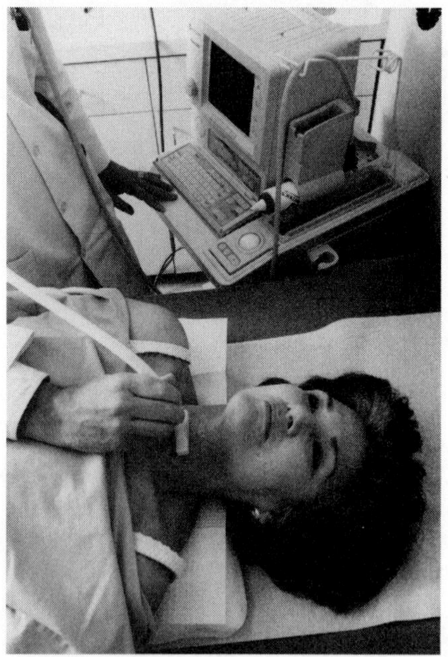

Figure 4.10. Patient having a thyroid ultrasound.

If a patient has an irregular thyroid gland, the examining physician may be unsure whether any nodules are present. An ultrasound picture of the thyroid gland will clarify the diagnosis. One thyroid nodule raises concern about thyroid cancer. In general, multiple nodules reduce the likelihood of cancer.

Thyroid ultrasound can also accurately determine the size of a nodule. A series of ultrasound measurements may be compared to see if a nodule is getting larger or smaller. In addition, the components of a thyroid nodule can be accurately described by thyroid ultrasound. For example, cystic structures have a different appearance than solid structures; completely fluid-filled thyroid cysts are less likely to be malignant than solid thyroid nodules. Thyroid ultrasound can also show if the windpipe (trachea) is being pushed out of its normal position (tracheal deviation) by an enlarged thyroid gland. Finally, thyroid ultrasound may detect recurrent thyroid cancer or cancerous lymph nodes in the neck of a patient who has had surgery for thyroid cancer.

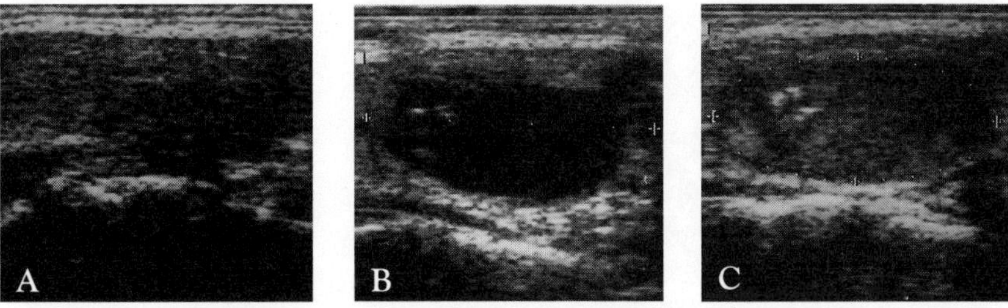

Figure 4.11. Thyroid ultrasounds (longitudinal view). (A) Normal thyroid. (B) Mostly cystic thyroid nodule (cystic area is dark). (C) Solid thyroid nodule.

Thyroid ultrasound is most useful as a diagnostic tool when performed by a physician who is familiar with the anatomy of the thyroid gland and who wants to answer a specific question about a particular patient. It may eliminate the need for further diagnostic studies, such as thyroid imaging and thyroid biopsy. On the other hand, thyroid ultrasound is not a substitute for thyroid biopsy in determining whether a thyroid nodule is benign or malignant.

Thyroid Biopsy

Ordinarily, when a patient has a thyroid nodule, a thyroid biopsy is performed to decide whether she needs surgery. A physician experienced in performing thyroid biopsies will obtain thyroid cells or tissue for analysis by a pathologist, a physician trained to determine whether cells and tissue are normal or abnormal.

Many times, a biopsy will eliminate the need for surgery, as is demonstrated in Figure 4.12. On the right of the picture are the charts of 120 patients who went directly to surgery without a preoperative needle biopsy; only thirteen patients were found to have cancer. The same number of cancers was also found in the twenty patients (charts on the left) whose preoperative needle biopsies yielded abnormal cells. Therefore, needle biopsies prevented unnecessary surgery in approximately 100 patients.

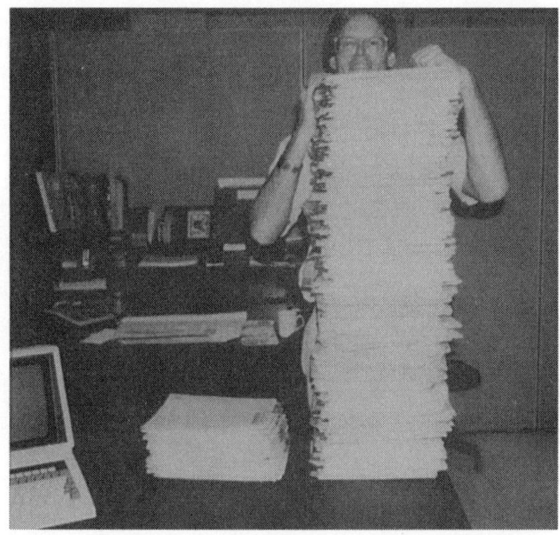

Figure 4.12. Charts of patients who had thyroidectomies. The difference between the stacks represents the number of unnecessary thyroid surgeries that could have been prevented with needle biopsies.

A fine needle aspiration biopsy (FNAB) is the most common type of thyroid biopsy. It is called a fine needle aspiration biopsy because the needle is very thin, much thinner than the needle used to draw blood from the arm. The neck may be anesthetized with a local anesthetic, and then a thin biopsy needle, with or without a syringe, is inserted into the thyroid gland. Up to ten needles may be introduced to obtain an adequate sample for evaluation by the pathologist. Pain is minimal, and complications are rare. Occasionally, cells cannot be obtained from a solid nodule by a fine needle aspiration biopsy, and a cutting needle biopsy (CNB) is performed. This procedure is essentially the same as the fine needle biopsy, except that a special cutting needle is used. At present, there is no substitute for a needle biopsy in determining, without surgery, whether a nodule is benign or malignant.

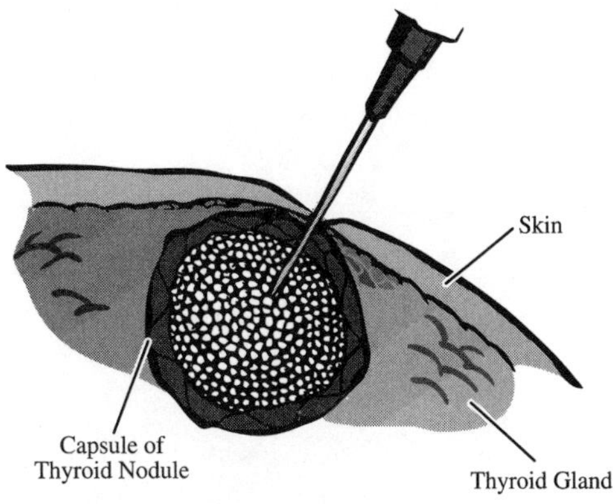

Figure 4.13. Fine needle aspiration biopsy.

Sometimes, either because a nodule may be in a difficult location or a patient's neck may be difficult to position correctly, the physician may not be able to easily perform a thyroid biopsy. In such circumstances, an ultrasound-guided thyroid biopsy may be performed using an ultrasound machine to guide the needle to the thyroid nodule. Ultrasound-guided thyroid biopsies are being performed more often because nodules that are difficult to feel are being discovered incidentally on x-rays taken for reasons other than suspected thyroid disease.

After a biopsy specimen is examined in the laboratory, a pathologist may report one of four diagnoses:

1. *Benign* (or *negative*)—65 to 75% of patients receive this result. Enough cells are present, the cells appear benign, and there is nothing to suggest cancer.

2. *Non-diagnostic* (or *unsatisfactory*)—Approximately 10% of the time, the number of cells is inadequate for the pathologist to determine whether the nodule is benign or malignant. A small number of benign cells may be present, but not enough for the pathologist to call the nodule benign. If the specimen is non-diagnostic, a patient might be asked to return for a second or third biopsy or even an ultrasound-guided biopsy.

3. *Malignant* (or *positive*)—In 5 to 10% of patients, the pathologist diagnoses cancer; sometimes he can specify the type of cancer.

4. *Suspicious* (or *inconclusive*)—In 10 to 15% of specimens, the cells have features suggestive of, but not diagnostic of, cancer. Inconclusive is not the same as a diagnosis of non-diagnostic or unsatisfactory.

Suspicious findings occur most often because cells from certain benign tumors (follicular adenomas) may look like cells from follicular cancers. Also, if there are many Hürthle cells (a distinctive variant of follicular cells) present—suggestive of a Hürthle cell tumor—the biopsy result will be categorized as suspicious. At present, the only way to determine whether a follicular tumor or a Hürthle cell tumor is benign or malignant is by surgery. Hopefully, newer techniques for analyzing biopsy specimens will make the distinction between benign and malignant follicular cells without surgery.

Thyroid Structure Tests

TEST	TO DIAGNOSE OR EVALUATE
thyroid imaging	nodules thyroid cancer aberrant thyroid tissue
thyroid ultrasound	presence and number of nodules characteristics of nodule(s) characteristics of a goiter presence of recurrent thyroid cancer presence of cancerous lymph nodes
thyroid biopsy	nodules

Some thyroidologists recommend a second biopsy, even when the first result is benign and the nodule has not increased in size. They recommend this because, occasionally, a second biopsy yields a different result than the first biopsy. On the other hand, an informal survey of 1,000 patients rebiopsied one to two years after their first biopsy found that the diagnosis changed from benign to suspicious in only five (0.5%) patients, and to malignant in none.

When selecting a pathologist, the referring physician must carefully consider the pathologist's experience in interpreting thyroid biopsies. One of the main functions of a physician is to ensure that the pathologist with whom he works is of the highest quality.

Other X-ray Procedures

Thyroid imaging (scanning), thyroid ultrasound, and thyroid biopsy usually provide all the information needed about thyroid structure. However, there are some circumstances in which information from additional procedures is needed. A substernal goiter is located behind the breastbone (sternum) and, therefore, a chest x-ray may be necessary to see if the trachea is pushed out of position or constricted by the goiter. An esophagram, or x-ray of the esophagus, may be ordered to see if an enlarged thyroid gland is compressing the esophagus and causing difficulty with swallowing. If a physician suspects that a goiter or a nodule has altered a patient's breathing or voice, then he may order a CAT scan of the neck and chest to see if the trachea or vocal cords have been affected. A chest x-ray, CAT scan, MRI, or PET (positron emission tomography) scan may also be performed on a patient with thyroid cancer to see if there has been any spread of the cancer to the chest or elsewhere.

Tests for Autoimmune Disease

Two common autoimmune diseases affect the thyroid gland—Hashimoto's thyroiditis and Graves' disease. Autoimmune diseases are characterized by the presence of autoantibodies circulating in the bloodstream. Antibodies are proteins formed by the immune system to protect the body against foreign chemicals, bacteria, or viruses. In an autoimmune disease, antibodies are formed against the patient's own tissues, and they are, therefore, called *auto*antibodies.

Hashimoto's thyroiditis is a chronic inflammation of the thyroid that leads to enlargement and eventual destruction of the thyroid gland. Antithyroid autoantibodies play a primary role in this disease. Antibodies to two thyroid components are of particular diagnostic value for Hashimoto's thyroiditis—thyroperoxidase (TPOAb) and thyroglobulin (TgAb) antibodies.

Graves' disease is an autoimmune disease that affects the thyroid gland, and, less often, the eyes and the skin. When the thyroid gland is affected, Graves' patients form antibodies to TSH receptors (thyrotropin receptor antibodies, or TRAb). A receptor is the specific site on a cell that selectively captures its corresponding hormone. The hormone fits in the receptor like a key in an ignition switch. When TSH receptors on thyroid follicular cells capture TSH, they combine to stimulate, or "ignite," thyroid hormone production. Some TRAb duplicate the function of TSH. They bind to receptors and stimulate thyroid hormone production, which, in turn, signals the pituitary gland to stop making TSH.

TRAb are measured by different methods that measure different properties of these antibodies, and, therefore, they may go by different names. For example, TRAb that stimulate and activate TSH receptors are called either thyroid-stimulating immunoglobulins (TSI) or thyroid-stimulating antibodies (TSAb). As mentioned above, these remarkable antibodies (TSI and TSAb) duplicate the function of TSH—they stimulate thyroid hormone production and secretion. Some physicians find TSI or TSAb levels useful in both the diagnosis of Graves' disease and in following the course of Graves' disease in patients treated with antithyroid drugs.

TRAb that inhibit the binding of TSH to its receptors are called either TSH-binding-inhibitory immunoglobulins (TBII) or TSH-stimulation-blocking antibodies (TSBAb). These antibodies (TBII and TSBAb) may be found in patients with either Hashimoto's thyroiditis or Graves' disease.

Tests for Autoimmune Thyroid Disease

TEST	TO EVALUATE
TPOAb	Hashimoto's thyroiditis
TgAb	Hashimoto's thyroiditis
TRAb	
TSI	Graves' disease
TSAb	Graves' disease
TBII	Hashimoto's thyroiditis and Graves' disease
TSBAb	Hashimoto's thyroiditis and Graves' disease

Other Related Tests

Thyroglobulin

Thyroglobulin (Tg) is a protein made exclusively by the thyroid gland. Thyroid hormones are bound to this protein within the colloid of the thyroid follicle (see Chapter 1). Thyroglobulin also circulates in the blood and can be measured with a blood test. A series of thyroglobulin measurements and the response of thyroglobulin to synthetic TSH (Thyrogen) injections are useful in following patients with differentiated thyroid cancers (see Chapter 11). Since thyroglobulin antibodies will interfere with the measurement of thyroglobulin, laboratories should also report the presence or absence of thyroglobulin antibodies when they report thyroglobulin measurements.

Synthetic TSH (Thyrogen®)

In addition to stimulating thyroglobulin, synthetic TSH (also called thyrotropin-alfa, recombinant human TSH, rhTSH, or Thyrogen) is used in some thyroid cancer patients to perform whole body scans without discontinuing thyroid hormone (see Chapter 11). It is expected that this synthetic TSH will also eventually be used to treat thyroid cancer patients with radioactive iodine without discontinuing their thyroid hormone.

Furthermore, synthetic TSH has potential as a diagnostic tool. During the next few years, synthetic TSH may be approved for the following diagnostic purposes:

- enhancement of thyroid tissue stimulation by TSH in a thyroid cancer patient undergoing a withdrawal scan
- enhancement of radioactive iodine uptake in a patient with a goiter and a low radioactive iodine uptake
- stimulation of suppressed thyroid tissue in a patient with unilateral radioactive iodine uptake in the neck
- evaluation of the function of the thyroid gland while a patient is taking thyroid hormone
- improvement of the diagnostic value of PET scans in a thyroid cancer patient

Sedimentation Rate

The sedimentation rate measures how rapidly proteins in the blood settle to the bottom of a small tube. This test helps to distinguish subacute thyroiditis from other causes of hyperthyroidism.

Calcitonin

Calcitonin is produced by C cells (parafollicular cells) in the thyroid gland; its function is not known. A marked elevation of calcitonin suggests the presence of an unsuspected medullary thyroid cancer (MTC), a thyroid cancer arising from the C cells. Therefore, some doctors recommend measuring calcitonin in all patients with thyroid nodules (see "Estelita's Story" on pages 91–94 and "Dick's Story" on pages 354–357). Calcitonin levels are also useful in following patients with known medullary cancer.

Tests that stimulate calcitonin may be helpful in both the diagnosis and follow-up of patients with medullary cancer. Intravenous infusions of either calcium (calcium infusion test) or a hormone called pentagastrin (pentagastrin test) can stimulate calcitonin, but, unfortunately, pentagastrin is not available in the United States at this time. In the calcium infusion test, calcium is given intravenously over a five-minute period. Blood samples for calcitonin are drawn immediately before the infusion begins and then at two-minute, five-minute, and ten-minute intervals.

Pregnant women should not have calcium infusion tests.

A small percentage of medullary thyroid cancers are familial, and they are occasionally part of a hereditary syndrome that includes tumors in multiple endocrine glands (multiple endocrine neoplasia type 2, or MEN 2). Family members of a patient with medullary cancer or MEN 2 may be screened for the presence of medullary cancer by the use of a single calcitonin measurement, a calcium infusion test, or, when available, a pentagastrin test.

Carcinoembryonic Antigen

Carcinoembryonic antigen (CEA) is another blood test useful for following some patients with medullary thyroid cancers and other non-thyroidal cancers such as colon cancer. In a patient with medullary cancer, CEA is measured preoperatively to determine if it is produced by the tumor. If the preoperative CEA level is elevated, this baseline measurement is compared with subsequent measurements of CEA.

Calcium

Calcium is an atomic element that is everywhere in the body. Calcium metabolism is regulated by parathyroid hormone produced by the parathyroid glands, which are located on the back of the thyroid gland. If the parathyroid glands are damaged during thyroid surgery, the result is hypocalcemia (low calcium in the blood). Therefore, calcium is measured multiple times following some thyroid surgeries, particularly those performed for thyroid cancer. On rare occasions, the large doses of radioactive iodine used to treat patients with thyroid cancer can damage the parathyroid glands.

Thyroid dysfunction may elevate calcium levels. Hypothyroidism and hyperthyroidism will both alter the rate at which bone, the major source of calcium in the body, is metabolized. This alteration can cause hypercalcemia (high calcium in the blood), a condition that should resolve once the thyroid problem is corrected. The most common cause of hypercalcemia, however, is hyperparathyroidism from a benign parathyroid tumor.

Prolactin

Prolactin, a hormone produced by the pituitary gland, is required for a woman to lactate (produce milk) and to breastfeed. The function of prolactin in males is unknown. A physician may refer a woman or a man to an endocrinologist for evaluation of an elevated prolactin or for a milky breast discharge (galactorrhea) since these abnormalities can be caused by hypothyroidism as well as by pituitary dysfunction. A man with a high prolactin level may also have growth of glandular breast tissue in one or both breasts (gynecomastia).

Genetic Testing

A test for a mutation of a gene called the RET proto-oncogene is available to diagnose multiple endocrine neoplasia type 2. Although Hashimoto's thyroiditis and Graves' disease are hereditary, there are no practical genetic tests available for determining susceptibility to these diseases. Nonetheless, one can envision the day when genetic testing for these and other thyroid diseases will be readily available.

Cholesterol and Homocysteine

Cholesterol is a known risk factor for heart disease. Homocysteine, an amino acid, is very likely another risk factor for heart disease. Hypothyroidism elevates both cholesterol and homocysteine levels. On the other hand, hyperthyroidism lowers cholesterol levels but does not have a significant effect on homocysteine levels.

Miscellaneous Blood Tests

Hypothyroidism and hyperthyroidism can cause other abnormal blood test results. Liver function tests, such as alkaline phosphatase, bilirubin, SGOT (AST), SGPT (ALT), and LDH, may be elevated by thyroid dysfunction. Anemia, a reduction in the number of red blood cells, may also occur. Muscle enzymes, such as creatine kinase, are frequently elevated in patients with hypothyroidism, while testosterone may be low in some men with hypothyroidism. These test results should return to normal once the patient's thyroid disease is successfully treated.

Interleukin-6 (IL-6) is one of many cytokines, or hormone-like proteins, that play an important part in the body's immune response. IL-6 is often elevated in patients with Type II amiodarone-induced thyrotoxicosis and can be useful for distinguishing it from Type I amiodarone-induced thyrotoxicosis.

Thyroid Screening Programs

Screening, an important tool in preventive medicine, is the process of detecting disease among people who do not have symptoms of a disease or who are unaware that they may have a disease. It differs from routine testing of patients who complain of a symptom or symptoms that may lead physicians to suspect particular disorders. The high incidence of thyroid disease, the existence of safe and effective treatments, and the ready availability and relatively low cost of accurate thyroid function tests have led to screening programs for thyroid disease in certain groups of patients.

Neonatal Screening

The signs and symptoms of congenital hypothyroidism are seldom apparent at birth; however, delay in treatment of a congenitally hypothyroid infant can cause irreversible brain damage. Therefore, screening for congenital hypothyroidism is performed on all newborns in the United States, Canada, Israel, Japan, Australia, New Zealand, and most countries in Europe.

Neonatal thyroid screening has led to a marked reduction in

cretinism (mental retardation and short stature due to hypothyroidism) and untreated hypothyroidism in newborns. The cost of screening and treating children for congenital hypothyroidism is far less than the long-term cost of caring for untreated children.

Screening Adults

There is a growing consensus among scientists and public health officials that, in addition to newborns, other groups of people should be screened for thyroid disease. Some physicians recommend screening groups of people known to be at an increased risk for thyroid disease—such as women over thirty-five, men and women over fifty-five, people with Down's syndrome, and people with autoimmune diseases, such as Type 1 diabetes.

Although screening programs for thyroid disease are effective, questions have been raised about their cost-effectiveness. A 1996 study examined the cost benefit of early thyroid disease detection and concluded that screening under certain circumstances was justified. Specifically, the authors of the study stated that measurement of TSH among adults thirty-five years of age or older every five years compared favorably to the cost of other well-recognized screening programs, such as mammograms for breast cancer.

Physicians agree that a measurement of TSH is the single most accurate screening test for thyroid dysfunction. When TSH results are abnormal, follow-up should include a physical examination, measurement of thyroid hormones, and, perhaps, a repeat TSH measurement. Physicians, insurance companies, and government agencies will be more likely to endorse screening for thyroid disease among selected groups of people as the cost of measuring TSH decreases.

Some physicians also recommend screening all pregnant women for the antithyroid antibodies characteristic of Hashimoto's thyroiditis because at least two-thirds of the cases of postpartum thyroiditis occur in women with Hashimoto's thyroiditis. High antibody levels are likely to identify many of the 5 to 9% of the women who will develop postpartum thyroiditis after delivery.

Patient Profiles

GAIL'S STORY

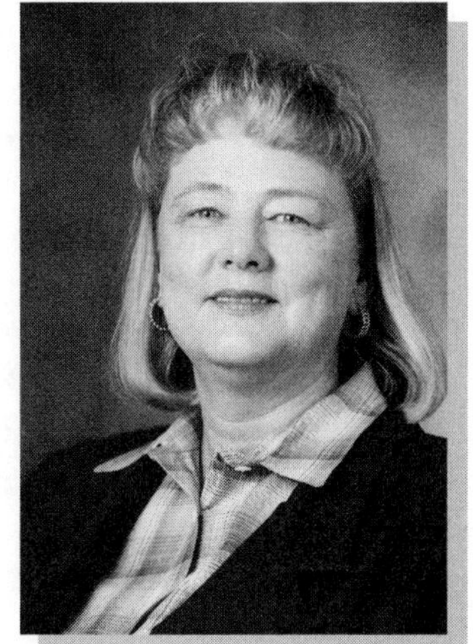

One day, Gail, a fifty-two-year-old retired teacher, was watching television and became interested in a local talk show featuring thyroid disease.

> The show interested me because my daughter had been diagnosed when she was sixteen with hypothyroidism.
>
> I saw [the endocrinologist who had diagnosed my daughter] demonstrating how to check your own thyroid on the show, so I thought I would try it. I felt a lump about the size of a pea.

Gail's situation was more unusual than most patients with thyroid nodules. In 1968, she was diagnosed with Ehlers-Danlos Syndrome (EDS), a rare disorder that causes extreme elasticity of connective tissues.

> As a child, my shoulders would separate, but no one knew why. It was diagnosed after my daughter was born. During my pregnancy, both hips dislocated. The orthopedic surgeon said that it couldn't be EDS—that only animals had it. But a skin biopsy proved him wrong.
>
> I've had multiple joint restructuring since then. I was also diagnosed with Crohn's disease in 1990. Even though I have these conditions, I try to stay as active

> as I can. I do water aerobics to keep my muscles toned. I believe that chronic illness is a matter of the mind.

Because of her health problems, Gail was very familiar with doctors and with medical and surgical procedures. She brought up the subject of her thyroid nodule with one of her physicians.

> You are your own advocate. If your intuition tells you something is wrong, you have to follow up on it. No one else will.
>
> As it happened, I had an appointment with [an ear, nose, and throat doctor, or ENT] to check for a possible hearing loss. At first, he couldn't feel [the thyroid nodule], and then he did. He sent me to a radiologist at [a major medical center] who did a fine needle aspiration biopsy and radioactive iodine scan. I also had blood work.
>
> The doctor said, "Everything indicates it's benign, but it's there and it's large." He said we could wait and observe or operate now. I chose to have the surgery. [My ENT] removed the right side of my thyroid.

Gail's nodule was benign. Shortly after surgery, Gail began taking 0.1 mg (milligram) of levothyroxine daily. Six weeks later, Gail resumed her active lifestyle, including water aerobics.■

TRINA'S STORY

Twenty-seven–year-old Trina is married and works as a special education teacher. In 1998, she began to experience symptoms that are all too familiar in her family.

> I was lethargic, short of breath, and had headaches for a month straight. I also had scant menstrual periods and a decreased sexual drive. My heart palpitated a lot. I'm 5'4" and usually weigh 120 pounds, but I lost

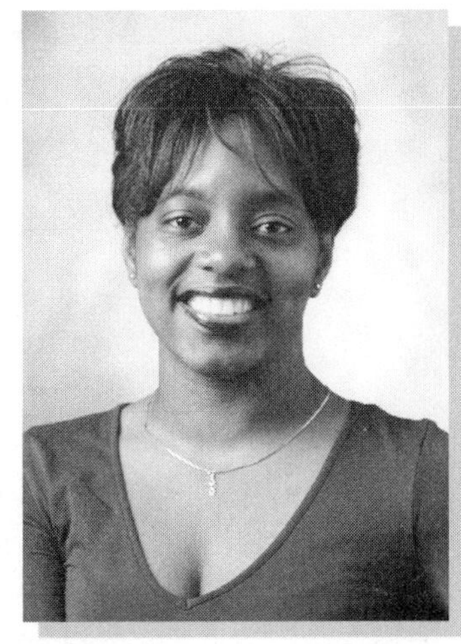

> down to 102 pounds. My mom noticed that my skin color changed; it got darker. I was working at the time and in school. I noticed when I walked from the car to class, I would get short of breath.
>
> I knew that thyroid disease ran in my family. My grandmother, an aunt, mom, and sister all have hyperthyroidism. I went to an endocrinologist right away. He drew my blood. It came back a week later, and he told me I had Graves' disease. He put me on antithyroid medication because he said I was too young for surgery. I can't remember why we didn't do radioactive iodine.
>
> I took the [antithyroid medication] for about four to five months. One day my mom took me to breakfast and noticed my neck was still kind of large. All of the other symptoms were better. She referred me to her endocrinologist.

Her mother's endocrinologist reviewed the pretreatment test results, which included an elevated free T_4 level and a low TSH level. Her initial radioactive iodine uptakes were high at 25% after four hours and 47% after twenty-four hours. These test results confirmed a diagnosis of hyperthyroidism.

Physical examination by her new endocrinologist revealed the presence of a thyroid nodule. A fine needle aspiration biopsy was done and was negative for cancer. Trina had become hypothyroid; therefore, the antithyroid medication was discontinued. Her TSI were positive, confirming the diagnosis of Graves' disease. Seven months later, her thyroid function test results were normal, but Trina developed new symptoms.

> I had problems with frequent urination, so I wanted

> to check my bladder. I went to a urologist, and he ordered an IVP. They injected me with [iodinated] dye. The results came back normal.

Trina returned for a follow-up visit with her endocrinologist three months after her IVP. He discovered that her TSH was below normal, and her 6-hour radioactive iodine uptake was now low at 0.8%.

> When I went for the thyroid scan at [my endocrinologist's] office, it came out black. They thought the machine was broken, and so they had it serviced. They called me back, and the scan still came out somewhat black. So they figured it was me. It was black because of the [iodinated] dye.
>
> I put it on a medical form at the urologist's office that I had Graves' disease, but he didn't ask me any questions about it. I didn't know that the dye they used could have an effect on my thyroid.
>
> My blood work showed that I was hyperthyroid, but [my endocrinologist] didn't put me on any medication. He said to wait a couple of months until the dye got out of my system. Now I'm not on thyroid medication of any kind.

Iodine, especially the large amounts in iodinated x-ray dyes, can interfere with thyroid function and thyroid function test results for a long time. Six months after her IVP, Trina's thyroid function test results returned to normal and her 6-hour radioactive iodine uptake was normal at 15.6%. Five months later, her thyroid function test results were still normal.■

SEYMOUR'S STORY

Seymour went to his optometrist for a routine eye examination in 1981. What his optometrist found was anything but routine. Seymour's wife Sharon recalls:

> The eye doctor said that there was something wrong with his [visual] field. He could see one line, and then he couldn't see it. One eye was affected. Seymour hadn't noticed any problems because his good eye was compensating for the bad one. His optometrist referred him to an ophthalmologist who sent him to a neurosurgeon. Within two weeks, Seymour had surgery to remove a pituitary tumor. They went in from the side of his head.
>
> Before the operation, the doctors asked him all kinds of questions. Are you having sex problems? No. Have your feet grown? No. Has your hat size increased? No. I guess most people with pituitary tumors have these problems, but not Seymour.

The pituitary gland is located just below the point where the nerves from each eye (optic nerves) cross before they connect to the rest of the brain. The pituitary gland is called the "master gland" because it controls the production of so many hormones, such as thyroid hormones, adrenal hormones, female hormones, and testosterone. Therefore, a patient with a pituitary tumor could experience problems, such as fatigue, and a decrease in libido (sex drive), depending on the location, size, and function of the tumor. If the tumor presses on the optic nerves, it could interfere with a patient's vision.

Seymour had a TSH-secreting pituitary tumor, which is very uncommon. Ordinarily, thyrotropin-releasing hormone from the hypothalamus and thyroid hormone from the thyroid gland regulate TSH secretion. Seymour's pituitary tumor was making inappropriate amounts of TSH independently of normal control mechanisms, which caused unusual, and possibly misleading, thyroid function test results. Once the cause of the unusual test results was identified, surgery was recommended. Sharon explains:

> The reason his tumor had to be removed was because

> the roots of it were wrapping around his optic nerve, and he would go blind without an operation. His doctor told us that pituitary tumors are usually benign. I think he said 90 to 95% were benign. I said, "Will you put that in writing?"
>
> Seymour did quite well after the operation. Afterwards, they gave him six weeks of radiation. My understanding was that it would kill the roots so that the tumor wouldn't come back. Seymour was a little tired after the radiation, but I think most people feel that way after having it.

At the insistence of his brother, Seymour and Sharon moved from Canada to Texas to be closer to his family. While there, he developed increasing headaches and decreasing libido with a low testosterone level. X-rays showed a recurrence of his pituitary tumor.

> Seymour was going for check-ups regularly to be sure his tumor hadn't come back. [Two] years after the first surgery, he had to have another operation. This time they went up above his gum line, through the back of his nose. He came out with a little patch under his nose.
>
> Seymour had to take prednisone and had hormone shots. The shots were to protect his sexuality, although he never had a problem with that. When he first started getting the shots, he went around with an erection for six weeks. We were hysterical about it; it was really funny. I would say, "You're walking around like some young boy."

Seymour's physicians discontinued his prednisone and started him on testosterone shots and levothyroxine shortly after his second surgery. His pituitary gland could no longer produce the hormones necessary to stimulate either his thyroid gland or his testes. Prior to his first surgery, his pituitary tumor was making too much TSH; now his pituitary gland was making hardly any.

> After we moved back to Canada, Seymour had to have surgery for a third time. This is the first time I heard them say this was an aggressive tumor—aggressive, meaning that it would return. Seymour was the type that if he didn't want to hear something, he didn't. He might have been told along the way that his tumor would keep growing back, but I never heard that until this time. So it was not until the third time that we realized it would continue to grow back. I don't understand why they gave him radiation the first time.

In 1995, an MRI indicated that Seymour had a different tumor in his brain; it was malignant.

> Seymour and I were separated at the time, but a friend told me that he was stumbling and falling and getting forgetful. My daughter noticed that he couldn't remember little things. It got to the point he didn't shower or shave. He didn't change shirts. I thought this couldn't be Seymour; he was always so neat and well-groomed.

> Then they found him in his room in a coma. He was having seizures. He was in the hospital two weeks. Fortunately, when he regained consciousness, he wasn't in any pain and didn't have to take pain medicine. He didn't remember that we were separated. He just wanted to go home, but the doctors said he would have to go to a nursing home. He didn't want that. At two in the morning I got a call from Seymour's sister that he had had another bad seizure. We rushed to the hospital, but he had already died. He was fifty-three years old.

Seymour had an unusual pituitary tumor, one that produced TSH. The TSH produced by the tumor initially caused confusion regarding his thyroid function test results, but his thyroid dysfunction was eventually corrected. On the other hand, while the treatment of his pituitary tumor was reasonably successful in that his vision and hormonal function were restored, he developed a fatal brain tumor, possibly as a result of his radiotherapy.■

JIM'S STORY

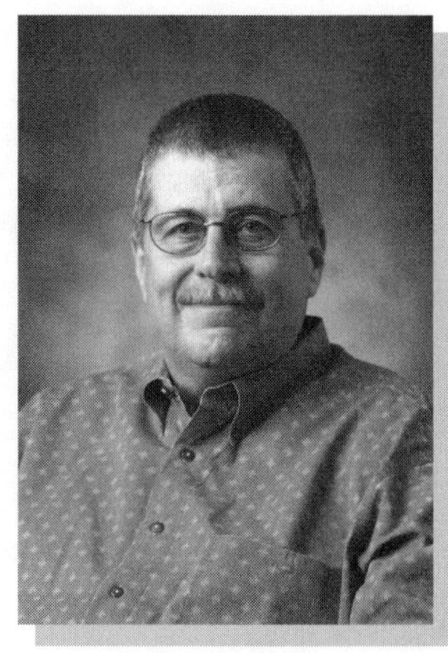

Forty-six-year-old Jim has an intimate and long-term relationship with the world of medicine. He has endured two aortic valve replacements, a mitral valve replacement, chronic ventricular tachycardia, ventricular fibrillation, multiple cardiac resuscitations, implantation of a cardioverter defibrillator, and atrial fibrillation. Throughout it all, Jim has persevered with a sense of humor and the love and support of his family. He has even parlayed his personal medical experiences into a career as a health care software consultant.

In 1998, shortly after having a cardiac defibrillator implanted for ventricular fibrillation, Jim went out of town on a business trip.

> My heart just took off. I went to the emergency room, and that's when they discovered I was suffering from atrial fibrillation, which is different from ventricular fibrillation. The doctors thought that the amiodarone I had started taking in 1996 for my heart condition had caused me to become hyperthyroid. [The doctor] shocked me back into sinus rhythm and put me on Tapazole [an antithyroid drug] three times a day.

The large amounts of iodine in amiodarone stimulated excessive thyroid hormone production (hyperthyroidism) that, in turn, caused atrial fibrillation. Therefore, Jim's physician discontinued the amiodarone when he prescribed the Tapazole. Unfortunately, Jim continued to suffer episodes of atrial fibrillation.

> The doctors shocked me back into sinus rhythm several times. When I was hospitalized again in July, an endocrinologist examined me; he and my cardiologist decided I needed to have my thyroid taken out. But I had to get my thyroid [hormone] levels down first.

Operating on Jim when he had elevated thyroid hormone levels would increase his risk of developing thyroid storm, a dramatic and life-threatening form of hyperthyroidism. In order to prepare Jim for his thyroidectomy, the endocrinologist placed him on a regimen of Tapazole, Perchloracap, and prednisone. At approximately the same time, Jim's cardiologist placed him on the heart transplant list.

> Between getting put on the list in July and December, I gained weight and had lots of problems with atrial fibrillation. My medications were adjusted to control my heart rate. My wife noticed that I had become very irritable, and I was very anxious.
>
> On December 9, I was sitting in a recliner watching television when my defibrillator delivered a shock. Let me tell you, it hurts! I felt dizzy just before it happened. Afterwards I was a little short of breath, and I could feel my heart rate had increased. Then [three days later] while I was in the grocery store shopping with my fourteen-year-old son, I turned to him and said, "I'm going out." I passed out and hit the ground; my head hit the pavement.

Jim's implanted defibrillator shocked him two times, and he was rushed to the hospital. His physicians decided that the time was right for a thyroidectomy. Although he was euthyroid, Jim was experiencing significant side effects from the high doses of prednisone necessary to control his hyperthyroidism. He could not continue his prednisone, and he could not resume his amiodarone. Therefore, in December, Jim had a total thyroidectomy.

> There was no real pain to speak of. I wasn't allowed to walk around because of my heart, but I was eating by that night. Compared to everything else I've been through, [having my thyroid removed] was nothing.
>
> I started taking [levothyroxine] the day after surgery. My thyroid levels stayed pretty much consistent. I really didn't feel any different. I was still anxious. Then I woke up one morning [one month after surgery] and felt different. I was back in sinus rhythm and have been since then. The thyroid surgery did the job. Once I was in sinus rhythm, they put me back on amiodarone.
>
> I take levothyroxine every day. I also have to take potassium and magnesium because I have problems keeping my electrolytes balanced. I can't take [levothyroxine] at the same time I take the magnesium, so I take it at noon.

Even though Jim no longer suffered from amiodarone-induced hyperthyroidism and atrial fibrillation, he continued to experience ventricular tachycardia. His implanted defibrillator "delivered a shock" when he had these episodes, as many as forty-eight in twenty days. He desperately needed a heart transplant. Because of his height, Jim had to wait until a large heart was available. Jim believes there is also another hurdle prospective organ recipients must overcome—a lack of communication and knowledge about organ transplants.

> People sign up to be organ donors, but they don't discuss it with their family. If the family is unaware of their loved ones' wishes, they might not sign the authorization necessary to donate organs.

Jim's patience and faith were rewarded in March 2001 when he received a new heart. He is also euthyroid on thyroid hormone replacement and is looking forward to a long, healthy life.■

ESTELITA'S STORY

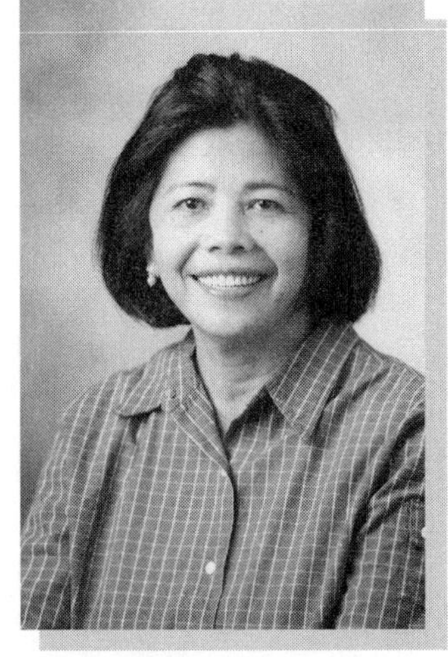

Forty-eight-year-old Estelita learned about thyroid cancer when two of her sisters were successfully treated for it years ago. Because of her family history, she was not shocked when she was also diagnosed with thyroid cancer, but she was surprised when she discovered that she had a different type of thyroid cancer.

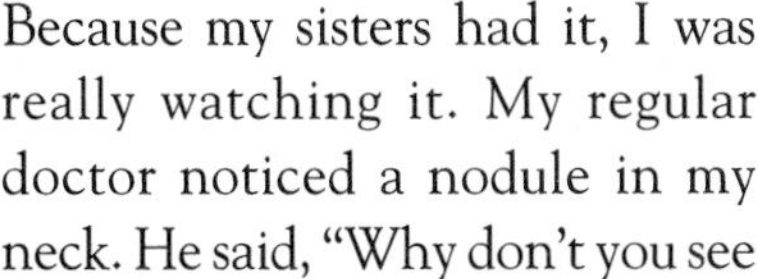

> Because my sisters had it, I was really watching it. My regular doctor noticed a nodule in my neck. He said, "Why don't you see [an endocrinologist]?" I took the [ultrasound] to [this endocrinologist]. He redid the ultrasound and confirmed that there were nodules. I wasn't really concerned because I had several nodules, and I knew that meant it was less likely that I had cancer. But [my endocrinologist] said that I needed a biopsy.

When Estelita's endocrinologist examined her thyroid, he found an irregular goiter with a 1.0-cm (centimeter) nodule in her right lobe. A thyroid ultrasound revealed a solid right lower lobe nodule and a mixed nodule midway in the back of her right lobe. Several very small nodules were also present in her left lobe. Both of the larger nodules were cold on scanning. Biopsy of the solid nodule yielded cells "suspicious for malignancy, papillary carcinoma type." In addition, her calcitonin was 23 pg/mL (picograms per milliliter) —normal calcitonin for women is less than 4 pg/mL.

> So [my endocrinologist] recommended that I have surgery. From that point on, it was like an emotional roller coaster. Just thinking about the possibilities, you know, is unthinkable!

> The surgeon removed just one lobe of my thyroid since the nodule was so little. The big nodule turned out to be nothing, but there was a smaller nodule [4 millimeters] that was medullary cancer. I'm just so glad they found that little nodule, thanks to a good pathologist. Of course, just hearing that you have cancer makes you shaky. All of a sudden, your whole life is changed.
>
> I called my sisters in the Philippines and asked that they get reports from their doctor about the type of cancer they had. Unless the pathologist in the Philippines made a mistake, the reports said that they had papillary cancer, not medullary.
>
> I asked [my endocrinologist] what I should do next. He said there were blood tests that can determine if I needed another surgery. I had a calcium infusion test. It showed that my calcitonin was up, meaning I needed another surgery.

One month after surgery, Estelita's calcitonin was 7 pg/mL; four months after surgery, it was 4 pg/mL. During a calcium infusion test, her calcitonin rose to 99 pg/mL . She did not have a mutation in her RET proto-oncogene, which indicated that a hereditary form of medullary thyroid cancer was unlikely.

> I was scheduled to go to the Philippines again to visit my family and asked if I could still make the trip. The doctors said to go ahead. I had the surgery a couple of weeks later. My surgeon took the other lobe out and found another small nodule with medullary cancer. It was even smaller than the last one.

Estelita's surgeon performed a left central compartment dissection but was unable to perform a right central compartment dissection. This time, the pathologist found a 2-millimeter medullary cancer. All removed lymph nodes were cancer-free.

I was in the hospital one night when I had the first surgery. This time I spent two nights. I was expecting it to be painful once the anesthesia was gone. I was surprised it wasn't. Although I lost a little of my voice after the first surgery, it came back after a few months. I got hoarse after the second surgery but not as bad as the first. My volume was affected but not too bad; it's normal now. I'm naturally kind of hoarse a little bit. I was up and about in a week and driving carpool. I didn't lift anything heavy and did light work for about three weeks.

I thought, oh my God, am I going to die? Knowing my cancer is different from my sisters makes me worry. I thought maybe the pathologist was wrong. My head was kind of spinning; I was wondering, what does this all mean? [My endocrinologist] says I'm probably cured. I only have a little thyroid tissue left. They also found nothing in my lymph nodes.

I go back for routine blood tests now. My calcium went really down after surgery, but this usually happens. I'm taking lots of calcium pills and have to wait to see if it gets better.

So I said what's next? If I die, I die. At some point it comes to that. All this uncertainty is difficult, but I am stronger now. Even if my calcitonin is high now, I try not to worry about it, but I still get some sleepless nights.

From my experience, I would say I went through shock first, then said that I have to be strong. After I got through the sobbing stage, I solved a lot. It's very, very crucial to have friends and support. There was always someone with me when I went to the doctor. I would tell people [diagnosed with thyroid cancer] that they just have to be strong and don't procrastinate. Just go

> ahead and do what needs to be done. It helps to go to doctors who know what they're doing. It gives you a lot of hope.
>
> The process is really exhausting—emotionally, physically, and financially. Having friends and their support made the process bearable. I feel like I have a new lease on life. I don't want to waste any day feeling bad. It's like I have an extension on life.

Although Estelita underwent two surgeries and lots of worry, now she is doing fine. She has a normal calcium level, and her calcitonin is less than 1.0 pg/mL.■

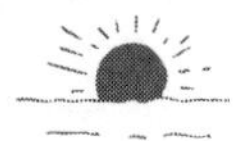

Chapter 5

WHAT IS HYPOTHYROIDISM?

Hypothyroidism is too little thyroid hormone in the blood; it is sometimes referred to as an underactive thyroid. This disease affects a minimum of six million Americans and one out of every 4,000 newborns. Women are much more likely to have hypothyroidism than men are.

Worldwide, iodine deficiency is the most common cause of hypothyroidism (see Chapter 2). The most common cause of hypothyroidism in the United States and other iodine-sufficient areas of the world is Hashimoto's thyroiditis (see Chapter 8). Regardless of the cause of hypothyroidism, treatment is safe, simple, and very effective.

Signs and Symptoms of Hypothyroidism

As can be seen from the list on page 96, there are many signs and symptoms of hypothyroidism. Individual hypothyroid patients may have none, some, or many of these signs and symptoms, depending upon the severity of their disease. These signs and symptoms are often present in other diseases as well. Even if patients have many of these signs and symptoms, they may not be hypothyroid. Therefore, hypothyroidism cannot be diagnosed by signs and symptoms alone; the diagnosis can only be confirmed after a thorough medical history, physical examination, and the appropriate laboratory tests.

Signs & Symptoms of Hypothyroidism

Hypothyroid patients may have none, some, or many of these signs and symptoms, depending upon the severity of their disease.

Patients may have many of these signs and symptoms and not be hypothyroid.

feeling slow or tired	constipation
feeling cold	numbness of hands
husky voice; hoarseness	muscle cramps
drowsiness during the day	slow heart rate
excessive sleeping	slow reflexes
poor memory	goiter
difficulty concentrating	elevated blood pressure
puffy face, especially under the eyes	elevated cholesterol
difficulty losing weight	milky breast discharge
decreased appetite	menstrual problems
hair loss	infertility
dry, brittle, and coarse hair	miscarriage
dry, coarse, flaky, yellow skin	loss of interest in sex
brittle nails	in children, delayed growth
sleep apnea	

Symptoms of Hypothyroidism

The most common complaints voiced by hypothyroid patients are fatigue, excessive sleepiness, memory loss, hair loss, and feeling cold (cold intolerance). Many times patients do not remember that they have a poor memory until they are reminded of it by a book like this or by someone who accompanies them to the doctor. Weight gain may occur, but it is minimal. Some patients may notice that they are having more trouble maintaining their usual weight (see Chapter 2).

When hair loss (alopecia) occurs, it may be a very discouraging experience. Hair loss can be caused by many things other than hypothyroidism, such as stress, hyperthyroidism, and, in women, too much male hormone. Hair lost from hypothyroidism will grow back within three to six months after successful treatment of hypothyroidism.

Hypothyroidism may cause menstrual abnormalities and infertility, although it is not the most common cause of either. A patient with hypothyroidism may have a milky breast discharge (galactorrhea), and the patient's interest in sex (libido) may decrease.

The symptoms of depression may overlap with, or be confused with, the symptoms of hypothyroidism. For example, fatigue, sleeping excessively, inability to concentrate, apathy, and poor memory may occur in both disorders. Furthermore, hypothyroidism can aggravate symptoms of depression, although it does not ordinarily cause depression. To determine whether patients have depression or hypothyroidism, their physicians may ask them to make the distinction between feeling sad and feeling tired. Similarly, physicians may ask their patients to make the distinction between losing interest in the activities of daily living and not having the energy to do them.

Both depression and hypothyroidism are common, especially in women. In addition, depression may be seen more often in patients with thyroid dysfunction than in euthyroid patients. Therefore, it is possible, and not at all unusual, for patients to have both hypothyroidism and depression.

Even when tests indicate normal thyroid function, some patients are reluctant to consider that they could be suffering from depression. Misconceptions and the social stigma erroneously attached to depression may make it a difficult diagnosis to accept. Nonetheless, if hypothyroid patients are also depressed, they will not get well without treating both their depression and their hypothyroidism.

Physical Signs of Hypothyroidism

A hypothyroid patient may notice her skin becoming dry and slightly yellow, her face becoming puffy, and her voice becoming hoarse. Galactorrhea may become apparent when the doctor applies pressure to the nipple. The doctor may note a goiter, a slow pulse rate, and perhaps an elevated blood pressure. Also, the patient's reflexes may be slow.

Once again, individual hypothyroid patients may have none, some, or all of these signs and symptoms, depending upon the severity of their disease. Furthermore, even if patients have many of these signs and symptoms, they may not be hypothyroid.

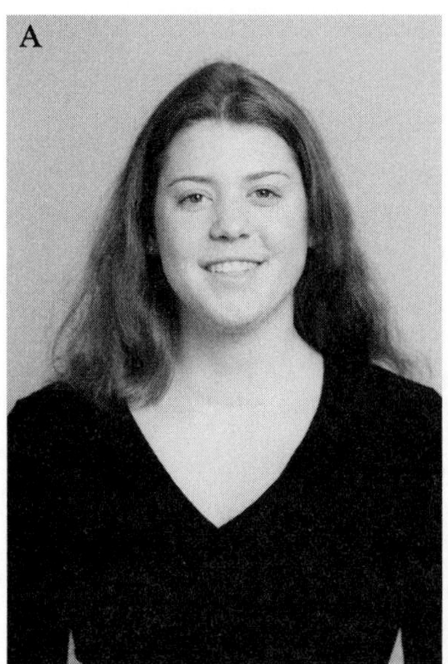

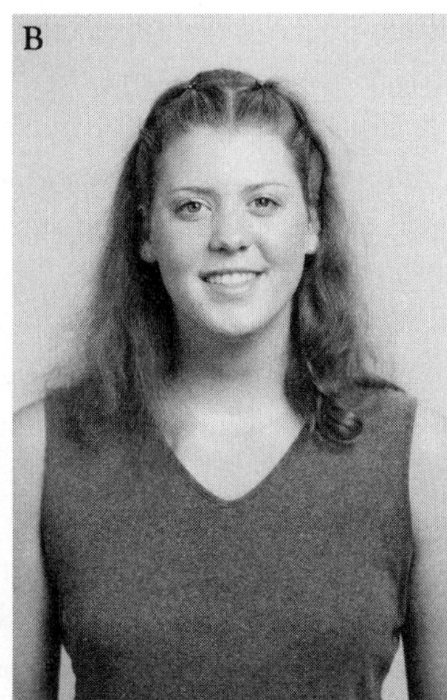

Figure 5.1. Thyroid cancer patient. (A) Hypothyroid six weeks after her thyroidectomy and the day after radioactive iodine therapy. Note the puffiness in her face. (B) Euthryoid on levothyroxine.

Laboratory Test Result Abnormalities Caused by Hypothyroidism

Abnormalities in laboratory test results other than thyroid function test results sometimes suggest the diagnosis of hypothyroidism to physicians. These abnormalities may include anemia (low red blood cell count), elevated liver function tests—SGOT or AST, SGPT or ALT, LDH, and alkaline phosphatase—high prolactin, high calcium (hypercalcemia), and elevated muscle enzymes, such as creatine kinase (CK). Low testosterone is also occasionally seen in hypothyroid men.

Of particular interest is the elevation of cholesterol that occurs in hypothyroid patients. Many patients are aware of a rise in their cholesterol levels, even if the levels are still within the normal range. Hypothyroidism can also cause hypercholesterolemia (high cholesterol), which is a risk factor for cardiovascular disease. Therefore, all patients with high cholesterol should have thyroid function tests. High cholesterol caused by hypothyroidism is reversible with successful treatment of the hypothyroidism. Elevation of homocysteine, an amino acid that may be another risk factor for cardiovascular disease, is also seen with hypothyroidism. Thyroid hormone replacement therapy reduces homocysteine levels in hypothyroid patients.

Causes of Hypothyroidism

Hypothyroidism may be *permanent* and require a lifetime of thyroid hormone replacement, or it may be *transient* (temporary) and require little, if any, treatment.

Causes of Hypothyroidism

Permanent Hypothyroidism	Temporary Hypothyroidism
Hashimoto's thyroiditis	subacute thyroiditis
radioactive iodine treatment	postpartum thyroiditis
removal of the thyroid gland	painless thyroiditis
congenital abnormalities	certain drugs
iodine deficiency	
radiation	
pituitary or hypothalamic dysfunction	
idiopathic (cause unknown)	

Causes of Permanent Hypothyroidism

The three most common causes of permanent hypothyroidism in iodine-sufficient areas of the world are discussed at great length elsewhere in this book. To learn more about each of these causes, refer to the chapters cited below:

- Hashimoto's thyroiditis, an autoimmune disease affecting 5% of the adult population, is the most common cause of hypothyroidism in the United States (Chapter 8).
- Radioactive iodine treatment of hyperthyroidism frequently results in permanent hypothyroidism (Chapter 7).
- Surgical removal of the thyroid gland (thyroidectomy) can also result in permanent hypothyroidism if sufficient thyroid tissue is removed (Chapter 10).

Iodine deficiency is the most common cause of hypothyroidism in the world. Since iodine has been added to table salt, milk, bread, and other foods, iodine deficiency is very uncommon in the United States. For that reason, it is unnecessary, and potentially harmful, for Americans to take kelp or any other iodine supplement.

Another cause of permanent hypothyroidism is congenital hypothyroidism, which occurs in approximately one of 4,000 live births. Common causes of congenital hypothyroidism are failure of the fetal thyroid gland to develop (agenesis) and enzyme deficiencies in the thyroid gland.

Therapeutic radiation is becoming a more common cause of hypothyroidism. For example, patients who have had radiation therapy to the neck and chest for Hodgkin's disease or other cancers are at high risk of developing hypothyroidism. On the other hand, people who were given radiation therapy twenty or more years ago for acne, ringworm, or other skin conditions or for enlargement of the thymus or tonsils are not likely to develop hypothyroidism, although they are more likely to develop thyroid nodules.

Children from Chernobyl who were exposed to radioactive fallout containing radioactive iodine must be carefully monitored for the development of hypothyroidism and, especially, thyroid nodules. Anyone who has a history of radiation exposure or treatment should have a thyroid examination and thyroid function tests annually. On the other hand, routine diagnostic x-rays do not cause either hypothyroidism or thyroid tumors, and should not be a cause for concern.

Pituitary or hypothalamic dysfunction also causes hypothyroidism. Hypothyroidism caused by a defective thyroid gland is called primary hypothyroidism, while hypothyroidism caused by the pituitary gland's failure to produce enough thyroid-stimulating hormone (TSH or

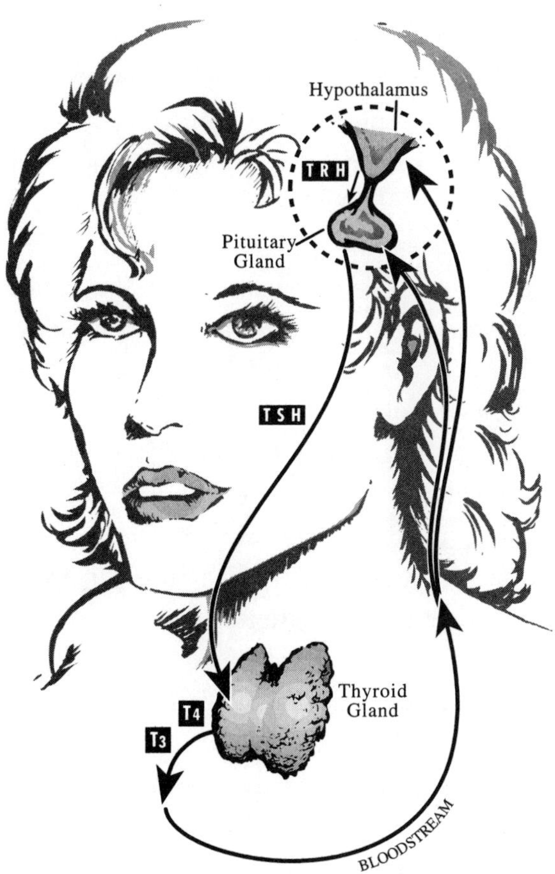

Figure 5.2. A defect in the hypothalamus, pituitary gland, or thyroid gland can cause hypothyroidism.

thyrotropin) is called secondary hypothyroidism. Failure of the hypothalamus to produce thyrotropin-releasing hormone (TRH) is called tertiary hypothyroidism. Together, secondary and tertiary hypothyroidism are referred to as central hypothyroidism. Central hypothyroidism is very uncommon and, ordinarily, is easily distinguished from primary hypothyroidism (see "Matilde's Story" on pages 119–120). Finally, if a patient has no obvious cause for hypothyroidism, the condition is called idiopathic hypothyroidism.

Causes of Transient (Temporary) Hypothyroidism

The most common cause of transient hypothyroidism is thyroiditis. Subacute thyroiditis, postpartum thyroiditis, and painless thyroiditis can cause temporary hypothyroidism (see Chapter 8). In most cases of transient thyroiditis, treatment with thyroid hormone replacement is not necessary. However, some patients with transient thyroiditis will develop permanent hypothyroidism and require a lifetime of thyroid hormone treatment.

Drugs may induce a temporary form of hypothyroidism. For example, up to 50% of patients taking lithium for various psychiatric disorders will become hypothyroid for as long as they take the drug. Interferon alpha, a drug used to treat patients with hepatitis C infection, can also cause temporary hypothyroidism, as well as other thyroid abnormalities.

Another drug that can cause temporary hypothyroidism is amiodarone, a very effective medication for the control of dangerous heart rhythm disturbances (arrhythmias). Amiodarone's high iodine content can cause abnormal thyroid function test results and, in a small number of patients, actual thyroid dysfunction. Approximately 5% of patients develop amiodarone-induced thyrotoxicosis (AIT), or amiodarone-induced hyperthyroidism. Additionally, about 7% of patients taking this drug develop amiodarone-induced hypothyroidism (AIH). Patients with Hashimoto's thyroiditis are more likely to develop amiodarone-induced hypothyroidism than those without Hashimoto's thyroiditis are. Other risk factors for the development of amiodarone-induced hypothyroidism include an elevated TSH level, a family history of thyroid disease, and a nodular goiter.

Tests for Hypothyroidism

An elevated TSH and a low free T_4 confirm the diagnosis of primary hypothyroidism. These test results, however, do not predict the severity of a patient's symptoms (see "Melissa's Story" on pages 122–125).

In addition to TSH and free T_4, antithyroid antibodies (TPOAb and TgAb) are commonly measured to determine if hypothyroid patients have Hashimoto's thyroiditis. It is important to make the diagnosis of Hashimoto's thyroiditis since this autoimmune disorder is hereditary, is associated with other autoimmune disorders, and virtually assures that hypothyroidism will be permanent.

Not all patients with elevated TSH levels are hypothyroid. Certain unusual conditions can cause elevation of TSH. For example, people with resistance to thyroid hormone, a rare hereditary disease, may have elevated TSH levels along with elevated thyroid hormone levels (see "Bob's Story" on pages 12–14). They may have symptoms of either hypothyroidism or hyperthyroidism, but most patients have only goiters and abnormal thyroid function tests. Since patients with resistance to thyroid hormone have unusual and confusing thyroid function test results, it is important that they are accurately diagnosed to avoid

Typical Test Results in Hypothyroid Patients

TSH	high
free T_4	low normal in subclinical hypothyroidism
TPOAb	positive in Hashimoto's thyroiditis negative in other causes
TgAb	positive in Hashimoto's thyroiditis negative in other causes

unnecessary treatment. The need for an accurate diagnosis also applies to patients with TSH-producing pituitary tumors who may have similarly misleading TSH test results (see "Seymour's Story" on pages 84–88).

Patients whose test results do not support the diagnosis of either hypothyroidism or subclinical hypothyroidism (see below) should not be treated with thyroid hormone. Some patients are treated for "low thyroid" even though their thyroid function test results are normal. This treatment is inappropriate, misleading, and potentially dangerous. If patients are treated for hypothyroidism and do not have it, then the true causes of their symptoms have been overlooked. Treatment with thyroid hormone should be reserved for patients with confirmed thyroid disease, not for patients with symptoms that *could* be thyroid disease.

Subclinical Hypothyroidism

Sometimes patients may have normal free T_4 with elevated TSH levels or elevated TSH levels in response to thyrotropin-releasing hormone (TRH test); this combination of test results is called subclinical hypothyroidism (mild thyroid failure). The term "subclinical" means that there are abnormal laboratory test results without any apparent symptoms. Unless physicians suspect the presence of thyroid disease or perform routine thyroid screening, subclinical hypothyroidism may go undetected.

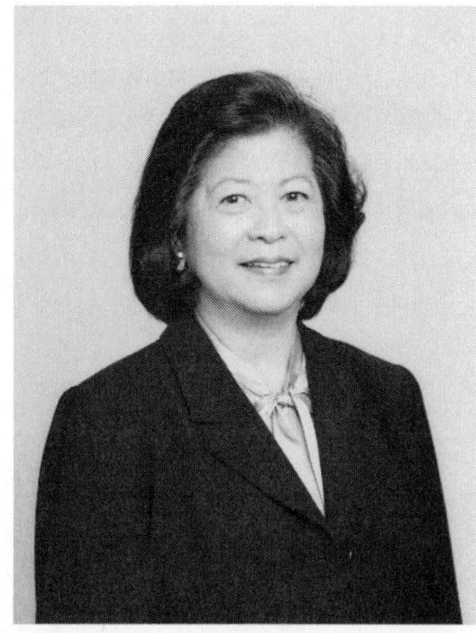

Figure 5.3. Postmenopausal women are more likely to develop subclinical hypothyroidism.

Women are more likely to develop subclinical hypothyroidism than men are (see "Kitty's Story" on pages 121–122). Approximately 6 to 11% of adult women and 3% of adult men have subclinical hypothyroidism, and the percentages increase as patients age. For example,

15% of women over age sixty and 8% of elderly men will develop it. In addition, patients who have Hashimoto's thyroiditis or Type 1 diabetes and patients who have had radioactive iodine treatment for hyperthyroidism are at higher risk of developing subclinical hypothyroidism than the general population is.

Physicians may also suspect subclinical hypothyroidism in patients with one or more of the following:

- elevated cholesterol levels
- goiter
- personal or family history of thyroid disease
- nonspecific complaints (in patients over age forty)
- unexplained, minimal weight gain
- depression unresponsive to treatment
- unexplained infertility

Causes of Subclinical Hypothyroidism

Generally, the causes of subclinical hypothyroidism and overt hypothyroidism are the same. An additional cause of subclinical hypothyroidism is inadequate treatment of previously diagnosed hypothyroidism. Some patients may be unable to take the recommended dose of levothyroxine because they have pre-existing heart conditions, or they may not consistently take their thyroid medication as prescribed. If hypothyroid patients do not have regularly scheduled follow-up visits that include TSH measurements, they may develop subclinical hypothyroidism, which will go undetected.

Treatment of Patients with Hypothyroidism

In many ways, treatment of hypothyroid patients represents the best that medicine has to offer. The definition of hypothyroidism is both clear and straightforward—deficiency of thyroid hormone. The treatment is equally clear and straightforward—thyroid hormone replacement. Brand-name levothyroxine is the drug of choice. Once the diagnosis of permanent hypothyroidism is confirmed, patients must take levothyroxine every day for the rest of their lives. For hypothyroid patients taking thyroid hormone replacement, the details of treatment with levothyroxine are very important. Therefore, hypothyroid patients should read and re-read the next chapter, "What is Levothyroxine Therapy?"

The onset of hypothyroidism is slow and insidious. Similarly, a full response to treatment occurs gradually and may take six weeks or longer. Therefore, hypothyroid patients should not expect immediate improvement, even if their initial dosage of levothyroxine is correct. Re-examination of patients and repeat thyroid function tests are ordinarily performed six to twelve weeks after initiation of therapy with levothyroxine. If adjustments of the dosage are made, patients will be examined and tested again in another six to twelve weeks. Once the correct dosage of levothyroxine is determined, physicians ordinarily see their hypothyroid patients

How to Take Levothyroxine

- Levothyroxine should be taken daily unless directed otherwise.
- If you miss a dose, you may "double up" the next day. If you miss more than one day, double up for as many days as necessary to catch up.
- Levothyroxine is best absorbed when it is taken:
    - on an empty stomach
    - with water only
    - one hour before or two hours after eating
    - one hour before taking any medications, vitamins, or supplements
    - four hours before taking iron or calcium
    - twelve hours before taking Questran® or Colestid®

at least once a year.

Treatment of Patients with Subclinical Hypothyroidism

Many endocrinologists believe that untreated subclinical hypothyroidism can adversely affect overall health and, therefore, should be treated. Potential reasons to treat patients with subclinical hypothyroidism may include one or more of the following:

- prevention of progression to overt hypothyroidism
- reduction and prevention of symptoms of hypothyroidism
- reduction of cholesterol levels
- reduction of cardiovascular disease risk
- improvement of heart function
- improvement in treatment of depression
- improvement of fertility
- prevention of intellectual impairment in children born to inadequately treated hypothyroid mothers

Patients may have elevated TSH levels for months or years before their T_4 levels fall below normal. However, their physicians may recommend that they begin levothyroxine therapy to prevent subclinical hypothyroidism from becoming overt, symptomatic hypothyroidism. Some patients with subclinical hypothyroidism are at higher risk of developing overt hypothyroidism than others are. Patients with the highest risk of developing overt hypothyroidism have TSH levels over 20 mU/L (milliunits per liter) and Hashimoto's thyroiditis with high antithyroid antibody levels. Older patients with subclinical hypothyroidism and Hashimoto's thyroiditis are four times more likely to progress to overt hypothyroidism than younger patients are.

The treatment of patients with subclinical hypothyroidism is the same as that of patients with overt hypothyroidism—levothyroxine therapy (see Chapter 6). Although, by definition, patients with subclinical hypothyroidism do not have symptoms of hypothyroidism, they may feel better after treatment with levothyroxine. They may not have noticed their symptoms until the symptoms were gone. Other patients do not notice any improvement in the way they feel. However, a detailed and sensitive assessment of such patients, performed in a research setting, demonstrated improvement in several areas. For example, tests done before and after treatment revealed improvement of dry skin, low energy, cold intolerance, memory, anxiety, and signs of depression.

Patients with subclinical hypothyroidism have higher total cholesterol levels and higher low-density lipoprotein (LDL, the "bad" cholesterol) levels than euthyroid patients do. However, the higher levels may still be in the normal range. Levothyroxine treatment of patients with subclinical hypothyroidism lowers both their total cholesterol and LDL levels.

It is unclear whether treating subclinically hypothyroid patients with levothyroxine to lower their total cholesterol and LDL reduces their risk of developing coronary artery disease. Further research will clarify the exact nature of the relationship between subclinical hypothyroidism, cholesterol, and cardiovascular risk. However, at least one study has demonstrated that subclinical hypothyroidism is a risk factor for the development of hardening of the arteries (aortic atherosclerosis) and heart attacks (myocardial infarction) in elderly women. Other detailed and sensitive studies, also conducted in a research setting, have demonstrated that patients with subclinical hypothyroidism have subtle impairments of heart function. These subtle changes in heart function are reversed by levothyroxine treatment.

As previously discussed, depression and hypothyroidism share many symptoms, and one disease may mask the other. Since abnormal thyroid function may be more common in patients suffering from depression, it is logical to test the thyroid function of depressed patients. Even mild thyroid failure can interfere with the treatment of depression. For example, antidepressants do not work as effectively in patients with subclinical hypothyroidism as compared to euthyroid patients who are depressed. Therefore, levothyroxine therapy is usually recommended for patients who are suffering from depression and have elevated TSH levels.

In summary, the advantages of treating subclinically hypothyroid patients with levothyroxine usually outweigh other concerns, such as the risk of causing subclinical hyperthyroidism, the cost of medication and follow-up, and the lack of patient commitment to taking a drug daily for a lifetime when there are few, if any, symptoms. The potential for improving cholesterol and LDL, reducing the risk of cardiovascular disease, decreasing symptoms, and preventing the development of overt hypothyroidism with levothyroxine therapy is very appealing.

Treatment of Patients with Amiodarone-Induced Hypothyroidism

Treatment of patients with amiodarone-induced hypothyroidism can be difficult for two reasons. First, many patients cannot discontinue amiodarone because it is often the only drug that can control their life-threatening arrhythmias. Second, even when amiodarone is discontinued, the residual iodine remains in the body for six months or more, continuing to affect thyroid function. For these reasons, patients with amiodarone-induced hypothyroidism must be evaluated frequently over a long period of time.

Although most patients taking amiodarone will not develop amiodarone-induced thyroid disease, it is important that all patients taking this drug have periodic thyroid function tests. The frequency of the testing depends upon factors such as age, pre-existing thyroid disease, and other medications. However, thyroid function tests should be done three months after starting amiodarone and then at least every six months for as long as patients take the drug. Patients should continue to have thyroid function tests every six months for two to three years after amiodarone is discontinued because the lingering iodine can affect thyroid function long after the drug is stopped.

Hypothyroidism and Pregnancy

A woman needs approximately 45% more T_4 during pregnancy to maintain a normal TSH level. Assuming she lives in an iodine-sufficient area, such as the United States, a pregnant woman without thyroid disease can meet this demand; her thyroid gland will automatically increase production of T_4 and T_3. However, the thyroid gland of a *hypothyroid* pregnant woman may not adequately increase production of these thyroid hormones. Therefore, even if she is taking levothyroxine, her TSH level may rise out of the normal range, indicating subclinical hypothyroidism.

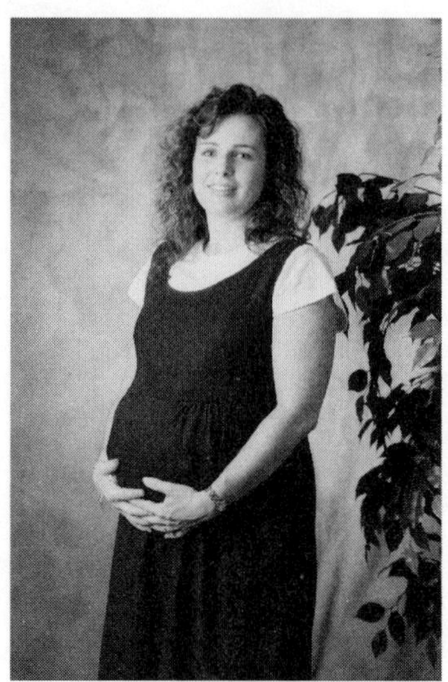

Figure 5.4. Pregnant patient on levothyroxine.

In order to prevent even mild hypothyroidism during pregnancy, a hypothyroid woman should have her TSH checked shortly before she becomes pregnant and, then again, within six weeks of conception. Her TSH should then be rechecked approximately every six weeks during the remainder of her pregnancy. It is not unusual for the dosage of levothyroxine to increase early in the pregnancy and then change several times before delivery. Once a pregnant woman delivers, her TSH should be rechecked three to four months later.

A hypothyroid woman should take her levothyroxine as prescribed during pregnancy to avoid the possibility of impairing her child's intelligence. One study looked into the impact of maternal hypothyroidism during pregnancy on childhood intellectual performance. Results indicated that the average IQ of children born to inadequately treated hypothyroid mothers may be four points lower than the average IQ of children born to mothers without hypothyroidism. The average IQ of children born to untreated hypothyroid mothers was seven points lower than the average IQ of children born to mothers without hypothyroidism. In addition, the frequency of children born with IQs below 85 increased when their mothers received no treatment for their hypothyroidism. The results of this study underscore the importance of maintaining adequate thyroid hormone levels in expectant mothers.

A hypothyroid woman should definitely continue taking her levothyroxine when she becomes pregnant for the following reasons:

- Levothyroxine, prescribed in the proper amounts, does not harm the fetus.

- Inadequately treated hypothyroidism is associated with an increased risk of miscarriage.

- A hypothyroid woman frequently requires more levothyroxine during pregnancy.

- A child's IQ may be reduced if its mother had inadequately treated hypothyroidism during pregnancy.

Iron supplementation is frequently prescribed during pregnancy, often in the form of prenatal vitamins. Since it interferes with levothyroxine absorption, iron should be taken at least two hours after taking levothyroxine.

Hypothyroidism in Children

Congenital Hypothyroidism

The signs and symptoms of congenital hypothyroidism are seldom apparent at birth; however, delay in treatment of congenitally hypothyroid infants can cause irreversible brain damage. Therefore, screening for congenital hypothyroidism is performed on all newborns in the United States, Canada, Israel, Japan, Australia, New Zealand, and most countries in Europe.

Congenital hypothyroidism occurs in one out of every 4,000 newborns. Among the 12 million newborns screened worldwide, approximately 3,000 new cases are found every year. Neonatal thyroid screening has led to a marked reduction in untreated congenital hypothyroidism and in cretinism (mental retardation and short stature due to hypothyroidism). Screening has also revealed differences in the incidence of congenital hypothyroidism in some groups of people. For example, in the state of Texas, there is a higher than average incidence of congenital hypothyroidism in newborns of Hispanic descent, as well as a lower incidence in African-American newborns, as compared to Caucasian newborns. The cost of screening and treating children for congenital hypothyroidism is

Signs & Symptoms of Congenital Hypothyroidism

Early Appearance

gestation longer than 42 weeks	low body temperature
generalized swelling and puffiness	swollen tummy
poor feeding	

Onset First Month

blue tint in fingers and toes	poor sucking ability
uneven skin tone	decreased frequency of bowel movements
respiratory distress	decreased activity
failure to gain weight	

Onset First Three Months

enlarged belly button	enlarged tongue
constipation	hoarse cry
dry, yellow skin	

far less than the long-term cost of caring for untreated hypothyroid children.

Acquired Childhood Hypothyroidism

Although the development of hypothyroidism in a child before puberty is uncommon, it does occur, especially if there is a family history of thyroid disease. A child's doctor needs to know if either the mother or father has a hereditary autoimmune disease, such as Hashimoto's thyroiditis or Graves' disease. The doctor will then pay particular attention to the child's thyroid examination.

The first signs that a child has hypothyroidism may be thyroid enlargement and a decline in growth rate. Most short children, however, do not have hypothyroidism. Tests for hypothyroidism are frequently

Signs & Symptoms of Acquired Childhood Hypothyroidism

Onset after 6 Months and before 3 Years of Age	
slow development of body length	enlarged tongue
coarse facial features	enlarged belly button
dry, yellow skin	swollen, tight muscles
hoarse cry	

Onset during Childhood	
goiter	swollen, tight muscles
delayed growth rate	constipation
delayed dental development	dry, yellow skin
delayed tooth eruption	generalized puffiness
muscle weakness	early sexual development

Onset during Adolescence	
goiter	generalized puffiness
delayed puberty	delayed dental development
delayed growth rate	delayed tooth eruption
constipation	milky discharge from breasts
dry, yellow skin	

performed on children who are overweight, but hypothyroidism does not cause obesity.

Diagnosing and treating hypothyroid children before puberty is somewhat more complicated than diagnosing and treating hypothyroid teens and adults. Children's growth and development must be carefully monitored. In childhood, the normal range for TSH and free T_4 varies with age. Levothyroxine dosage must be adjusted more frequently in growing children than in teenagers or mature adults. For all these reasons, pediatric endocrinologists are usually consulted in the management of hypothyroid infants or children. Once hypothyroid children have gone through puberty and growth has ceased, treatment is essentially the same as that of adults.

Hypothyroidism in Older Patients

The signs and symptoms of hypothyroidism may be difficult to detect in older patients. Fatigue, diminished memory, hair loss, and skin changes are features common to both aging and hypothyroidism. Furthermore, thyroid gland examinations may be more difficult in older patients.

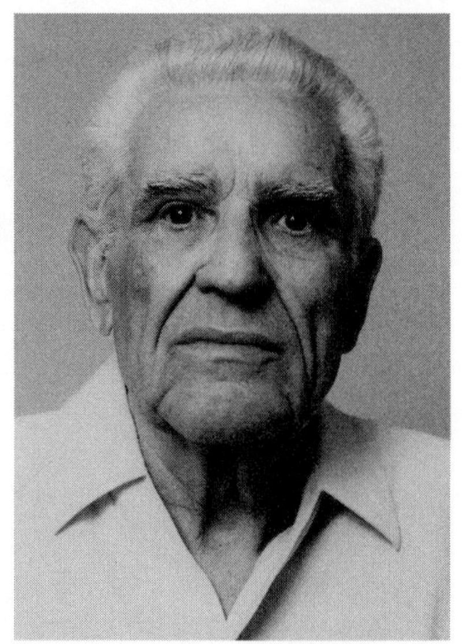

Figure 5.5. Elderly hypothyroid man.

Similarly, some older hypothyroid patients may be difficult to treat. They are more likely to be forgetful or have heart disease that prevents adequate thyroid hormone replacement. Use of a pillbox allows both patients and, when necessary, their caregivers to see if levothyroxine and other medications have been taken as prescribed. Older patients are also more likely to take multiple medications, some of which may interfere with thyroid hormone absorption.

The incidence of Hashimoto's thyroiditis, the most common cause of hypothyroidism in the United States, increases markedly with age, especially in women. As many as 24% of women between fifty-five and sixty-four years of age will have positive antithyroid antibodies. In other words, by the time women are sixty-five years old, they have a one in four chance of having Hashimoto's thyroiditis. Subclinical hypothyroidism affects 15% of women over sixty years of age and 8% of older men.

The possibility of thyroid dysfunction in any symptomatic older patient must be kept in mind for the following reasons:

- Hashimoto's thyroiditis is common in older patients.
- Subclinical hypothyroidism is common in older patients.
- Hypothyroidism is often undiagnosed in older patients.
- Hypothyroidism can cause symptoms that are mistakenly attributed to aging.

Hypothyroidism can contribute to the senility of elderly patients. Since hypothyroidism is one of the more common *treatable* causes of senility in aging patients, any senile patient should be checked for hypothyroidism. Furthermore, for all of the above reasons, consideration also should be given to screening all *asymptomatic* older patients for hypothyroidism.

Treatment of Hypothyroid Patients with Coronary Artery Disease

Patients with untreated or incompletely treated coronary artery disease and hypothyroidism require special care. Hypothyroidism tends to relieve symptoms of coronary artery disease, such as angina pectoris (chest pain) by reducing demands on the heart. Correction of hypothyroidism increases demands on the heart and, therefore, may worsen symptoms of coronary artery disease.

For this reason, coronary artery disease is frequently corrected with medications or surgery prior to full replacement therapy with thyroid hormone. Once the coronary artery disease is successfully treated, full replacement dosages of levothyroxine can be prescribed.

In some situations, the coronary artery disease cannot be completely corrected; therefore, the patient's hypothyroidism may not be completely treated either. When this situation occurs, the patient should be started on a low dose of levothyroxine, such as 0.025 mg (milligrams) a day. The dosage can then be increased by 0.025 mg every five to six weeks, until either the hypothyroidism is corrected or the patient develops worsening heart symptoms. If symptoms do develop, the dosage of levothyroxine is reduced.

Surgery in Hypothyroid Patients

Hypothyroid patients who take adequate thyroid hormone replacement generally do well when they have surgery. However, if these patients are unable to eat or drink for several days following surgery, they will require levothyroxine either intravenously or by intramuscular injection. Under these circumstances, they will need no more than 80% of their usual dose of levothyroxine since that is approximately the amount absorbed when taken orally.

Some studies have shown that inadequately treated or untreated hypothyroid patients have increased risk of minor surgical complications. Ordinarily, hypothyroid patients may proceed with urgent surgery as long as their physicians monitor them closely for these complications. On the other hand, when surgical procedures are elective, it may be prudent for hypothyroid patients to postpone surgery until they become euthyroid.

Severely hypothyroid patients require very careful preoperative evaluations before proceeding with any surgery, as surgery can precipitate myxedema coma.

Myxedema Coma

Patients with undiagnosed hypothyroidism and noncompliant hypothyroid patients who do not take their levothyroxine for months at a time may develop myxedema coma. Myxedema coma is an uncommon, life-threatening condition characterized by progressively worsening signs and symptoms of hypothyroidism until the patients become comatose. It is often precipitated by surgery, a severe infection, or any other serious illness.

Patients with myxedema coma are treated in the Intensive Care Unit. They often require respirators to help them breathe and intravenous levothyroxine. Since hypothyroidism is easily diagnosed, and, in compliant patients, effectively treated with levothyroxine, myxedema coma should rarely occur.

Screening Patients for Hypothyroidism

Screening, an important tool in preventive medicine, is a process for detecting disease among people who do not have symptoms of a disease or who are unaware that they may have a disease. It is not the same as routine testing of patients who describe a symptom or symptoms that may lead physicians to suspect a particular disorder. The high incidence of hypothyroidism, its safe and effective treatment, and the ready availability and relatively low cost of accurate thyroid function tests make screening people for hypothyroidism very worthwhile.

As previously mentioned, screening newborns for congenital hypothyroidism has been very successful and widely accepted. There is a growing consensus among scientists and public health officials that other groups of people also should be screened for thyroid diseases. Some physicians recommend screening groups of people known to be at increased risk of developing thyroid disease, such as women over thirty-five, men and women over fifty-five, people with Down's syndrome, and people with autoimmune diseases, such as Type 1 diabetes.

Health care costs have been the subject of debate among medical professionals, insurance companies, government agencies, and politicians for a long time. In particular, the cost-effectiveness of screening for thyroid disease has been questioned. One study examined the cost benefit of early thyroid disease detection and concluded that screening under certain circumstances was justified. Specifically, they stated that measurement of TSH every five years in adults thirty-five years of age or older compared favorably to the cost of other well-recognized screening programs, such as mammograms for breast cancer.

For all the reasons previously discussed in "Hypothyroidism and Older Patients," it would seem especially logical to screen all older adults for hypothyroidism by measuring their TSH levels. Unfortunately, Medicare does not yet cover the cost of a screening TSH test. On the other hand, Medicare has recognized the importance of, and pays for, screening tests for other diseases that affect the elderly, such as bone density measurements for osteoporosis. Therefore, advocacy groups, such as the American Association of Retired People (AARP), and the medical community can argue that Medicare should also cover screening for thyroid disease for the following reasons:

- Thyroid disease is at least as prevalent in the elderly as osteoporosis.
- TSH testing is much less expensive than a bone density measurement.
- Screening for hypothyroidism in adults is cost-effective.
- Treatment of thyroid disease is very effective.
- Treatment of thyroid disease is safe, simple, and inexpensive.
- TSH testing is readily available and accessible.

Physicians agree that measurement of TSH is the single most accurate indicator of thyroid dysfunction. When TSH test results are abnormal, follow-up should include a physical examination, measurement of thyroid hormones, and, perhaps, a repeat TSH measurement. As the cost of measuring TSH decreases, physicians, insurance companies, and government agencies will be more likely to endorse screening for thyroid disease among selected groups of people.

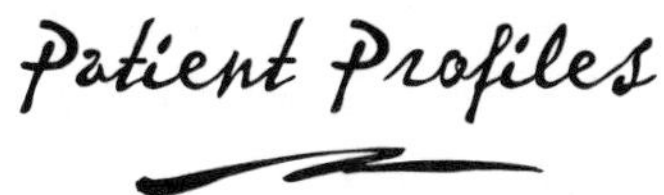

MATILDE'S STORY

Matilde is a forty-eight-year-old wife and mother who lives in Mexico. She comes to the United States every three months for medical care and to shop. In 1997, when her weight went from 104 to 125 pounds and her energy level dropped, she went to an endocrinologist.

> I was always tired. I wanted to sleep all the time. If I sat down, I fell asleep. I had no energy to do anything. I was too tired to even go shopping! I had gained weight, and so I thought that was the reason I was tired.
>
> When I got sick, my family was concerned because they worried about the medicines that doctors might prescribe. I had received the wrong medicines before.
>
> My doctors did tests for months. I was concerned with what might be wrong with my body, my health. The answer was not immediately forthcoming. It was a long wait.

When Matilde went to the endocrinologist, he felt a small goiter. Her laboratory test results showed that her free T_4 and free T_3 levels were low. Unlike the typical test results in patients with primary hypothyroidism, her TSH level was also low and could not be stimulated by thyrotropin-releasing hormone. She had a normal thyroxine-binding globulin, high antithyroid antibody levels, and no detectable antibodies to TSH. An MRI of her pituitary gland and the remainder of her pituitary function were normal. These laboratory results and x-rays confirmed the diagnosis of central hypothyroidism (inadequate TSH stimulation of the thyroid gland).

Central hypothyroidism is a very uncommon form of hypothyroidism. Typically, a defective thyroid gland causes hypothyroidism, but Matilde's thyroid gland was not the cause of her hypothyroidism. She became hypothyroid because of an isolated deficiency of TSH.

As discussed in Chapter 1, thyroid hormone production is part of a feedback mechanism. If the hypothalamus does not produce thyrotropin-releasing hormone, the pituitary gland cannot produce TSH. If there is no TSH, the thyroid gland cannot make thyroid hormones. Because both the pituitary gland and the hypothalamus are part of the central nervous system, hypothyroidism caused by a defect in either is called central hypothyroidism.

> I knew no one who had thyroid disease—no friends, no relatives. I knew what the thyroid gland was, but I didn't realize how important it was.
>
> When I got the diagnosis, I was relieved to know it was a problem that could be treated; it wasn't like cancer. I was so relieved to know what was wrong with me that I started feeling better right away. I started taking [levothyroxine], and, in a few weeks, I was better. After I started feeling better, I started walking more. Just by moving around more, it didn't take long to lose weight. I'm not back to my original weight, but you can't blame everything on your thyroid.
>
> I would advise everyone to check with an endocrinologist once a year. Women go to a gynecologist and a dentist once a year—not because something is wrong, but to be sure nothing is. Why not check on the thyroid, too?

Matilde's story highlights the importance of having a complete medical evaluation, by an experienced physician, of unusual thyroid function test results. A TSH measurement is normally the best test to diagnose and follow patients with hypothyroidism. However, TSH measurements are not useful in following patients with central hypothyroidism. Now that she is euthyroid on levothyroxine, Matilde enjoys her trips to the United States more than ever, especially her shopping. ■

KITTY'S STORY

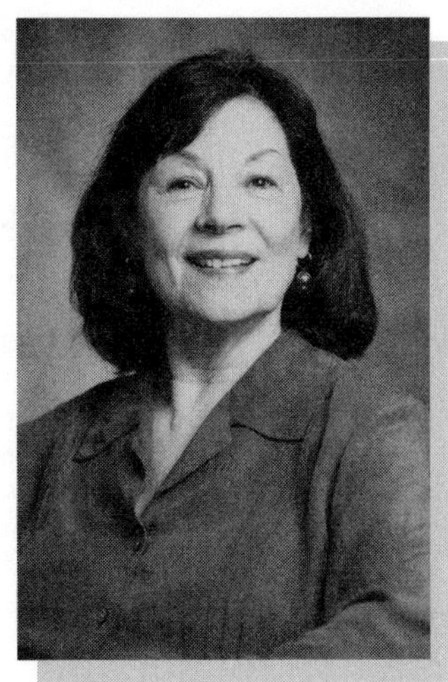

Originally from Amsterdam, Kitty has lived in the United States for thirty years.

> I never thought about my thyroid. Then about five years ago, I developed some hoarseness. I went to [an ear, nose, and throat doctor, or ENT], and he said I had a [thyroid] nodule and referred me to [an endocrinologist]. I couldn't see the nodule, but I could feel it.

The endocrinologist measured her thyroid hormone levels and ordered a thyroid scan and a thyroid ultrasound. These tests revealed that Kitty had Hashimoto's thyroiditis, normal thyroid function, and a cold nodule. More surprising to Kitty was the fact that she had been born with only half of a thyroid gland (hemiagenesis).

> I was not experiencing any symptoms, or I had dismissed any symptoms I might have had. My hair was falling out a little more than usual. I had more trouble losing weight. My skin was dry, and I felt sluggish, but I thought it all part of the normal process of aging.

A fine needle aspiration biopsy of the thyroid nodule was negative. To suppress the growth of the thyroid nodule, Kitty's endocrinologist prescribed levothyroxine. Kitty did not notice any difference in the way she felt so, on her own, she decided to stop taking her levothyroxine. Two years later, Kitty's TSH was slightly elevated at 4.81 mU/L. Kitty had developed subclinical hypothyroidism.

> After I stopped taking my thyroid pills, I did feel a little more fatigued and slightly depressed, but my children were leaving home, and I attributed my symptoms to that. Then I read about how important it was to treat mild thyroid deficiency, and, two years

> later, my doctor put me back on [levothyroxine]. This time I really noticed the difference the medication made. In addition to losing five pounds, I also felt a definite change in the overall quality of my life.

When Kitty realized the difference that thyroid disease could make and that it tended to run in families, she talked with her daughter and wrote her sisters and nieces living in Europe.

> I told them about the symptoms of hypothyroidism and to watch out for them. I am really worried about my niece who has had two miscarriages. The government health plan she's under says you must have three miscarriages before they will test you for thyroid disease or any other possible cause.
>
> I'm spreading the word. I think women should be sure to be tested even if they have minor complaints—the earlier the better. If they are diagnosed with thyroid disease, they should warn their relatives, especially the women in their families.

Despite being born with only half a thyroid gland, which was then attacked by antithyroid antibodies, and developing both subclinical hypothyroidism and a benign thyroid nodule, Kitty leads a full and productive life—as long as she takes her levothyroxine.■

MELISSA'S STORY

When Melissa, at twenty-five, started forgetting things and gaining weight, she attributed it to the stress of getting a divorce.

> I thought I was going nuts and needed to see a shrink, but one day I noticed that my right eye was swelling. I also had double vision. I went to an optometrist. He said, "You might have a brain tumor," and walked out of the room! I was in shock. He sent me to an

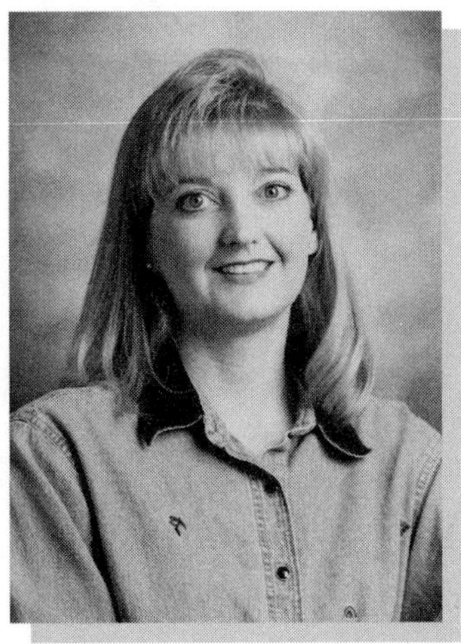

> ophthalmologist who did a MRI to rule out a brain tumor. He said, "I think you have Graves' disease," and referred me to an endocrinologist. It was the end of 1994. Instead of radioactive iodine, he opted for PTU [an antithyroid drug]. He explained that I could get a sore throat from it. He also said I had both Graves' disease and Hashimoto's thyroiditis.

After her doctor doubled her dosage of PTU to treat her Graves' disease, Melissa developed a sore throat and returned to her endocrinologist.

> I thought I had the flu, but he said, "No, you have agranulocytosis." My white blood count was 600, and I had a 104° fever. He wrote the diagnosis down on a piece of paper and said that I needed to see my family doctor.
>
> I went home and called my family doctor, but I couldn't get an appointment right away. Two or three days later, when I went to see him, he said, "This can't be right; you'd be dead!" But he didn't do blood work. He said it must be the flu and gave me an antibiotic and sent me home.
>
> While I was shopping for cold medicine in K-Mart, I almost passed out. My son was with me, so I took him to his dad's and went home and got in bed.
>
> When my fever got to 105°, I went to the emergency room, but they didn't know what to do. My endocrinologist was at a conference, out of reach. I stayed in the hospital four or five days. I got blisters in my mouth and nose and my eyes. It was awful! I think they had me on

> about ten antibiotics.
>
> When I went home, I was feeling weak and not sleeping well at night. At first, I was afraid if I went to sleep, I wouldn't wake up. Then I just couldn't sleep. It was hard; I couldn't really care for my son who was three years old at the time. He had to stay with my mother. I missed work for two months.

Unhappy with her endocrinologist, Melissa asked her family doctor to refer her to someone else. After explaining the various treatment options to Melissa, her new endocrinologist recommended radioactive iodine treatment. In January of 1996, Melissa took 15 millicuries of radioactive iodine to treat her Graves' disease. By April of that year, she was hypothyroid and began taking levothyroxine.

> I wish I had opted for iodine the first time. I think I would have if I had really been educated about the options. I was scared about it at first; I thought my hair would fall out or something.
>
> I don't remember having any symptoms of hypothyroidism after taking the radioactive iodine, but [my endocrinologist] monitored my blood every month. Within maybe three months, I started taking [levothyroxine].

Several years after her successful treatment, Melissa remarried and became pregnant.

> I had no trouble getting pregnant. I think the first time we tried I got pregnant! We had to increase my [levothyroxine] several times during the pregnancy because my thyroid levels fluctuated. I was concerned that the [levothyroxine] would affect the baby, but a specialist did a sonogram on the baby's thyroid and said he was fine.
>
> A month before the baby was born, my father died,

> and, a month after the baby was born, I had gallbladder surgery. A month after my surgery, my grandfather passed away. There was a lot of stress in my life. Anyway, I don't know why—I just stopped taking my [levothyroxine].

When Melissa went to her endocrinologist for her routine follow-up visit, her TSH was very high, over 150 mU/L, and her free T_4 was very low, less than 0.2 ng/dL (nanograms per deciliter).

> When I went back to see [my endocrinologist], all the tests came back out of whack, but I felt fine. He said my TSH was really high. I started taking [levothyroxine] again because of the blood work. I didn't feel any better afterwards; I felt the same.

> Before all this, I didn't know that anybody in my family had thyroid disease. Then I found out that a year before I was diagnosed, a male cousin had a goiter removed. And my grandmother said, "Well, you know your granddaddy's sister had thyroid problems all her life."

> My advice ... is don't go to just any Joe Blow on your HMO—go to a highly recommended doctor. Pay the extra; it's worth it.

Just like Melissa, many hyperthyroid patients eventually become hypothyroid. Even though Melissa had a dramatic encounter with hyperthyroidism, her story offers two important lessons about hypothyroidism. First, if a hypothyroid patient stops taking her levothyroxine, she will become hypothyroid again. Second, a patient can have a very high TSH level and not have many symptoms of hypothyroidism. The converse is also true—a patient can have a modestly elevated TSH level and have many symptoms of hypothyroidism. In either case, a patient should not stop taking levothyroxine without her doctor's recommendation. ■

ONE MORE "TAIL"

Thyroid disease in humans is the primary focus of this book. However, some readers, especially pet owners, might find it interesting that animals, particularly dogs and cats, develop thyroid disease, too. Dogs are more likely to develop hypothyroidism, and cats are more prone to hyperthyroidism (see Appendix B: "One Last 'Tail' ").

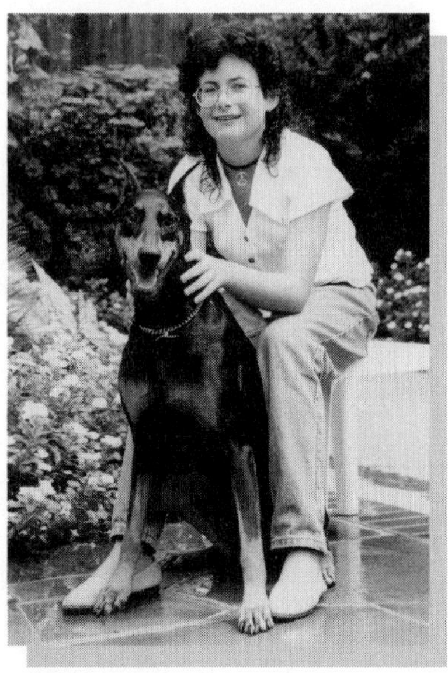

Pretty girl with hypothyroid dog

If a dog becomes overweight, sedentary, and loses hair, a veterinarian may suspect that the dog is hypothyroid. The veterinarian may measure the dog's T_4, T_3, free T_4, and TSH to confirm the diagnosis. When hypothyroidism is confirmed, dogs take the same medication as humans—levothyroxine.

According to Dr. Brian Poteet, a veterinary radiologist, "Hypothyroidism is a problem, but not a huge problem [in dogs]. The real problem is that it is over-diagnosed." When a dog gets sick from nonthyroidal illness, the results of the dog's thyroid function tests can be misleadingly low. Therefore, a veterinarian may assume that the dog's thyroid gland is causing the dog's illness when, in fact, something else is wrong. Dr. Poteet says, "Many dogs are supplemented if they need it or not. It won't do that much harm, but the real problem is that a veterinarian can miss what is really wrong with the dog."■

> As fate would have it, I have had three Doberman Pinschers, and all of them have been hypothyroid. Curiously, dogs require a much larger dose of levothyroxine than humans. At one point, my sixty-pound Doberman took 900 micrograms of levothyroxine daily, approximately *fifteen times* the dosage needed to treat a sixty-pound human. Somehow, it seems only appropriate that a thyroidologist would have hypothyroid dogs!

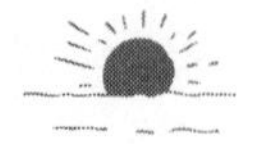

Chapter 6

WHAT IS LEVOTHYROXINE THERAPY?

In 1891, Dr. George R. Murray first demonstrated that hypothyroid patients benefited from injections of sheep thyroid. No one knew what the active ingredient in thyroid extract was until 1915, when Nobel laureate E. C. Kendall identified "thyroxin." In 1926, Sir Charles Harington identified the correct chemical structure of the active ingredient of thyroid extract and renamed it "thyroxine."

Until the 1950s, thyroxine preparations were not as effective as desiccated (dried and powdered) animal thyroid glands because they were not well absorbed and because they were also difficult to produce in large quantities. Therefore, from the late 1890s until the 1950s, desiccated animal thyroid was the primary source of thyroid hormone replacement. In 1958, the first well-absorbed synthetic (man-made) thyroxine tablets, formulated as sodium levothyroxine, became commercially available in the United States. Today, the preferred preparation for thyroid hormone treatment is brand-name synthetic sodium levothyroxine, also called levothyroxine, L-thyroxine, or T_4.

Levothyroxine therapy is indicated for all patients with hypothyroidism. The most common cause of hypothyroidism in the United States is Hashimoto's thyroiditis. In addition, nearly a million people have taken radioactive iodine to treat their hyperthyroidism, and, consequently, most of them have become hypothyroid.

Under certain circumstances, levothyroxine may also be indicated for patients with the following thyroid problems:

- goiter
- solitary thyroid nodule
- multinodular goiter
- thyroid cancer
- thyroiditis
- hyperthyroidism treated with antithyroid drugs

Some depressed patients without thyroid disease may be treated with levothyroxine to enhance the effectiveness of their antidepressants. Otherwise, levothyroxine is not indicated for patients without thyroid disease. Specifically, patients with fatigue, obesity, or infertility should not be treated with levothyroxine unless they also have a confirmed diagnosis of hypothyroidism.

T_4 and Not T_3

Even though thyroxine was identified and isolated as the active ingredient of thyroid extract from sheep, pigs, and oxen, scientists suspected that an even more potent substance was also present. In 1952, Jack Gross, M.D., Ph.D., and Rosalind Venetia Pitt-Rivers, Ph.D., discovered triiodothyronine (T_3), the more potent ingredient of thyroid extract. We now know that the thyroid gland in humans also produces both T_4 and T_3.

Synthetic levothyroxine (T_4) is preferred over triiodothyronine (T_3) for the treatment of patients with thyroid disease. The thyroid gland is the sole source of T_4 and the source of only 10 to 20% of T_3. The remaining 80 to 90% of T_3 comes from conversion of T_4 to T_3 by organs such as the liver, kidneys, brain, and skin. In other words, the body itself breaks down T_4 to produce the amount of T_3 it needs.

When a patient begins to take levothyroxine, the level of T_4 rises and becomes stable over a five-week period. From then on, the level of T_4 in the blood changes very little after each pill—the level of T_4 is slow to rise and slow to fall. On the other hand, when a patient regularly takes T_3, the level of T_3 in the blood tends to rise and fall rapidly over a period of hours after each pill. In addition, since T_3 is much more potent than T_4, a patient may experience symptoms of hyperthyroidism for several hours after taking a substantial dose of T_3.

Indeed, patients taking thyroid hormone preparations containing *substantial* amounts of T_3 may prefer them to preparations containing only T_4. Their reasons vary, but many patients say that it is easier to maintain their weight and that they have more energy when they take this combination of thyroid hormones. However, these benefits may come at a price—patients are often hyperthyroid for several hours each day. Hyperthyroidism predisposes these patients to osteoporosis, heart rhythm disturbances, and, possibly, a shorter life span. Substituting one disease for another is not desirable.

One recent scientific study of thirty-three hypothyroid patients suggested that adding a *small* amount of T_3 and reducing the dosage of T_4 may have improved their mood and neuropsychological function. The prospect of improved thyroid hormone replacement is very exciting; however, the quality of the study has been questioned. These results will have to be confirmed by other scientists in larger and better studies before thyroid hormone replacement with T_3 can be recommended.

Commercially available thyroid hormone preparations made from animal thyroid glands invariably contain T_3 and, as noted above, should not be used. Another reason to avoid these animal thyroid hormone preparations is the difficulty in preparing tablets that have exactly the same amount of thyroid hormones in each tablet. On the other hand, brand-name synthetic levothyroxine generally can be relied upon to have the stated amount of T_4 in each tablet.

Brand Name vs. Generic Levothyroxine

Currently, there are four well-tested brand-name synthetic levothyroxine preparations available for the treatment of thyroid patients—Levothroid, Levoxyl, Synthroid, and Unithroid. Although they are generally reliable and produce predictable results, they are not identical.

There are some differences in the manufacturing, composition (fillers and dyes), and absorption among these preparations. For this reason, it is preferable for patients to take the same brand-name levothyroxine consistently. If a change is made from one brand-name levothyroxine to another, thyroid function test results should be checked six or more weeks later to confirm that the patients are still getting the right amount of levothyroxine.

Levothyroxine tablets are color-coded, although different manufacturers utilize different color schemes. The table below provides a list of available strengths and colors for each of four brand-name levothyroxine tablets. (Since the Food and Drug Administration—the FDA—is now reviewing some levothyroxine products, these colors could change.) All the brand-name pills are round, except for Levoxyl, which is shaped somewhat like a thyroid gland. One way patients can confirm that their prescriptions have been filled correctly is by checking the color of

Levothyroxine Tablet Colors
as of October 2003

STRENGTH	LEVOTHROID®	LEVOXYL®	SYNTHROID®	UNITHROID®
25 mcg/0.025 mg	orange	orange	orange	peach
50 mcg/0.05 mg	white	white	white	white
75 mcg/0.075 mg	gray	purple	violet	purple
88 mcg/0.088 mg	mint green	olive	olive	olive
100 mcg/0.1 mg	yellow	yellow	yellow	yellow
112 mcg/0.112 mg	rose	rose	rose	rose
125 mcg/0.125 mg	purple	brown	brown	tan
137 mcg/0.137 mg	blue	dark blue	turquoise	(not made)
150 mcg/0.15 mg	light blue	blue	blue	blue
175 mcg/0.175 mg	turquoise	turquoise	lilac	lilac
200 mcg/0.2 mg	pink	pink	pink	pink
300 mcg/0.3 mg	lime green	green	green	green

dispensed pills; errors do occur (see "Sue's Story" on pages 147–149 and "Christine's Story" on pages 357–360).

Physicians can prescribe either brand-name or generic levothyroxine. If physicians want their patients to take a specific brand of levothyroxine, they will either write a prescription or call a pharmacist with verbal orders to dispense the prescribed brand. Therefore, if the words "Levoxyl," "Synthroid," "Unithroid," or "Levothroid" do not appear on the prescription label, then it is likely that patients are getting generic levothyroxine preparations. Furthermore, if only the words "sodium levothyroxine" or "levothyroxine" are on the label, then it is also likely that patients are getting generic rather than brand-name preparations.

Each state decides whether, and under what circumstances, pharmacists may substitute generic levothyroxine for a brand-name product without informing prescribing physicians. Furthermore, some physicians' contracts with health care providers permit the health care providers to substitute generic medications for brand-name products without informing prescribing physicians. Therefore, patients should be aware that they might not get exactly what their doctors ordered, and that their doctors might not be aware of the change either.

There are several reasons many physicians recommend brand-name over generic preparations of levothyroxine, including:

- quality control
- stability of manufacturer
- variety of available dosages

In the past, there has been less quality control in the production of generic levothyroxine than in brand-name levothyroxine. New FDA regulations may eliminate this discrepancy, although manufacturers of generic levothyroxine are "generally not required to include preclinical (animal) and clinical (human) data to establish safety and effectiveness."

Even if manufacturers of generic levothyroxine are now meeting the same production standards as the manufacturers of Synthroid, Unithroid, Levothroid, and Levoxyl, there are other reasons to prefer name brands. Generic manufacturers have no name recognition and may come and go in the marketplace more often than long-standing manufacturers of brand-name levothyroxine. For this reason, pharmacists may no longer be able to get generic levothyroxine from the same manufacturer. Furthermore, when substitution of generic for brand-name levothyroxine is permitted, pharmacists may select generic levothyroxine from any manufacturer—and it doesn't have to be the same manufacturer each time they refill the prescription. Therefore, when generic levothyroxine is prescribed, patients unknowingly may take preparations whose properties are not the same as their previously dispensed levothyroxine.

Another important factor to consider is that each brand-name manufacturer of levothyroxine offers eleven to twelve strengths from which physicians may choose. On average, a patient's levothyroxine dosage is changed once every three years. A change in dosage occurs even more often when levothyroxine treatment is initiated or when a hypothyroid patient becomes pregnant. Therefore, it is important that the prescribed drug is available in as many strengths as possible. Since many generic manufacturers offer a limited range of dosages, there is a higher likelihood of being switched from one manufacturer to another when generic drugs are prescribed.

Cost Factors

Patients may worry about the cost of taking levothyroxine over a lifetime. Levothyroxine is relatively inexpensive, especially when compared to many other drugs available today. For example, a three-month supply of brand-name levothyroxine will cost roughly between $25 and $50.

Levothyroxine is so inexpensive that patients might consider buying it themselves rather than using their insurance at the pharmacy. Typically, patients using insurance plans pay a flat rate, or co-pay, for each prescription they have filled, regardless of the actual cost of the medication. Many insurance plans also limit the number of pills that may be dispensed from a pharmacy. For example, a plan may only allow a thirty-day supply of levothyroxine to be dispensed at a time. If the co-pay for a thirty-day supply of generic levothyroxine is $10, patients will spend $30 for ninety pills and will have to go to the pharmacy three times. These patients could spend the same or less if they paid full price for 100 pills of certain name brands of levothyroxine, and they could avoid extra trips to the pharmacy.

There are other advantages to requesting 100 tablets of levothyroxine at a time. Manufacturers package levothyroxine several ways, including sealed and dated bottles of 100 pills. Because the bottles are sealed and have never been opened, the pills have not been exposed to light, humidity, and air, and, therefore, are less likely to deteriorate and lose potency. In addition, sealed bottles provided by manufacturers often contain a desiccant (that funny little thing that often gets in the way when you're trying to get your pills out), which absorbs moisture. Expiration dates on the bottles indicate how long the medicine will be potent. When pharmacists buy medicines in larger bottles—containing 1,000 pills for example—the tablets dispensed from the bottom of the bottles may be less potent because they've been on the shelf in unsealed bottles for an unspecified period of time. The question of potency does not arise if the pills come in sealed and dated bottles. One final advantage of having the original manufacturer's label on the bottles is the elimination of the possibility that the pharmacist accidentally packaged the wrong drug.

Finally, some people assume that generic levothyroxine is much cheaper than the name brand, but that is not always the case. For example, if switching between manufacturers of generic tablets introduces a new variable, then more frequent test result abnormalities might occur. Whenever there are test result abnormalities, more laboratory tests, at increased costs, are required. The increased costs of additional tests and doctor visits may offset any savings from using generic as opposed to brand-name levothyroxine.

Safety and Effectiveness of Levothyroxine

Levothyroxine has been prescribed, in one form or another, for more than one hundred years. As previously mentioned, synthetic levothyroxine has been widely used since the 1950s. At that time, the

FDA did not require an approved New Drug Application (NDA) before a synthetic levothyroxine drug product was introduced into the American market. On August 14, 1997, the FDA reversed its position and stated that there was:

> ...new information showing significant stability and potency problems with orally administered levothyroxine sodium products. Also, these products fail to maintain potency through the expiration date, and tablets of the same dosage strength from the same manufacturer vary from lot to lot in the amount of active ingredient present. This lack of stability and consistent potency has the potential to cause serious health consequences to the public. Manufacturers who wish to continue to market orally administered levothyroxine sodium products must submit new drug applications. [The] FDA has determined that orally administered levothyroxine sodium products are medically necessary, and accordingly the agency is allowing current manufacturers 3 years to obtain approved NDA's.

The FDA went on to say:

> ... no currently marketed orally administered levothyroxine sodium product has been shown to demonstrate consistent potency and stability and, thus, no currently marketed orally administered levothyroxine sodium product is generally recognized as safe and effective.

As of the writing of this book, the FDA has approved Synthroid, Levoxyl, Unithroid, and five other levothyroxine products. While awaiting FDA approval of its New Drug Application, the manufacturer of Levothroid gradually scaled back and, ultimately, eliminated its distribution on August 14, 2003, as required by the FDA. The remaining stock of Levothroid can still be sold by pharmacies. Since the approval process for Levothroid is still underway, Levothroid may eventually return to the marketplace. In the meanwhile, the approved versions of some levothyroxine products could differ slightly from their previously marketed versions. Physicians, therefore, may need to adjust dosages for some patients, even if the same brand of levothyroxine is prescribed.

In summary, the FDA is stating that, without an approved New Drug Application, they cannot attest to the safety and effectiveness of an individual levothyroxine product. Patients should not interpret the new FDA requirements to mean that currently marketed levothyroxine products are unsafe and ineffective. Furthermore, patients should not stop taking their levothyroxine or switch to another brand without first discussing it with their doctors.

Dosage

The exact dosage of levothyroxine required by patients must be individually determined. The initial dosage prescribed by physicians is based on an educated guess. Many factors alter the choice of the initial dosage of levothyroxine. For example, hypothyroid patients with severe coronary heart disease may be started on very low dosages of levothyroxine with small increases every five to six weeks.

Patients who have had their thyroid glands completely removed by surgery may require considerably more levothyroxine than other hypothyroid patients who have some residual thyroid function. Pregnant women and women taking estrogens for contraception or for treatment of menopause may also require higher initial dosages. Other drugs, such as phenytoin, carbamazepine, and rifampin increase the metabolism of levothyroxine; therefore, patients taking these drugs may require slightly higher dosages of levothyroxine.

Taking extra levothyroxine will not make the symptoms of hypothyroidism go away any faster, and it may be harmful. In his heavyweight boxing match against Larry Holmes in 1980, Muhammad Ali learned about the harmful effects of taking too much thyroid hormone. Ali was incorrectly diagnosed as having hypothyroidism, and thyroid pills were inappropriately prescribed. Ali, thinking that he was a big man and could take a big dose, took two or three times the prescribed amount. At the time of the bout, he experienced fatigue and muscle weakness that, in part, was due to taking too much thyroid hormone. He was badly beaten.

Some patients may be tempted to take extra levothyroxine to lose weight. Thyroid hormone can cause weight loss—but only if taken in excess. People who take excessive thyroid hormone to lose weight become hyperthyroid. Much of the weight hyperthyroid patients lose is muscle mass, not fat. In addition to losing muscle mass, these patients risk losing their hair, developing irregular heartbeats, and experiencing other unpleasant symptoms.

Patients should not take more or less levothyroxine than prescribed without a physician's recommendation.

Nonprescription Drugs, Iodine, and Levothyroxine

The labels on some nonprescription cold and flu preparations state that the drugs should not be taken if patients have thyroid disease. This warning does not apply to patients taking levothyroxine in prescribed amounts.

There are, however, many over-the counter preparations containing either iodine or thyroid hormones, or both, that will interfere with levothyroxine therapy and should not be taken. These preparations can both aggravate thyroid disorders and alter thyroid function test results. Consequently, problems arise when physicians prescribe levothyroxine based on misleading test results caused by over-the-counter products.

Unfortunately, over-the-counter iodine and thyroid supplements are readily available on the Internet, in health food stores, and in some grocery and drug stores. Many well-intentioned patients erroneously assume that supplementing their diets with natural products will help their thyroid problems; however, these products will not help. When patients search the Internet for information on thyroid disease, they are likely to see advertisements and links to sites selling natural products for thyroid dysfunction, weight loss, or energy. Very few sites list the ingredients or the amounts of the ingredients in these products. Therefore, patients cannot possibly know what they are taking—and neither can the physicians writing levothyroxine prescriptions.

Similarly, products from health food stores may not be adequately labeled. The labels on a variety of supplements contain terms such as "thyroid" or "thyro," leading some consumers to assume the products contain thyroid hormone. A closer look will show that few of these supplements actually list thyroid tissue as an ingredient. If they do, they usually do not state the source or the amount of the thyroid hormone in the products. Typically, iodine from kelp is among the ingredients listed on the labels of these products. The recommendations stated on some labels may range from 450 to 600 mcg of iodine daily, well above the minimum 150 mcg of iodine recommended by the World Health Organization for nonpregnant adults. Since the average daily intake of iodine in the United States is already 300 to 500 mcg, supplementing the typical American diet with iodine is unnecessary and potentially harmful.

Iodine is also found in certain prescription medications. In most cases, there are iodine-free substitutes available for medications

Substances* Containing Iodine

amiodarone
- Cordarone®
- Pacerone®

iodoquinol
- Yodoxin®
- Vytone®

kelp

potassium iodide
- KI Syrup®
- Pediacof Syrup®
- Pima Syrup®
- SSKI® (Lugol's solution)

povidone-iodine douches
- Betadine® Medicated Douche
- Massengill® Medicated Douche

povidone-iodine topical ointments
- Betadine® Ointment

x-ray dyes
- CAT scans
- IVPs
- myelograms
- arteriograms

* *This list contains some, but not all, of the substances containing iodine that may affect thyroid patients.*

containing iodine; however, sometimes an iodine-free substitute is not available. For example, some patients cannot discontinue amiodarone, a very effective iodine-rich medication for the control of dangerous heart rhythm disturbances (arrhythmias). Some x-ray dyes also contain large amounts of iodine. These dyes can affect thyroid function test results and, occasionally, thyroid function for many months. CAT scans, arteriograms, intravenous pyelograms (IVPs), heart catheterizations, and myelograms are x-ray procedures that typically use injectable dyes with iodine.

In summary, patients should inform their physicians when they have had any procedures with iodinated dye within the preceding year. Furthermore, patients should not take over-the-counter products containing iodine or thyroid hormones but, if they do, they should tell their physicians.

When to Take Levothyroxine

Successful treatment with levothyroxine requires that patients take it as directed by their physicians. Levothyroxine should be taken daily. Inexpensive plastic pillboxes may be helpful for patients who forget to take their daily medications. A pillbox with seven compartments, each marked with the day of the week, may be filled weekly and placed in a convenient location (see Figure 6.1). If a pill is forgotten, a patient may take it the next day or at the end of the week when the omission is detected, even though literature from pharmacists and from the United States Pharmacopeia (USP) recommends skipping a missed dose. Although "doubling up" may be done with levothyroxine, it should not be done with other medications without first checking with a physician.

Some patients do not take their levothyroxine daily although their physicians have told them to do so. Physicians may then suggest that some chronically noncompliant patients take their total weekly dose of levothyroxine once a week. However, physicians have to take into account the possibility that patients who cannot remember to take a pill once a day may also not remember to take seven pills once a week.

Levothyroxine is best absorbed when taken with water and on an

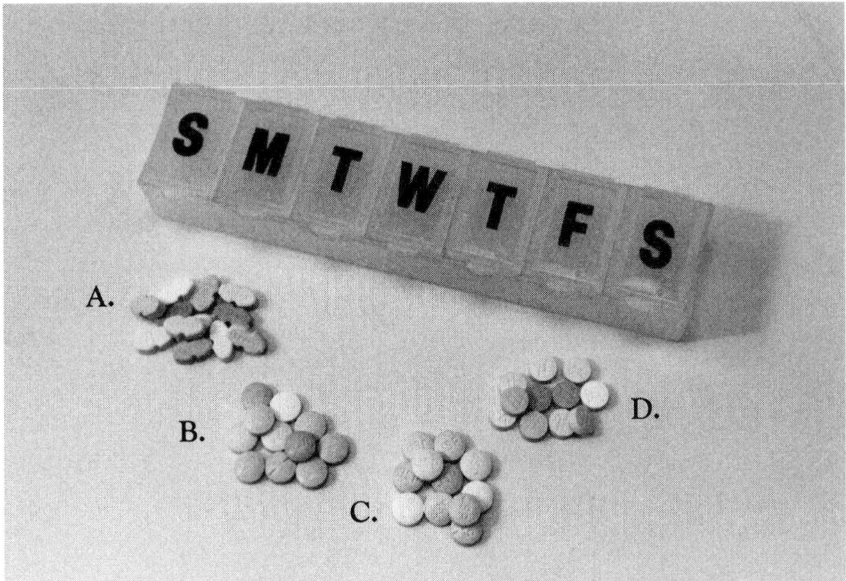

Figure 6.1. Pillbox and levothyroxine. (A) Levoxyl (note the shape). (B) Synthroid. (C) Unithroid. (D) Levothroid.

empty stomach, either one hour before or two hours after a meal. Taking levothyroxine this way is recommended because levothyroxine absorption is decreased by some foods, such as those containing large amounts of either fiber or soybean products (for example, tofu and soy milk). Synthetic fiber substitutes, such as FiberCon, do not interfere with levothyroxine absorption, but the effect of products containing natural fiber, such as psyllium, is unknown (see "Ken's Story" on pages 145–147).

In addition to food, certain drugs and supplements may interfere with levothyroxine absorption. Calcium supplements, such as Tums, Os-Cal, Citracal, and Viactiv, can interfere with the absorption of levothyroxine. Similarly, Feosol, Fergon, prenatal vitamins, and other preparations containing large amounts of iron will alter levothyroxine absorption. Therefore, patients should take their levothyroxine two hours before taking calcium or iron. Other drugs, such as sucralfate (Carafate) and antacids, may also interfere with levothyroxine absorption. Certain drugs used in the treatment of hypercholesterolemia (high cholesterol), such as Questran and Colestid, may have an even more profound effect on levothyroxine absorption. Therefore, they should be

Other Substances* Affecting Thyroid Patients

5-fluorouracil (5-FU)
aluminum hydroxide
- Maalox®
- Mylanta®

amphetamines
- Adderal®

androgens
- Androderm®
- Androgel®
- Depo®-Testosterone
- Testoderm®

beta-blockers
- atenolol (Tenormin®)
- propranolol (Inderal®)

calcium
- Maalox®
- Os-Cal®
- Viactiv®

carbamazepine
- Tegretol®

cholestyramine
- Questran®
- Cholybar®

clofibrate
- Atromid-S®

colestipol hydrochloride
- Colestid®

danazol
- Danocrine®

estrogens
- birth control pills
- Premarin®

fiber
furosemide
- Lasix®

grapefruit juice
heparin
heroin
interferon alfa
- Rebetron®

iron
- Feosol®
- Fergon®
- prenatal vitamins

l-asparaginase
- Elspar®

lithium
- Duralith®
- Eskalith®
- Lithobid®

mefenamic acid
- Ponstel®

methadone
perphenazine
- Etrafon®
- Trilafon®

phenytoin
- Dilantin®

raloxifene **
- Evista®

rifampin
SSRI's
- Celexa®
- Paxil®
- Prozac®
- Zoloft®

salicylates
salsalate
- Disalcid®

slow-release niacin (nicotinic acid)
- Slo-Niacin®

soy products
steroids
- Decadron®
- Deltasone®

sucralfate
- Carafate®

tamoxifen
- Nolvadex®

thalidomide

** This list contains some, but not all, of the substances affecting thyroid patients and some, but not all, of the name brands of those substances.*

*** There is contradictory evidence about the effect of raloxifene on thyroid function test results.*

taken at least four hours, and preferably twelve hours, after levothyroxine.

Patients who have had most of their small intestine surgically removed, or patients who have severe gastrointestinal diseases, may not be able to absorb levothyroxine. In these rare cases of levothyroxine malabsorption, patients might be treated with either intramuscular or intravenous levothyroxine.

How to Take Levothyroxine

- Levothyroxine should be taken daily unless directed otherwise.
- If you miss a dose, you may "double up" the next day. If you miss more than one day, double up for as many days as necessary to catch up.
- Levothyroxine is best absorbed when it is taken:
    - on an empty stomach
    - with water only
    - one hour before or two hours after eating
    - one hour before taking any medications, vitamins, or supplements
    - four hours before taking iron or calcium
    - twelve hours before taking Questran® or Colestid®

Follow-Up Visits

After patients begin levothyroxine therapy, their physicians will perform physical examinations and request thyroid function tests every six to twelve weeks until the correct dosage is determined. Once physicians determine that their patients are taking the correct dosage of levothyroxine, they will ordinarily see them at least once a year for a routine follow-up visit. On average, a patient's maintenance dosage of levothyroxine is changed once every three years for one reason or another. These reasons include:

- pregnancy
- estrogen replacement therapy for menopause
- birth control pills containing estrogen
- drugs or food interfering with absorption
- drugs, iodinated dyes, and over-the-counter supplements interfering with thyroid function or tests
- aging
- noncompliance
- the variable nature of the underlying thyroid disease
- changes in the prescribed brand-name levothyroxine
- decrease in potency of stored levothyroxine
- malabsorption of levothyroxine (rare)

Levothyroxine and Hypothyroidism

The onset of hypothyroidism is slow and insidious. Similarly, a full response to treatment occurs gradually and may take six weeks or more. Hypothyroid patients should not expect immediate improvement, even if the initial dosage of levothyroxine is correct.

Re-examination of patients and repeat thyroid function tests are usually performed six or more weeks after initiation of therapy with levothyroxine. If an adjustment of the dosage is made, patients will be re-examined in another six or more weeks. Ordinarily, once physicians determine their patients are taking the correct dosage of levothyroxine, they will see these patients at least once a year for routine follow-up.

When the diagnosis of permanent hypothyroidism is confirmed, patients must take levothyroxine for the rest of their lives.

Levothyroxine Therapy for Pregnant or Breastfeeding Hypothyroid Women

Even if hypothyroid patients become pregnant, there is no reason for them to stop taking levothyroxine without a physician's recommendation. In fact, discontinuing levothyroxine during pregnancy may be harmful. Women with inadequately treated hypothyroidism have an increased risk of miscarriage as well as an increased risk of impairing the intellectual development of their children. Finally, even though breastfeeding mothers should not take certain medications, levothyroxine can be taken safely while breastfeeding.

Patients Taking Thyroid Hormone Who May Not Need It

Occasionally, physicians suspect that some patients taking thyroid hormone are not actually hypothyroid and, therefore, do not need to take thyroid medication. For example, patients may have been started on thyroid hormone many years ago for an abnormal basal metabolic rate (BMR) or a low basal body temperature, two notoriously unreliable tests for hypothyroidism.

In order to determine if these patients actually need thyroid hormone treatment, physicians may advise them to stop taking their thyroid hormone for three weeks. If patients are genuinely hypothyroid, their TSH levels will be elevated three weeks after they stop taking thyroid hormone. On the other hand, if their TSH levels are not elevated, it is likely that they do not now, and never did, need thyroid hormone. Fortunately, if patients with normal thyroid glands have been taking thyroid hormone unnecessarily for years or even decades, their thyroid function will usually be normal within eight weeks of discontinuing thyroid hormone.

Sometimes patients are reluctant to stop taking their thyroid hormone. Some patients have taken thyroid hormone for such a long time that they have become psychologically dependent upon it. These patients may be afraid that they will experience severe symptoms, such as loss of energy or weight gain, within days of stopping their medication, particularly if they have been taking a medication containing T_3.

If patients have been taking only levothyroxine, it is very unlikely that they will experience symptoms within the first few days after discontinuing the medication—even if they are actually hypothyroid. On the other hand, if patients have been taking only short-acting T_3, they may experience symptoms within the first few days after discontinuing the medication, whether they are hypothyroid or not. Either way, if their thyroid glands are functioning normally, their TSH levels generally will be normal three weeks after discontinuing their thyroid medication.

Levothyroxine and Osteoporosis

There have been many articles written about one potential side effect of taking too much levothyroxine—osteoporosis. Osteoporosis is a thinning of the bones that predisposes patients to fractures; osteopenia is a milder form of bone mineral loss. The diagnoses of osteopenia and osteoporosis are made by measuring the bone density of both the spine and the hip, common fracture sites in osteoporotic patients.

Many patients, especially postmenopausal women, are concerned that taking *any* amount of levothyroxine will cause osteoporosis. However, patients taking the *proper* amount of levothyroxine do not have an increased risk of developing osteoporosis. Early studies suggested that taking *too much* levothyroxine could cause osteoporosis, but later studies have contradicted this conclusion. Nonetheless, it is always preferable to take the proper amount of any medication rather than too little or too much.

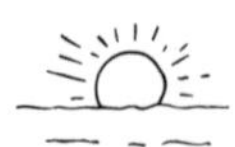

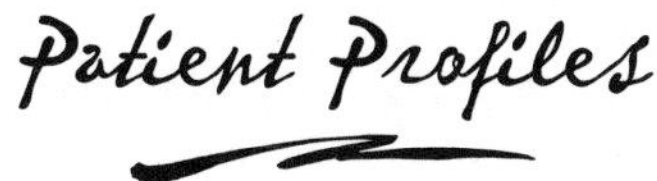

KEN'S STORY

Back in the '70s, Ken, a college professor, who had always suffered with allergy problems, couldn't shake a persistent sore throat.

> I had a really bad sore throat for a very long time, and [my internist] couldn't figure out anything causing it. Throat cultures turned out negative. I found myself getting very emotional about it. I was also very tired and tripping over things all the time. Finally, someone suggested that I see an ENT [ear, nose, and throat doctor], and that's what I did.

Ken's parents reminded him that he had radiation of his thymus when he was a child, and, after watching a television show about the impact of early radiation on babies and young children, they were concerned that he might be at an increased risk for thyroid cancer. Ken mentioned his history to his ENT who ordered a thyroid scan.

> I went for the scan; it was a two-day procedure. I remember sitting in the waiting area with the other patients on the second day. They dismissed everybody but me! Finally, a doctor saw me and said that there were no signs of cancer but that my thyroid was three times larger than a normal thyroid. I had thyroiditis, and it had reduced my thyroid [hormone] levels.
>
> They gave me a small amount of [levothyroxine]. There was such a dramatic difference very quickly. I had more energy and was getting so much done at work that my secretary threatened to flush my thyroid pills down the toilet.
>
> After a year, I got off thyroid medication. But then

> they found out that my thyroid levels were still low. They kept increasing the dosage [of levothyroxine]. I thought something was really wrong since I had to take so much thyroid [hormone].
>
> Then I started getting sick a lot. I had zero resistance. Almost every month, I got sick with a viral infection of some sort. I was having the symptoms of hypothyroidism. I went to an endocrinologist. My TSH [thyroid-stimulating hormone] level was very high. Basically, I had no thyroid function. He didn't understand how I could even function.
>
> He went through all the things I did. I was taking Metamucil and Per Diem [psyllium] every day. He said that they were interfering with the absorption of my thyroid medicine. He told me not to take any of these laxatives within two hours of taking my thyroid medicine.

In addition, his endocrinologist became concerned when he learned about Ken's history of radiation to his thymus as a child.

> He suggested surgery because he was so worried about the thymus x-rays. He sent me for an ultrasound, and [the technician] thought she saw something. I decided to get a second opinion. I went to [another endocrinologist], and he redid the ultrasound and never saw anything. He said I didn't need an operation, and I walked out of there very happy.

When Ken went to the second endocrinologist, he took a copy of his previous laboratory results with him. They confirmed that he had Hashimoto's thyroiditis.

> I switched to [another brand-name levothyroxine] that was absorbed better and take bulk laxatives now only in the evening.

> Another secondary problem I had [when I was hypothyroid] was that I had fallen in love and had no sexual function. Getting my thyroid level fixed helped that.

Like many other patients, Ken's thyroid disease is not an isolated incident in his family.

> My dad had hyperthyroidism and took the iodine cocktail. My wife also takes thyroid [hormone], and I suggested that she get it checked.

Because he had seen a physician and took his levothyroxine as prescribed, Ken assumed thyroid dysfunction could not be the source of his fatigue and diminished sex drive. He was unaware that certain substances, such as laxatives, can interfere with levothyroxine absorption, resulting in inadequately treated hypothyroidism.

> Just knowing you have a thyroid problem is not enough. I didn't understand something else I was doing was affecting it. It was a surprise to me because I didn't dream it was a thyroid problem because I was taking my thyroid [medication].

Taking levothyroxine on an empty stomach, with water only, prevents some unpleasant and unanticipated consequences and ensures that your medicine is completely absorbed. Patients should not take anything else, including over-the-counter supplements and natural products, with their levothyroxine.■

SUE'S STORY

Sue is a forty-five-year-old wife and mother of five children. She was thirty years old when she became pregnant for the first time. During the third month of her pregnancy, Sue's obstetrician discovered that she had Hashimoto's thyroiditis and was hypothyroid.

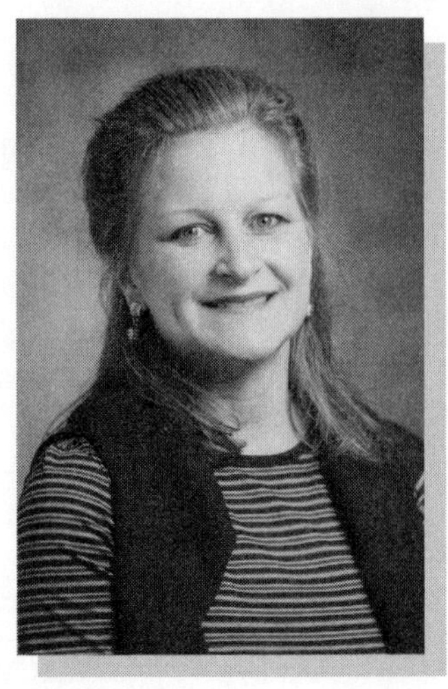

> I knew something was up before I was diagnosed, but I associated sleeping a lot with the move to Houston and the hot weather. I had maybe two periods a year, and they were very heavy. They were never regular until I started taking [levothyroxine].

As is the case with many thyroid patients, Sue had a family history of thyroid disease. She also discovered that she had one more thing in common with some patients suffering from autoimmune thyroid diseases—an increased risk of developing another autoimmune disease.

> I have a sister who is hypothyroid, and my father says he's borderline. When I was thirty-five, I found out that I had ITP [idiopathic thrombocytopenic purpura], an autoimmune disease similar to lupus. It affects my platelet count.

After years of uneventfully taking her levothyroxine, Sue shared another experience that many other thyroid patients have encountered.

> In December of 1999, I had a prescription for [levothyroxine] filled at [a national pharmacy chain]. I took it for several months before I found out they had given me too little. I really didn't feel bad, but I have children and would have dismissed any feelings of fatigue.

Sue's prescription was for 0.1 mg (milligrams) of levothyroxine. Her pharmacist gave her 0.088 mg instead of the prescribed amount. When Sue came in for her routine follow-up visit, she was nine weeks pregnant and had developed subclinical hypothyroidism with a mildly elevated TSH of 5.96 mU/L.

> I still go to the same drugstore, but I look at the color of the pills they give me before I leave the store. I think all patients should learn what color their [levothyroxine] is and, for that matter, what all their medicines look like. You can't blame the pharmacy for everything; you have to take some responsibility, too.

Pharmacists can make mistakes. Check the name, strength, and color of the actual levothyroxine pills. They might not be the right dosage—they might not even be levothyroxine! ■

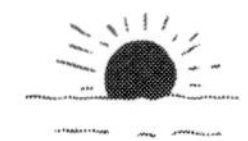

Could It Be My Thyroid?

Chapter 7

WHAT IS HYPERTHYROIDISM?

Hyperthyroidism is too much thyroid hormone in the blood; it is sometimes referred to as an overactive thyroid. Hyperthyroidism affects approximately 2.5 million Americans, and women are more likely to have it than men are.

The most common cause of hyperthyroidism in the United States is Graves' disease. In other parts of the world, toxic autonomously functioning thyroid nodules and toxic multinodular goiters are more common causes of hyperthyroidism. Regardless of the cause of hyperthyroidism, effective treatment is available.

Signs and Symptoms of Hyperthyroidism

As can be seen from the list on page 152, there are numerous signs and symptoms of hyperthyroidism. Hyperthyroid patients may have none, some, or many of these signs and symptoms, depending upon the severity of their disease. Patients may also have many of these signs and symptoms and not be hyperthyroid. Therefore, hyperthyroidism cannot be diagnosed by signs and symptoms alone. The diagnosis can only be confirmed after a thorough medical history, physical examination, and the appropriate laboratory tests.

Symptoms of Hyperthyroidism

Hyperthyroid patients most commonly voice complaints of fatigue, nervousness, irritability, increased sweating, feeling hot all the time (heat intolerance), insomnia, racing heart, hair loss, and poor memory. Many

Signs & Symptoms of Hyperthyroidism

Hyperthyroid patients may have none, some, or many of these signs and symptoms, depending upon the severity of their disease.

Patients may have many of these signs and symptoms and not be hyperthyroid.

fatigue	increased number of bowel movements
nervousness	shortness of breath
irritability	heart murmur
feeling hot	goiter
increased perspiration	osteoporosis
moist, wet, red palms	smooth skin
difficulty sleeping	generalized itching
fast, strong, or irregular heart beat	fingernails separating from nail beds
poor memory	swollen fingertips
inability to concentrate	swollen lymph glands
sudden mood swings	retracted eyelids
"racing mind"	infertility
delusions of grandeur	miscarriages
tremor	menstrual problems
hair loss	decreased or increased sexual interest
weight loss, in spite of an increased appetite	in men, slight swelling of breasts
muscle weakness	

times patients do not realize that they have a poor memory or an inability to concentrate, or that they have become very difficult to live with, until it is pointed out to them in a book like this or by someone who accompanies them to the doctor. If patients experience a change in libido (interest in sex), it is usually decreased; however, there are exceptions (see "Patrick's Story" on pages 200–202).

Another common symptom in hyperthyroid patients is weight loss, in spite of an increased appetite. A few, and often frustrated, hyperthyroid patients gain weight because the increase in their appetite exceeds the increase in their metabolic rate. As one patient succinctly put it, "It's not fair!" On the other hand, overweight patients who lose weight effortlessly from hyperthyroidism are often overjoyed. However, the weight lost is primarily from muscle as opposed to fat, and is frequently accompanied by muscle weakness. Muscle weakness from hyperthyroidism is characterized by an inability to climb stairs or to get up from a deep couch. Other patients may experience difficulty in holding their arms up while brushing their hair or teeth.

When hair loss (alopecia) occurs, patients may also become very frustrated. Stress, hypothyroidism, and, in women, too much male hormone may also cause hair loss. Hair loss due to hyperthyroidism is temporary; the hair will grow back within three to six months after the patients have been successfully treated.

Hyperthyroid patients who develop either shortness of breath from muscle weakness or palpitations (a racing and pounding heart) may think that they have developed a heart condition. In hyperthyroid patients with otherwise healthy hearts, palpitations and shortness of breath neither signify the presence of heart disease nor pose a danger to the heart.

The symptoms of hyperthyroidism in older patients may be somewhat different than those in younger patients. For example, apathy may be the only symptom of hyperthyroidism in patients over sixty years of age. This situation occurs often enough that it has been given its own name, apathetic hyperthyroidism.

Physical Signs of Hyperthyroidism

In examining hyperthyroid patients, physicians may note the following signs: rapid heartbeat, tremor of the hands, warm and moist skin, brisk reflexes, and a goiter (enlargement of the thyroid gland). Sometimes they may also detect a heart murmur. Muscle wasting may be visible, and muscle weakness may be demonstrated when patients have difficulty rising from a squatting position.

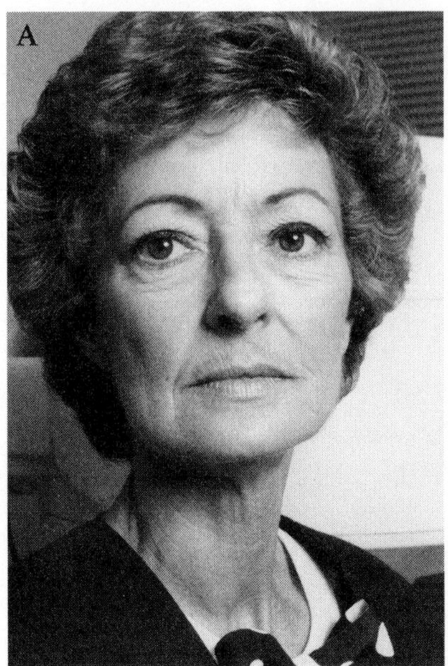

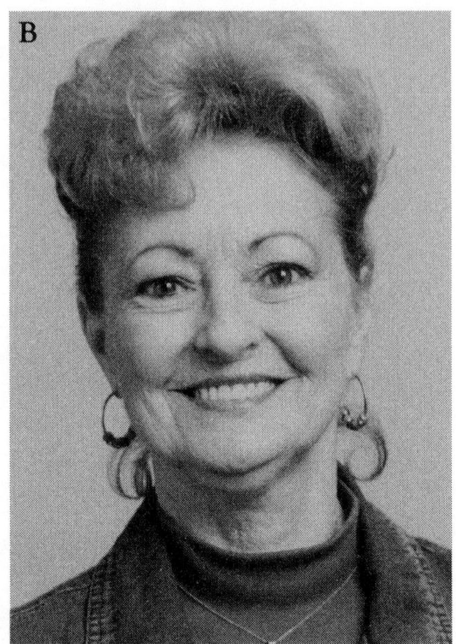

Figure 7.1. Before and after pictures of hyperthyroid woman. (A.) Note the asymmetrical goiter and thin face. (B) Several years after treatment with radioactive iodine.

Eye Changes and Hyperthyroidism

Hyperthyroidism may be associated with retraction of the upper eyelids, giving patients the appearance of staring. Excess thyroid hormone in the blood causes this effect by stimulating the activity of the muscles that open the eyelids. Eyelid retraction may occur regardless of the cause of hyperthyroidism and often, but not always, resolves as the hyperthyroidism is controlled.

On the other hand, the eye changes seen *only in patients with Graves' disease* may be much more troubling (see "Debbie's Story" on pages 202–208). When patients have Graves' disease, consultation with an ophthalmologist is recommended because the eye changes may be too subtle to be detected by routine physical examination. For example, glaucoma (increased pressure in the eye) can only be detected by measuring the pressure in the eyes. When eye changes are present, a baseline eye examination is very useful for detecting progression or improvement of the eye disease.

The eye changes seen in patients with Graves' disease are called

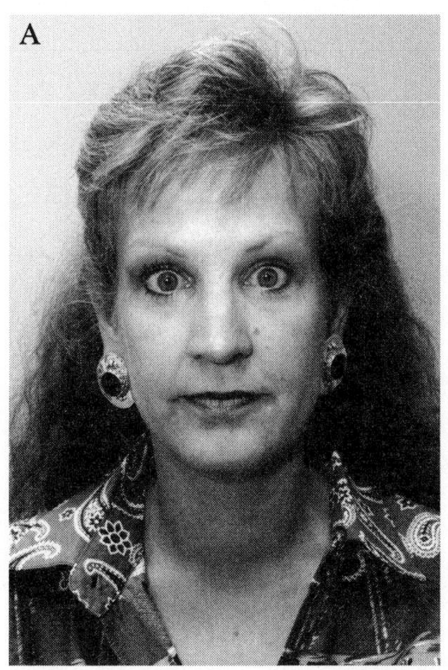

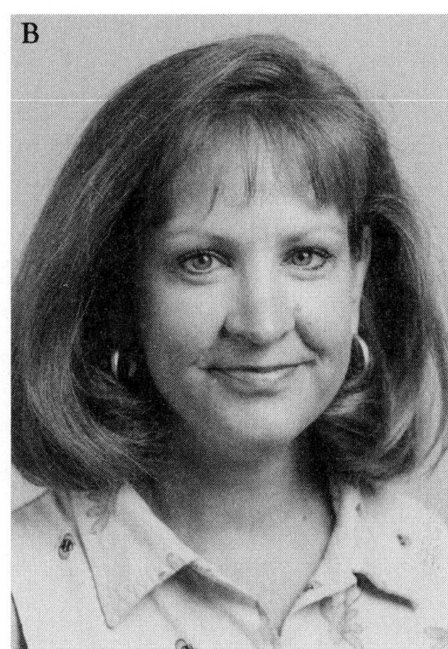

Figure 7.2. Before and after pictures of hyperthyroid patient with a goiter. (A) Note her goiter and the retraction of her eyelids. (B) Her goiter is much smaller, and her eyelids are no longer retracted.

many different names, such as Graves' eye disease, Graves' ophthalmopathy, Graves' orbitopathy, thyroid eye disease, and endocrine ophthalmopathy. For simplicity's sake, and to avoid confusing readers, the term "Graves' eye disease" is used throughout this book except where noted. Approximately 50% of the patients with Graves' disease develop eye disease, but the eye changes may be so subtle that patients are unaware of them. Severe eye involvement occurs in less than 5% of patients with Graves' disease.

There are several groups of people at increased risk of developing Graves' eye disease. Smokers and women are more likely to develop it. In addition,

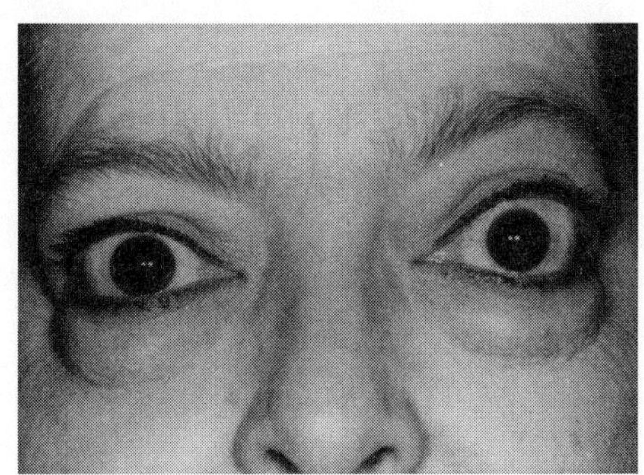

Photograph Courtesy of James R. Patrinely, M.D., Houston, Texas

Figure 7.3. Bilateral upper eyelid retraction and left lower eyelid retraction. Moderate puffiness of all eyelids.

Graves' Eye Disease

Signs and Symptoms	Cause
dryness gritty feeling redness sensitivity to light	mild inflammation incomplete blinking
tearing swelling pain	moderate to severe inflammation incomplete closure of eyes while sleeping
protrusion of the eyeball glaucoma	inflamed eye muscles or fat behind the eye
double vision	inflamed and improperly aligned eye muscles
loss of vision	pressure on optic nerve from swollen tissue

some studies have indicated that Caucasians may be at greater risk for Graves' eye disease than some other ethnic groups are. Furthermore, there are groups of people at increased risk for *severe* Graves' eye disease—smokers and men over age sixty. Therefore, smokers with Graves' hyperthyroidism can decrease their risk of developing Graves' eye disease if they stop smoking. Similarly, if smokers with Graves' eye disease stop smoking, their eye disease is less likely to become more severe.

Another important point to remember about Graves' eye disease is that it is not caused by thyroid dysfunction. Graves' disease is an autoimmune disease that can affect the eyes, the thyroid gland, or both—although not necessarily at the same time. Thus, Graves' hyperthyroidism

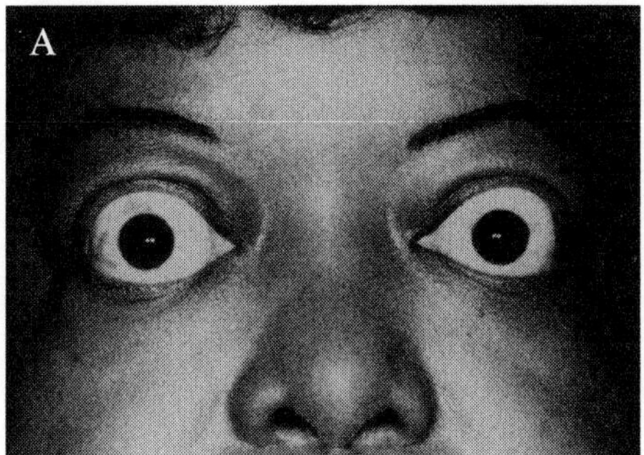

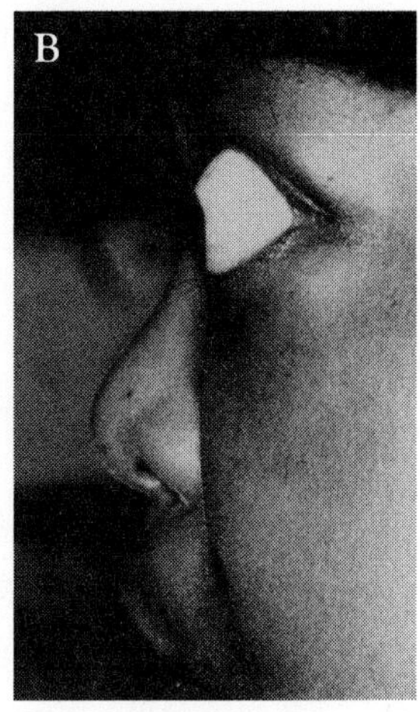

Photographs Courtesy of James R. Patrinely, M.D., Houston, Texas

Figure 7.4. Patient with severe exophthalmos. (A) Front view. (B) Side view.

may improve with therapy, while Graves' eye disease stays the same or gets worse. Proof that Graves' eye disease and hyperthyroidism are relatively independent of one another comes from the observation that patients may develop eye disease in the absence of hyperthyroidism. When Graves' eye disease occurs in patients with normal thyroid function, it is called euthyroid Graves' disease.

Symptoms of Graves' eye disease may include a feeling of irritation or sand in the eyes, double vision (diplopia), and excessive tearing. Inflammation and swelling behind the eye may cause actual protrusion of the eyeball from the orbit. When this protrusion occurs, it is called exophthalmos, or proptosis. Exophthalmos is measured, not surprisingly, by an exophthalmometer.

Graves' eye disease usually affects both eyes, although each eye may be affected to a different degree. In some cases, only one eye is affected. When the eye changes are severe, there may be marked swelling of the eye(s), impaired eye movement, corneal ulceration, glaucoma, and, in extreme cases, loss of vision.

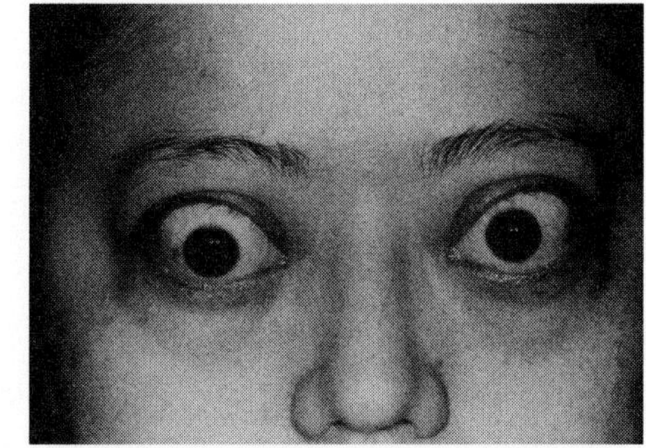

Photograph Courtesy of James R. Patrinely, M.D., Houston, Texas

Figure 7.5. Patient with ocular misalignment from Graves' eye disease. The right eye is turned down compared to the left eye.

Fortunately, these severe changes occur infrequently, but, when they do occur, consultation with an ophthalmologist is essential.

Changes in the Skin and Nails

Patients with hyperthyroidism from any cause may have changes in their skin characterized by warm, moist, red palms, smooth skin (particularly over the elbows), and separation of the fingernails from the nail beds (onycholysis). Occasionally, patients may experience generalized itching (pruritus). Some patients, particularly African-Americans, may note darkening of their skin. These changes are usually reversible with successful treatment of hyperthyroidism.

On the other hand, only those patients with hyperthyroidism from Graves' disease are at risk for the uncommon changes in the skin referred to as Graves' dermatopathy (disease of the skin). A few patients with Graves' dermatopathy will develop acropachy, a disease that includes elevation of the nail beds, soft-tissue swelling of the hands and feet, and, on x-ray, new bone formation. Most patients with Graves' dermatopathy will develop a thickening of the skin called myxedema. Myxedema appears most commonly on the shin (tibia), in which case, it is called pretibial myxedema (see "Kym's Story" on pages 208–211). Similar to the course of Graves' eye disease, the course of Graves' dermatopathy is independent of the course of hyperthyroidism. Sometimes a biopsy is necessary to confirm that skin changes are actually those of Graves' dermatopathy. However, dermatologists are reluctant to perform biopsies since the biopsy sites may not heal very well.

Interestingly, the word "myxedema" applies to both hyperthyroid and hypothyroid patients since, under the microscope, the skin of patients with Graves' dermatopathy looks similar to the skin of patients with hypothyroidism. The term "myxedema" was originally used to describe deposits of certain material beneath the swollen skin of hypothyroid patients. Although they look the same under the microscope, the skin of hypothyroid patients and the skin of patients with Graves' dermatopathy behave differently. Therefore, hypothyroid patients may be myxedematous, while hyperthyroid patients with Graves' dermatopathy may have pretibial myxedema.

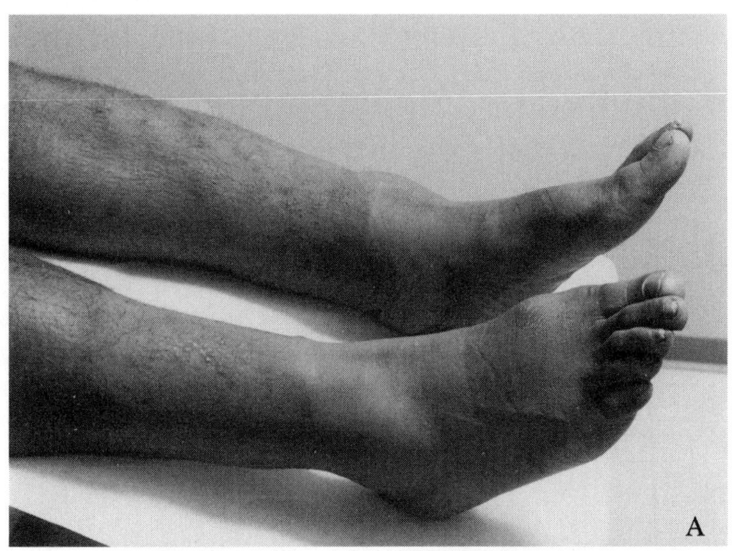

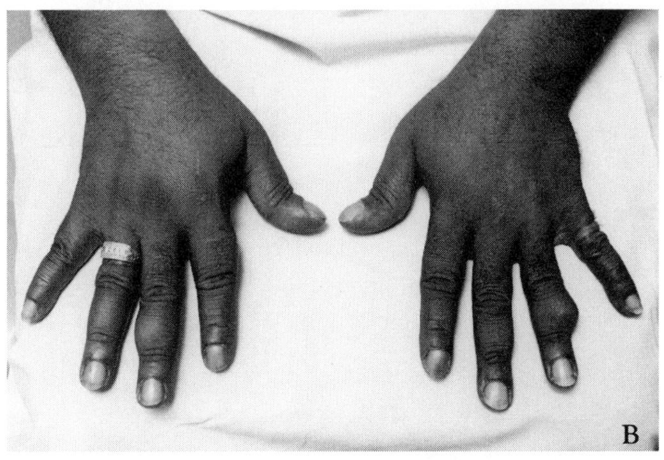

Figure 7.6. Myxedema. (A) Pretibial area. (B) Hands.

Abnormal Laboratory Test Results Caused by Hyperthyroidism

Liver function tests—SGOT (AST), SGPT (ALT), bilirubin, and LDH—may be elevated in hyperthyroid patients. Alkaline phosphatase, an enzyme found in both bone and the liver, is frequently elevated even when liver function tests are normal. Hypercalcemia (high calcium) occurs occasionally. Hyperthyroidism also lowers cholesterol.

Causes of Hyperthyroidism

Broadly speaking, there are four causes of hyperthyroidism—thyroid overstimulation, thyroid nodules, thyroid disruption, and miscellaneous causes.

Causes of Hyperthyroidism

Thyroid Overstimulation	Thyroid Nodules	Thyroid Disruption	Miscellaneous
Graves' disease	toxic autonomously functioning thyroid nodule (TAFTN)	subacute thyroiditis	T_4 or T_3 overdose
excess hCG	toxic multinodular goiter (TMNG)	postpartum thyroiditis	struma ovarii
pituitary tumor		painless thyroiditis	
iodine excess		radiation-induced thyroiditis	
		acute suppurative thyroiditis	

Thyroid Overstimulation: Graves' Disease

The most common cause of hyperthyroidism in the United States is Graves' disease, named after Dr. Robert Graves, a nineteenth century physician. Graves' disease is an autoimmune disease characterized by some or all of the following: hyperthyroidism, goiter, eye changes, and skin changes. Autoimmune diseases are characterized by the presence of autoantibodies circulating in the bloodstream. Antibodies are proteins formed by the immune system to protect the body against foreign chemicals, bacteria, and viruses. In an autoimmune disease, antibodies are formed against the body's own chemicals. These antibodies are technically called autoantibodies. Nonetheless, they are often simply referred to as antibodies.

Antibodies may be formed against a receptor, the specific site on a cell that captures a chemical. In Graves' disease, antibodies are formed against the receptors on thyroid follicular cells that capture thyroid-stimulating hormone (TSH). Remarkably, some of these antibodies duplicate the function of TSH and stimulate the thyroid gland to produce and secrete more thyroid hormone than normal.

Some physicians find tests for TSH receptor antibodies (TRAb) useful in both the diagnosis of Graves' disease and in following the course of Graves' disease in pregnant patients or in patients treated with antithyroid drugs. Other types of TSH receptor antibodies can be found in both Graves' disease and Hashimoto's thyroiditis, a common autoimmune disease that frequently causes hypothyroidism. The sensitivity of tests for these antibodies is continually increasing. Increased sensitivity of tests translates into an increased ability to accurately diagnose autoimmune thyroid disease.

Autoimmune diseases, such as Graves' disease and Hashimoto's thyroiditis, tend to run in families and are much more common in women. It is not unusual for several generations of women to have either Graves' disease and hyperthyroidism or Hashimoto's thyroiditis and hypothyroidism. Patients who have Graves' disease should tell members of their families—especially their mothers, daughters, sisters, aunts, and nieces—about their condition so that they are aware that there is a hereditary thyroid disease in the family. At least 50% of patients with Graves' disease will have the antibodies found in Graves' disease, as well as the antibodies characteristic of Hashimoto's thyroiditis.

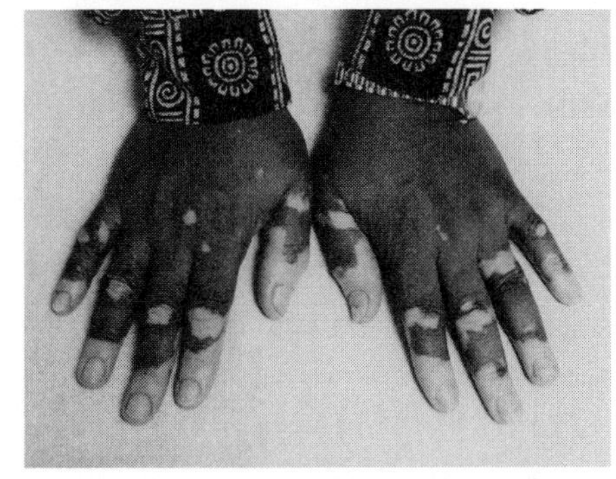

Figure 7.7. Vitiligo.

Other autoimmune conditions, such as vitiligo (a patchy loss of skin pigmentation) and prematurely gray hair are seen frequently in patients with Graves' disease. More serious autoimmune diseases, such as myasthenia gravis, rheumatoid arthritis, systemic lupus erythematosus, and Type 1 diabetes, are seen with only a slightly increased frequency in patients with Graves' disease as compared to patients without Graves' disease.

Thyroid Overstimulation: Human Chorionic Gonadotropin (hCG)

An uncommon cause of hyperthyroidism is excessive secretion of human chorionic gonadotropin (hCG), a hormone that is produced by the placenta during a normal pregnancy. The highest levels of hCG are found at ten to twelve weeks of pregnancy. A portion of the hCG molecule is so similar to TSH that it, too, stimulates the thyroid gland to produce thyroid hormone. However, hCG stimulation of the thyroid gland does not ordinarily produce enough thyroid hormone to cause hyperthyroidism. Nonetheless, in up to 20% of normal pregnancies, hCG stimulation may produce enough thyroid hormone to temporarily suppress TSH and, much less often, elevate free T_4 in the first trimester. These laboratory findings (an elevated free T_4 and a low TSH) in a normal pregnancy are sometimes referred to as gestational transient hyperthyroidism, gestational thyrotoxicosis, or gestational hyperthyroxinemia. Since hCG levels are normally higher when there are multiple fetuses, gestational transient hyperthyroidism is more likely to occur when a woman is carrying more than one baby.

Hyperthyroidism may also occur in a woman with hyperemesis gravidarum. Hyperemesis gravidarum is an exaggerated and severe form of the nausea and vomiting that may occur during a normal pregnancy. It is characterized by persistent vomiting, more than a 5% weight loss, dehydration severe enough to require intravenous fluids, and ketosis, a metabolic abnormality found in people who do not have adequate nutrition. Interestingly, the hCG level is higher and the hCG has more thyroid-stimulating activity in a woman with hyperemesis gravidarum than in a woman with an uncomplicated pregnancy. Treatment of a woman with hyperemesis gravidarum often involves one or more hospitalizations for intravenous fluids, drugs to control vomiting, and, when the symptoms of hyperthyroidism are severe, antithyroid drugs. The vomiting usually subsides by the sixteenth to twentieth week of pregnancy as the hCG levels come down.

Two types of abnormal fertilization events can cause very high hCG levels—hydatidiform mole and choriocarcinoma. A hydatidiform mole in the uterus leads to a defective pregnancy and, sometimes, to a malignant tumor called choriocarcinoma. Both a mole and a choriocarcinoma can produce sufficient hCG to cause hyperthyroidism. Treatment of a patient with a hydatidiform mole requires complete removal of the mole from the uterus. Surgery is also the treatment for a patient with choriocarcinoma; sometimes chemotherapy may be necessary, too. A patient with symptomatic hyperthyroidism from either a hydatidiform mole or a choriocarcinoma may also be treated with beta-blockers and antithyroid drugs.

Hyperthyroidism from excessive secretion of hCG occurs uncommonly in males. The usual source of excessive hCG secretion in hyperthyroid men is a testicular tumor. Fewer than twenty such cases of "toxic testicle" have been described in medical literature.

Thyroid Overstimulation: Pituitary Tumor

A relatively rare kind of pituitary tumor may produce TSH in excessive amounts and cause hyperthyroidism (see "Seymour's Story" on pages 84–88). TSH-secreting pituitary tumors account for less than 1% of all cases of hyperthyroidism. Since low TSH levels characterize all other causes of hyperthyroidism, a normal or elevated TSH level and elevated thyroid hormone levels in a hyperthyroid patient may indicate the presence of a TSH-secreting pituitary tumor.

Visual field defects and galactorrhea (a milky breast discharge) in a hyperthyroid patient also suggest the presence of a TSH-producing pituitary tumor. Treatment often involves surgery to remove the tumor, drugs to reduce TSH secretion, and beta-blockers to control the symptoms of hyperthyroidism.

Thyroid Overstimulation: Iodine-Induced Hyperthyroidism

Ingestion of excessive iodine can occasionally induce hyperthyroidism (Jod-Basedow's disease) in susceptible patients, particularly ones with long-standing multinodular goiters. Many well-intentioned patients erroneously assume that supplementing their diet with natural products will help them when, in fact, these products may contain excessive and potentially harmful amounts of iodine. Unfortunately, these products are readily available on the Internet, in health food stores, and in some grocery and drug stores. Labels on some of these products recommend iodine (usually from kelp) in amounts that may cause or worsen hyperthyroidism. The recommendation on some labels for a daily consumption of 450 to 600 mcg (micrograms) of iodine is well above the minimum 150 mcg of iodine recommended by the World Health Organization for a nonpregnant adult. Since the average daily intake of iodine in the United States is already 300 to 500 mcg, supplementation with iodine is unnecessary and potentially harmful.

Iodine is also found in various oral and topical medications (see table below). In most cases, there are iodine-free substitutes available for medications containing iodine; however, sometimes an iodine-free substitute is not available. For example, some patients cannot discontinue amiodarone, a very effective iodine-rich medication for the control of dangerous heart rhythm disturbances (see "Jim's Story" on pages 88–90).

Substances* Containing Iodine

amiodarone
- Cordarone®
- Pacerone®

iodoquinol
- Yodoxin®
- Vytone®

kelp

potassium iodide
- KI Syrup®
- Pediacof Syrup®
- Pima Syrup®
- SSKI® (Lugol's solution)

povidone-iodine douches
- Betadine® Medicated Douche
- Massengill® Medicated Douche

povidone-iodine topical ointments
- Betadine® Ointment

x-ray dyes
- CAT scans
- IVPs
- myelograms
- arteriograms

* *This list contains some, but not all, of the substances containing iodine that may affect thyroid patients.*

Iodine-induced hyperthyroidism may also occur weeks to months after exposure to x-ray dyes with iodine (see "Trina's Story" on pages 82–84). CAT scans, arteriograms, intravenous pyelograms (IVPs), heart catheterizations, and myelograms are x-ray procedures that typically use injectable dyes containing iodine. The amount of iodine used in these procedures may be thousands of times greater than the amount a person might eat in a typical day. On the other hand, the injectable dyes used for MRIs do not contain iodine and, therefore, do not affect thyroid function.

All in all, it is best to avoid over-the-counter supplements and foods, such as kelp, that contain excessive amounts of iodine. Drugs and x-ray dyes with large amounts of iodine should also be avoided unless they are absolutely necessary.

Toxic Autonomously Functioning Thyroid Nodules and Toxic Multinodular Goiters

Autonomous function describes the function of a part of the thyroid gland that acts independently of normal control mechanisms. Ordinarily, TSH from the pituitary gland and thyroid hormone from the thyroid gland work in a feedback mechanism, much like a thermostat and an air conditioner (see Figure 7.8). When thyroid hormone production goes down, the pituitary gland (thermostat) senses it and secretes additional TSH. The additional TSH stimulates the thyroid gland (air conditioner) to bring production of thyroid hormones back to normal. When thyroid hormone production increases, TSH production decreases, and thyroid hormone production is reduced to normal. If a thyroid nodule fails to turn off its production of thyroid hormone, despite suppression of TSH production, it is referred to as an autonomously functioning thyroid nodule.

- When a thyroid nodule functions autonomously and produces sufficient thyroid hormone to cause hyperthyroidism, it is referred to as a toxic autonomously functioning thyroid nodule (TAFTN). Not all autonomously functioning thyroid nodules become toxic autonomously functioning thyroid nodules.

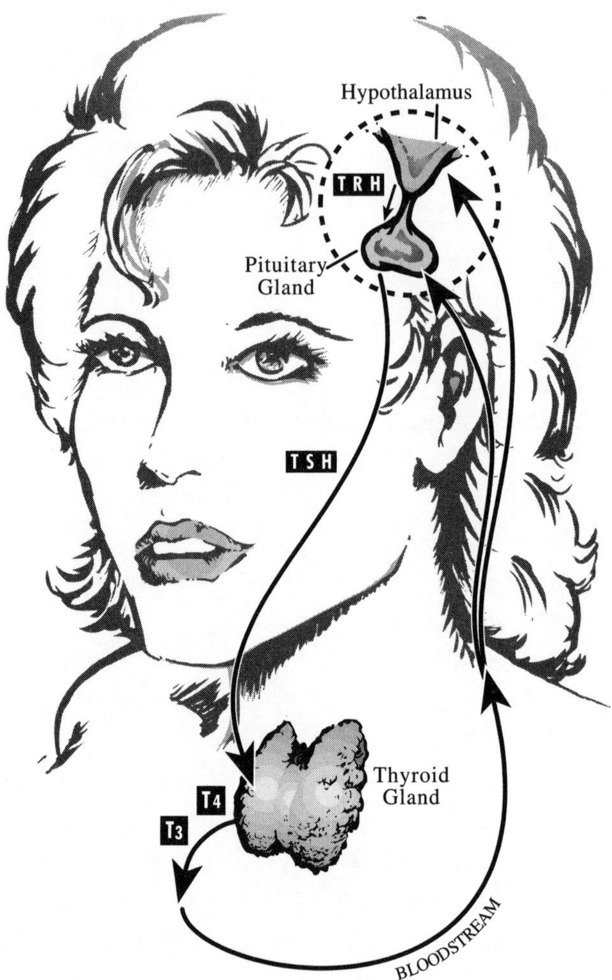

Figure 7.8. Feedback mechanism: hypothalamus, pituitary gland, and thyroid gland.

- When a multinodular thyroid gland with one or more autonomously functioning thyroid nodules produces sufficient thyroid hormone to cause hyperthyroidism, it is referred to as a toxic multinodular goiter (TMNG).

An autonomously functioning thyroid nodule is indicated by an increased uptake of radioactive iodine by the nodule. Since uptake of radioactive iodine is greater in the autonomously functioning thyroid nodule than in the surrounding tissue, it is referred to as a hot nodule.

Thyroid Disruption

A disrupted thyroid gland releases stored thyroid hormone into the bloodstream. Technically, this condition should be called thyrotoxicosis, not hyperthyroidism. Hyperthyroidism is defined as excessive *production* of thyroid hormone by the thyroid gland. A damaged (disrupted) thyroid gland does not produce too much thyroid hormone; it simply cannot control the *release* of stored thyroid hormone. "Thyrotoxicosis" is the all-encompassing term for disorders that result in too much thyroid hormone in the bloodstream, regardless of the source of the thyroid hormone.

When there is too much thyroid hormone in the bloodstream from Graves' disease, the condition may be called either hyperthyroidism or thyrotoxicosis. On the other hand, when there is too much thyroid hormone in the bloodstream from disruption of the thyroid, it should only be called thyrotoxicosis. Some of the literature available to the public, however, uses these two terms interchangeably, which may confuse readers. For simplicity's sake and to avoid confusion, the term "hyperthyroidism" is used throughout this book except where noted.

Disruption of the thyroid gland is seen in certain types of thyroiditis, including:

- subacute thyroiditis
- postpartum thyroiditis
- painless thyroiditis
- radiation-induced thyroiditis
- acute suppurative thyroiditis

These forms of hyperthyroidism are transient (temporary). Thyroiditis is discussed in detail in Chapter 8.

Miscellaneous Causes

Infrequently, patients may take too much thyroid hormone as a suicidal gesture. More commonly, patients erroneously, accidentally, or intentionally take too much thyroid hormone for other reasons. Physicians may sometimes inappropriately give patients thyroid hormone to promote weight loss or to increase energy. When physicians prescribe enough thyroid hormone to cause thyrotoxicosis, the patients are said to have iatrogenic thyrotoxicosis. Occasionally, patients either take too much thyroid hormone without realizing that they are doing so, or they intentionally take too much thyroid hormone and hide this fact from their physicians. In either case, the resulting condition is called factitious thyrotoxicosis.

Many well-intentioned patients erroneously assume that treating themselves with natural products is safe and effective when, in fact, these products may contain excessive and potentially harmful amounts of thyroid hormone. If patients search the Internet for information on thyroid disease, they are likely to see advertisements and links to sites selling natural thyroid products for thyroid dysfunction, weight loss, or energy. Very few sites list the ingredients, or the amounts of the ingredients, in these products. Labels on many products available in health food stores, and in some grocery and drug stores, often do not clearly state their ingredients. Therefore, patients cannot actually know what they are taking, and neither can their physicians.

The labels of some products found in health food stores may contain either the term "thyroid" or "thyro." These labels infrequently list the source, amount, or type of thyroid hormone in the products. These types of products, however, often contain thyroid hormones in amounts sufficient to either cause or worsen hyperthyroidism. Therefore, patients should avoid self-medicating with over-the-counter thyroid products.

One of the most unusual stories about accidental ingestion of too much thyroid hormone occurred in the Midwest. The reason for this small epidemic of hyperthyroidism was not immediately apparent. The team of medical scientists, however, who were sent to investigate the epidemic quickly discovered the cause. While harvesting neck muscles from cattle for meat, the slaughterhouse workers also harvested thyroid glands. Consequently, the people who ate this beef also ingested huge amounts of thyroid hormone and became hyperthyroid. The people most

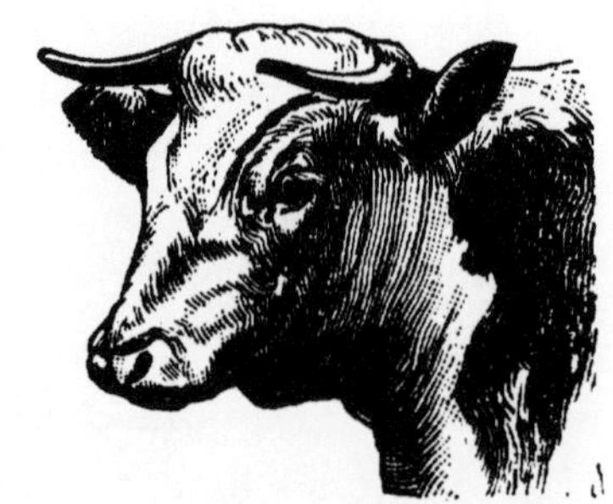

severely affected were those meat-packing plant workers who had taken the tainted meat home with them.

Another unusual cause of hyperthyroidism is struma ovarii. In this rare condition, thyroid tissue is found in the ovary. On even rarer occasions, this thyroid tissue produces enough thyroid hormone to cause hyperthyroidism. Most doctors, including endocrinologists, practice a lifetime without ever seeing a patient with a struma ovarii.

Tests for Hyperthyroidism

Most patients with hyperthyroidism will have typical symptoms, elevated thyroid hormones, and low TSH. Some patients with suppressed TSH will have neither symptoms of hyperthyroidism nor elevated thyroid hormones; these patients have subclinical hyperthyroidism.

Thyroid-Stimulating Hormone

Thyroid-stimulating hormone is suppressed in all hyperthyroid patients except for patients with TSH-producing tumors of the pituitary gland. However, not all patients with low TSH levels are hyperthyroid. For example, some older patients will have low TSH levels without being hyperthyroid, and many critically ill patients with nonthyroidal illnesses will also have low TSH levels. A thyrotropin-releasing hormone (TRH) test is sometimes necessary to confirm that the TSH is truly suppressed.

Thyroid Hormones

Most hyperthyroid patients will have high free T_4 and high free T_3. Ordinarily, only free T_4 is measured because this test is more readily available. On the other hand, in some hyperthyroid patients, only free T_3—and not free T_4—is elevated. This finding is seen more often in a patient with an autonomously functioning thyroid nodule or a toxic multinodular goiter than in a patient with Graves' disease. Furthermore, it is particularly important to measure free T_3 before making the diagnosis of subclinical hyperthyroidism.

Occasionally, a patient will have elevated thyroid hormone levels and a high TSH level. This combination of test results suggests the presence of a TSH-producing pituitary tumor. However, in the absence of signs and symptoms of hyperthyroidism, it is more likely that resistance to thyroid hormone is the cause of these unusual test results. Resistance to thyroid hormone is a rare hereditary condition characterized by the inability of various organs to fully respond to thyroid hormone (see "Bob's Story" on pages 12–14).

Thyroid Autoantibodies

Autoantibodies to the TSH receptor (TRAb) are usually found in patients with Graves' disease. These antibodies are measured by different methods and, therefore, may go by different names (see Chapter 4).

Occasionally, it is difficult to distinguish between the different causes of hyperthyroidism. For instance, Graves' disease may sometimes be confused with toxic multinodular goiter. When this confusion arises, a test that is positive for TSH receptor antibodies may be very helpful since it is diagnostic of Graves' disease. TSH receptor antibodies are also useful in confirming the diagnosis of Graves' disease when patients have only eye signs and symptoms without hyperthyroidism (euthyroid Graves' disease).

Unlike TSH receptor antibodies, positive antithyroid antibodies (TPOAb and TgAb) are not diagnostic of any specific cause of hyperthyroidism. Nonetheless, they are positive in at least 50% of patients with Graves' disease, postpartum thyroiditis, and painless thyroiditis.

Radioactive Iodine Uptake and Thyroid Imaging

The radioactive iodine uptake (RAIU) is essential in distinguishing among different causes of hyperthyroidism. The amount of radioactive iodine taken up by the thyroid gland is invariably suppressed in disruptive forms of hyperthyroidism, whereas it is elevated in Graves' disease. Thyroid imaging may also be very useful in distinguishing among Graves' disease, a toxic autonomously functioning thyroid nodule, and a toxic multinodular goiter. Examples of the thyroid image in each of these conditions are shown in Figure 7.9.

Radioactive iodine uptake and thyroid imaging may be misleading if a patient has had certain diagnostic tests within the preceding six to twelve weeks. For example, a patient having a CAT scan, myelogram, IVP, or arteriogram may be given x-ray dyes that contain large amounts

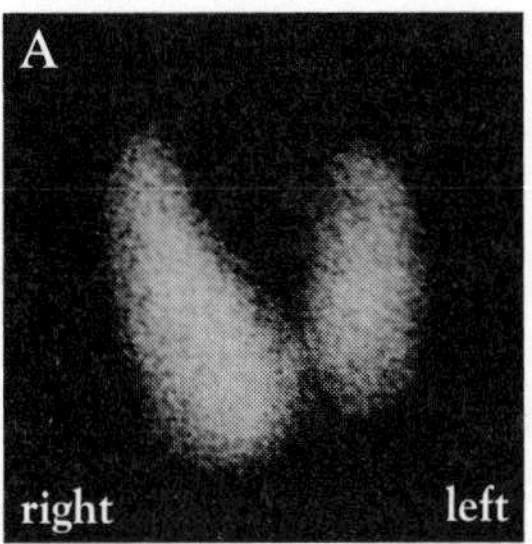

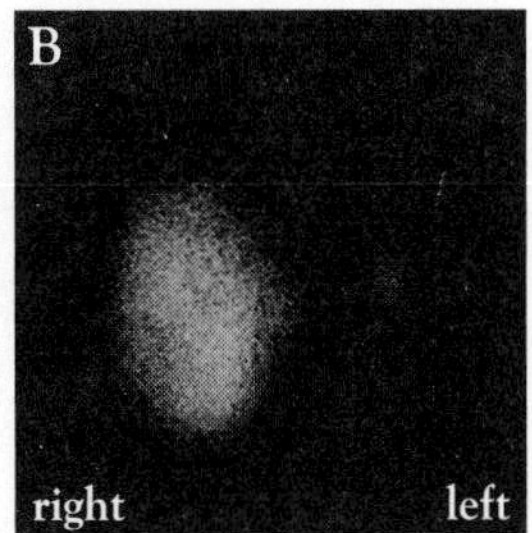

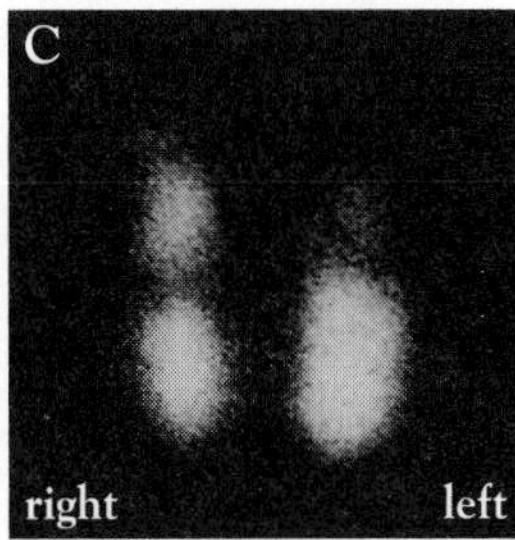

Figure 7.9. Thyroid images of hyperthyroid patients. (A) Graves' disease. (B) Toxic autonomously functioning nodule in right lobe; the left lobe and isthmus are suppressed. (C) Toxic multinodular goiter.

of iodine. The large amount of iodine given for these types of x-ray procedures dilutes the small amount of radioactive iodine given for the radioactive iodine uptake or thyroid imaging, making interpretation of these tests difficult. Therefore, whenever possible, a patient should postpone elective x-rays using iodinated dyes until after the radioactive iodine uptake or thyroid imaging is completed (see "Karen's Story" on pages 211–217).

Pregnant women should never take radioactive iodine.

Although radioactive iodine used for diagnostic testing does not harm an adult, it could harm a fetus. Therefore, if a patient has any doubt whether she is pregnant, any test using radioactive iodine should be delayed. Prior to performing any test involving radioactive materials, physicians will question a patient at length about the possibility of pregnancy.

Sedimentation Rate

The sedimentation rate measures how rapidly proteins in the blood settle to the bottom of a small laboratory tube. This test helps to distinguish subacute thyroiditis from other causes of hyperthyroidism.

Thyroglobulin

Thyroglobulin (Tg) levels will be elevated in all patients with hyperthyroidism except in patients who have taken too much thyroid hormone.

Usual Test Results in Some Forms of Hyperthyroidism

TEST	GRAVES' DISEASE	TAFTN AND TMNG	SUBACUTE THYROIDITIS	PAINLESS THYROIDITIS	PITUITARY TUMOR
TSH	low	low	low	low	high
free T_4, free T_3	high	high	high	high	high
RAIU	high	high or normal	low	low	high
TRAb	positive or negative	negative	negative	negative	negative
TPOAb, TgAb	positive or negative	negative	negative	positive or negative	negative
sedimentation rate	normal	normal	high	normal	normal

Interleukin-6

Interleukin-6 (IL-6) is one of many cytokines, or hormone-like proteins, that play an important part in the body's immune response. IL-6 is often elevated in patients with a particular type of hyperthyroidism caused by amiodarone, a drug used to treat heart rhythm disturbances.

Subclinical Hyperthyroidism

Patients with low TSH levels and normal levels of T_4 and T_3 have subclinical hyperthyroidism. The term "subclinical" refers to the absence of the signs and symptoms of a disease. In practice, it may be difficult to confirm the absence of signs and symptoms of hyperthyroidism. For example, physicians with extensive experience in the diagnosis of thyroid disease may identify subtle signs and symptoms of hyperthyroidism that less experienced physicians might overlook. Furthermore, some patients complain about even the mildest of symptoms while other patients are stoic, rarely acknowledging the presence of any symptoms. For these reasons, subclinical hyperthyroidism is a diagnosis based solely on the laboratory findings of a low TSH level and normal thyroid hormone levels.

The causes of subclinical hyperthyroidism are as varied as the causes of overt hyperthyroidism. In addition, all patients taking levothyroxine are at risk for subclinical hyperthyroidism if they take too much thyroid hormone. The prevalence of subclinical hyperthyroidism is uncertain since the definition of subclinical hyperthyroidism depends, in part, on the definition of low TSH. A reasonable guess would be that less than 2% of the adult American population has low TSH.

Progression from subclinical hyperthyroidism to overt hyperthyroidism is relatively uncommon (see "Jennifer's Story" on pages 217–219). Nonetheless, abnormalities in musculoskeletal, neuropsychological, and cardiovascular function have prompted consideration of treatment of patients with subclinical hyperthyroidism. Patients with subclinical hyperthyroidism, especially postmenopausal women, may have reduced bone density. In addition, disturbances of sleep and cognitive function may occur more frequently in patients with subclinical hyperthyroidism. Finally, these patients have an increased risk for a serious heart rhythm disturbance, atrial fibrillation, as well as a reduced exercise tolerance and other, more subtle, abnormalities of their heart function. Indeed, a recent study demonstrated that subclinically hyperthyroid patients over sixty years of age had an increased mortality rate during the ten years following an initial finding of low TSH levels; the primary cause of the increased number of deaths was heart disease.

Confirmation of the Diagnosis of Hyperthyroidism

Ordinarily, the diagnosis of hyperthyroidism is confirmed by the presence of the typical signs and symptoms, a low TSH level, and elevated thyroid hormone levels. A low TSH level with normal thyroid hormone levels is diagnostic of subclinical hyperthyroidism. A radioactive iodine uptake and thyroid imaging are instrumental in distinguishing among the different causes of hyperthyroidism. This distinction is critical since some types of hyperthyroidism, such as Graves' disease, are permanent and require definitive therapy, while other types are temporary and respond to symptomatic treatment and the passage of time.

Treatment of Patients with Hyperthyroidism: General Considerations

The treatment of patients with hyperthyroidism depends upon both the cause and the severity of the disease. Patients with temporary forms of hyperthyroidism due to disruption of the thyroid gland require only symptomatic treatment and the passage of time. Most patients will recover from disruptive forms of hyperthyroidism without definitive treatment, as discussed in Chapter 8.

In almost all cases, patients with permanent forms of hyperthyroidism, such as Graves' disease, toxic autonomously functioning thyroid nodules, and toxic multinodular goiters, require definitive treatment. Infrequently, Graves' hyperthyroidism disappears without any treatment; this phenomenon is called a spontaneous remission. There is no way of predicting which patients will have spontaneous remissions or how long the remissions will last. Unfortunately, spontaneous remissions of Graves' hyperthyroidism do not occur often enough to warrant postponing treatment.

Certain drugs are used to treat only the symptoms of hyperthyroidism without having a significant effect upon the function of the thyroid gland; they simply make patients feel better. For example, some patients with hyperthyroidism experience insomnia and severe anxiety. Sleeping medications and drugs for anxiety may be prescribed to relieve these symptoms until the hyperthyroidism is controlled. Similarly, beta-blockers, such as Inderal, Corgard, and Tenormin, will slow down the heart rate and reduce the tremor seen in hyperthyroid patients.

Beta-blockers have also been used successfully and safely to treat the symptoms of hyperthyroidism during pregnancy. However, beta-blockers cross the placenta, and the use of some beta-blockers, such as

Inderal, throughout pregnancy may be harmful to the fetus and the newborn. Fortunately, the symptoms of most hyperthyroid women will not be severe enough to require beta-blockers for the entire pregnancy.

Patients with asthma cannot take certain beta-blockers since these drugs can cause severe and, occasionally, fatal bouts of asthma.

TREATMENT OF PATIENTS WITH GRAVES' HYPERTHYROIDISM

In considering treatment options for patients with Graves' hyperthyroidism, it is helpful to bear in mind the following:

- Symptoms of untreated hyperthyroidism from Graves' disease may wax and wane over a period of months or years.
- Often, the end result of *untreated* Graves' hyperthyroidism is hypothyroidism—the thyroid gland "burns out" after ten to twenty years.
- The course of Graves' eye disease and the course of Graves' hyperthyroidism are independent of one another. The eye disease charts its own course, even with successful treatment of the hyperthyroidism.

The three basic treatment options for patients with Graves' hyperthyroidism are:

- radioactive iodine (I^{131})
- antithyroid drugs
  - propylthiouracil (PTU)
  - Tapazole (methimazole)
- surgery (thyroidectomy)

Radioactive Iodine

The majority of endocrinologists in the United States prefer radioactive iodine to treat patients with Graves' hyperthyroidism. In 1941, Dr. Saul Hertz in Boston and Dr. Joseph Hamilton in Berkeley were the first physicians to treat hyperthyroid patients with radioactive iodine. The popularity of radioactive iodine for the treatment of Graves' disease has grown rapidly since then because it is simple, effective, relatively inexpensive, and safe.

Many patients ask how it is possible to ablate (destroy) the thyroid gland with radioactive material without harming any other part of the body. The thyroid gland actively takes up significantly more iodine than any other part of the body; the salivary glands are the only other glands that take up any iodine at all. Therefore, administered radioactive iodine is taken up almost exclusively by the thyroid gland. The overactive thyroid gland gets the full impact of the radiation, while the rest of the body is unaffected.

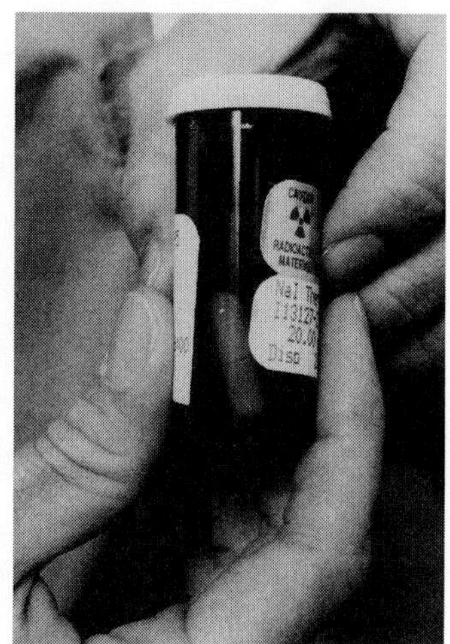

Figure 7.10. Radioactive iodine capsule for treatment of hyperthyroidism.

Patients sometimes have fears and misconceptions about radioactive iodine treatment because they do not understand what they will be expected to do or how it will affect them. The following statements are intended to clarify some of these issues:

- Radioactive iodine is usually given in liquid or capsule form.
- It is tasteless.
- Side effects are rare.
- Because radioactive iodine passes into breast milk, breastfeeding mothers are asked to wean their babies before treatment.

- It typically takes six weeks before thyroid hormone production is noticeably reduced.
- In most cases, patients become hypothyroid within three to six months after treatment.
- In more than 90% of patients, only one treatment is required. If patients are still hyperthyroid six months later, they will need a second dose of radioactive iodine.
- (Radioactive iodine will not make patients glow in the dark!)

Pregnant or breastfeeding women should not take radioactive iodine.

It may seem radical to destroy the thyroid gland with radioactive iodine. However, even when patients do not receive treatment, hypothyroidism usually occurs within one or two decades after the onset of Graves' hyperthyroidism because the thyroid gland eventually "burns out" (see "Kym's Story" on pages 208–211). With this realization in mind, ablation of the thyroid gland with radioactive iodine does not seem nearly as radical. In fact, some physicians believe that the preferred result of radioactive iodine treatment is hypothyroidism within six months. To achieve this result, they give most patients a relatively large dose of radioactive iodine. The subsequent development of hypothyroidism within three to six months of this treatment eliminates a prolonged follow-up period and frequent doctor visits.

Prior treatment with antithyroid drugs may influence the outcome of radioactive iodine treatment. The success rate of radioactive iodine treatment may depend on which antithyroid drug is used and when it is stopped. Tapazole (methimazole) can be stopped five to fourteen days before radioactive iodine treatment without affecting the outcome. On the other hand, the success rate of a single dose of radioactive iodine is reduced in patients who stop taking their PTU (propylthiouracil) as long as two months before their radioactive iodine treatment.

Some physicians give "cold" iodine to patients five days or so after administering radioactive iodine, usually in the form of potassium iodide (SSKI), five drops daily, until the patients' free T_4 levels are normal. This form of iodine is called "cold" to distinguish it from "hot" (radioactive) iodine. Cold iodine given after radioactive iodine may reduce thyroid hormones to lower levels more quickly than radioactive iodine alone. However, patients do not necessarily have fewer symptoms or benefit in any significant way as a result of taking cold iodine. Furthermore, although cold iodine following radioactive iodine is safe, a few patients may develop rashes.

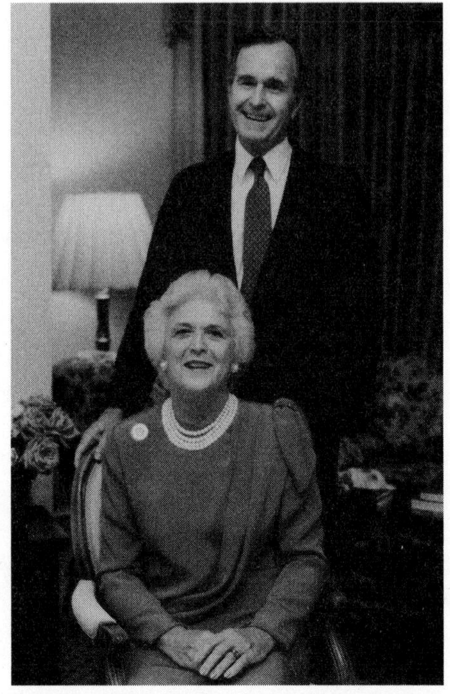

Figure 7.11. Former President and Mrs. George H. W. Bush each took radioactive iodine for Graves' disease.

Physicians, looking for a response to therapy and the development of hypothyroidism, will see their patients approximately every six weeks following radioactive iodine treatment. Patients should be aware of the signs and symptoms of hypothyroidism (see Chapter 5) and tell their physicians when they appear. Once the diagnosis of hypothyroidism is confirmed, levothyroxine therapy is started (see Chapter 6).

The transition from hyperthyroidism to hypothyroidism could be very dramatic—patients may be both relieved and frustrated. The relief comes from the disappearance of symptoms of hyperthyroidism, and the frustration comes from the appearance of symptoms of hypothyroidism. In particular, hair loss and weight gain may be very disconcerting. Patients may have lost hair while they were hyperthyroid; then, they may lose even more hair when they become hypothyroid. If the hair loss is the result of *only* a change in thyroid status, the hair will grow back once thyroid hormone levels have been normal for several months. Weight gain is less predictable and depends upon several factors, including diet, exercise, the amount of weight lost while hyperthyroid, and the adequacy of levothyroxine therapy once patients become hypothyroid.

Safety of Radioactive Iodine

Safety is one of the biggest concerns patients have about radioactive iodine. Radioactive iodine is one of the best-studied drugs used in the United States. Most studies of hyperthyroid patients treated with radioactive iodine have demonstrated the following:

- Radioactive iodine does not cause cancer.
- Radioactive iodine does not cause infertility.
- Radioactive iodine does not cause birth defects or cancer in children born to women who were treated prior to becoming pregnant.

Radioactive iodine not taken up by the thyroid gland is excreted in urine and saliva. There is no evidence that the small amount of radioactive iodine excreted in urine and saliva is harmful. Nonetheless, prudent nuclear medicine experts have recommended a wide variety of precautions. While these recommendations are sometimes confusing and inconsistent, it may be appropriate to take a few simple, precautionary measures. For example, immediately after drinking and eating, patients should rinse out their glasses, cups, and other utensils. The toilet should be flushed immediately after use, and the rim of the bowl should be wiped dry, if necessary.

Radiation from radioactive iodine travels only a short distance from the boundary of the thyroid gland and is not harmful to family members or co-workers. Nonetheless, it may be prudent to avoid holding infants or young children close to the neck for the first three or four days after radioactive iodine treatment; some patients have someone else care for their small children during this time.

Pregnant or breastfeeding women should not take radioactive iodine.

Even though radioactive iodine does not cause birth defects or cancer in children born to women who were treated prior to becoming pregnant, women should avoid becoming pregnant until their thyroid hormone levels are normal. Both hypothyroidism and hyperthyroidism are associated with a decreased pregnancy rate and an increased risk of miscarriage. In most patients treated with radioactive iodine, hypothyroidism occurs within three to six months, and euthyroidism is usually achieved within three months of starting levothyroxine. Therefore, it may be advisable for women to delay pregnancy for six to twelve months after taking radioactive iodine.

The effect of radioactive iodine on the progression of Graves' eye disease is controversial (see "Ed's Story" on pages 219–221). Most, but not all, studies suggest that radioactive iodine therapy, more often than surgery or antithyroid drug therapy, is associated with the appearance or worsening of Graves' eye disease. Steroids, such as prednisone, may prevent worsening of mild Graves' eye disease in patients treated with radioactive iodine. The benefits of prednisone have to be carefully weighed against the risks of developing serious side effects from steroids.

Less than 1% of patients treated with radioactive iodine will develop radiation-induced thyroiditis. Radiation-induced thyroiditis is characterized by pain in the area of the thyroid gland, which may last up to three weeks. The pain usually responds within a few days to treatment with nonsteroidal anti-inflammatory drugs, such as ibuprofen (Motrin or Advil).

Since iodine crosses the placenta, women must be certain that they are not pregnant before taking radioactive iodine for either diagnostic or therapeutic purposes. While there are limited data on the effects of radioactive iodine on the fetus, some very tentative conclusions have been reached. These conclusions are based on studies of children who were in the womb when atomic bombs were dropped on Hiroshima and Nagasaki, and on other studies of children born to mothers who were accidentally given radioactive iodine while pregnant.

These studies suggest that the risk to the fetus from the isotope of radioactive iodine (I^{123}) used in the radioactive iodine uptake test is so small that the question of terminating the pregnancy need not arise. On the other hand, when calculating the risk to the fetus from a therapeutic dose of radioactive iodine (I^{131}) given to a hyperthyroid pregnant woman, her physician must take into account the stage of pregnancy, the dosage of radioactive iodine, and the radioactive iodine uptake of the mother.

Although almost all of the small number of pregnancies in hyperthyroid women treated with radioactive iodine while they were pregnant have proved to be uncomplicated, the question of termination of the pregnancy is likely to come to mind. Treatment options other than termination, however, are available. The choice of treatment in this situation is difficult and must be individualized.

Antithyroid Drugs

Antithyroid drugs, such as propylthiouracil (PTU) and Tapazole, block the thyroid gland's ability to produce thyroid hormone and may affect the underlying autoimmune process as well. Up to 30% of patients who take antithyroid drugs will become euthyroid and remain euthyroid indefinitely after they stop taking these medicines. In other words, these patients will be in remission. Women over forty years of age with small goiters and mild hyperthyroidism have the best chance of going into remission. The highest success rate may occur in patients who take antithyroid drugs continuously for one to two years, or sometimes longer. Nonetheless, more than 70% of patients treated with antithyroid drugs will become hyperthyroid again once the drugs are discontinued. When hyperthyroidism recurs following discontinuation of antithyroid drugs, consideration should be given to treatment with either radioactive iodine or surgery. Some patients may elect to resume antithyroid drugs and to take them indefinitely (see "Joe's Story" on pages 221–224).

When considering antithyroid drugs as a treatment option for hyperthyroidism, here are some other factors to take into account:

- Normal thyroid function is usually achieved within six to eight weeks after starting antithyroid drugs.

- Antithyroid drugs sometimes have to be taken every eight hours when they are first prescribed.

- Antithyroid drugs have to be taken daily for months, or even years, to achieve a remission.

- Some patients complain that antithyroid drugs have an unpleasant smell and taste.

- Follow-up visits are frequent since the response to antithyroid drugs is somewhat unpredictable.

- Minor side effects, such as skin rashes, gastrointestinal distress, and joint pains, occur in up to 6% of patients.

- More serious side effects, such as a temporary destruction of white blood cells (agranulocytosis), occur in less than 1% of patients. Sore throat and fever may be the first indications of agranulocytosis (see "Melissa's Story" on pages 122–125).

- Antithyroid drugs can have toxic effects on the liver. These effects are usually reversible, but they are occasionally fatal. Fatal liver reactions occur more frequently with PTU than with Tapazole.

If patients taking Tapazole or PTU develop sore throats and fevers, they should stop taking their antithyroid drugs immediately and call their doctors.

Some older studies suggested that the remission rate from antithyroid drugs was higher in patients treated by the block-replace method. In the block-replace method, patients are given high enough doses of antithyroid drugs to make them hypothyroid (block) and are then given sufficient levothyroxine to restore them to the euthyroid state (replace). More recent studies have not confirmed higher remission rates in patients treated with antithyroid drugs plus levothyroxine, as compared to patients treated with antithyroid drugs alone. Nonetheless, it is sometimes easier to maintain euthyroidism using antithyroid drugs and levothyroxine together, rather than using antithyroid drugs alone.

Pregnancy and Antithyroid Drugs

Since pregnant women should not take radioactive iodine, treatment options for hyperthyroid Graves' patients who are pregnant are limited to:

- surgery in the second trimester when risk to the fetus is lowest
- observation
- antithyroid drugs

Most pregnant hyperthyroid patients want to avoid surgery, if possible. These are the factors that may influence which option is chosen:

- ◆ Hyperthyroid patients have an increased risk of miscarriage.
- ◆ Graves' hyperthyroidism tends to improve spontaneously during pregnancy.
- ◆ The fetal thyroid gland does not develop before the tenth or eleventh week of pregnancy.
- ◆ Antithyroid drugs cross the placenta and, in high doses, can cause fetal hypothyroidism and enlargement of the fetal thyroid gland.
- ◆ Pregnant hyperthyroid Graves' patients tend to require dosages of antithyroid drugs that are low enough not to cause problems in the fetus.

Each patient must be individually evaluated before a treatment option is recommended. In general, a pregnant patient with mild hyperthyroidism and few symptoms will be observed. Antithyroid drugs are more likely to be prescribed for a patient with many symptoms and marked elevation of thyroid hormones (see "Karen's Story" on pages 211–217). Physicians prefer PTU over Tapazole because PTU is thought to be less likely to cause a birth defect of the scalp called aplasia cutis. Although recent studies have been contradictory, PTU remains the antithyroid drug of choice for pregnant patients.

A hyperthyroid pregnant woman can usually be treated with lower dosages of antithyroid drugs than a nonpregnant woman can. Ordinarily, with these lower dosages, there are no adverse effects on the fetus, and the hyperthyroidism is controlled. The goal of treatment is to keep the mother's free T_4 in the high normal range to reduce the risk of fetal hypothyroidism. The mother's TSH level may remain low for several weeks or months after her free T_4 level returns to normal. In general, however, a low maternal TSH level is better for the fetus than a low maternal free T_4 level. Frequent monitoring of thyroid function test results is necessary to be sure that adequate control of the hyperthyroidism is achieved without excessive amounts of antithyroid drugs. Therefore, a physician may ask a pregnant patient taking antithyroid medication to return monthly.

Breastfeeding and Antithyroid Drugs

Antithyroid drugs pass into breast milk and can affect a breastfed baby's thyroid function. Previously, PTU had been the preferred antithyroid drug for hyperthyroid nursing mothers since it does not appear in breast milk in as high concentrations as Tapazole. However, more recent studies have demonstrated the safety of up to 20 mg (milligrams) per day of Tapazole in nursing mothers. A dosage of less than 200 mg of PTU per day in a nursing mother does not usually affect the baby's thyroid function. However, a breastfed baby should have thyroid function tests every three to four weeks for as long as its mother is taking either Tapazole or PTU.

Surgery for Graves' Disease

Treatment of hyperthyroid patients with surgery (thyroidectomy) has a long tradition in America. Beginning in the early part of the twentieth century, many of the most famous medical institutions in the United States, such as the Mayo, Cleveland, and Lahey Clinics, built their reputations on their success with thyroid surgery. When antithyroid drugs first became available in the 1950s, the number of thyroidectomies began to diminish. Once radioactive iodine was shown to be both safe and effective, the number of thyroidectomies dropped dramatically.

Radioactive iodine is now the treatment of choice for patients with Graves' hyperthyroidism in the United States, but thyroidectomy still has a place (see Chapter 10). Candidates for thyroid surgery include:

- pregnant patients in their second trimester
- patients who have thyroid nodules suspicious for cancer
- patients who have coexisting problems for which surgery in the neck is necessary
- patients with either severe Graves' eye disease or vision in only one eye who have not responded to antithyroid drugs and want to avoid possible worsening of their Graves' eye disease from radioactive iodine
- patients with very large goiters

Thyroidectomies during pregnancy are uncommon. When surgeons perform thyroidectomies on pregnant patients with Graves' disease, they prefer to do so during the second trimester for two reasons. First, the chances of surgery causing a miscarriage are slightly less during the second trimester than during the first trimester. Second, the chances of surgery causing premature labor are slightly less during the second trimester than during the third trimester.

Hypothyroidism commonly occurs after a thyroidectomy for

Graves' hyperthyroidism. The more thyroid tissue that is removed, the more likely patients are to develop hypothyroidism after surgery. Conversely, hyperthyroidism may recur after thyroid surgery, even though surgeons ordinarily remove 90 to 95% of the overactive thyroid gland. The remaining 5 to 10% of the gland may be stimulated by TSH receptor antibodies (TRAb) and grow again. If the stimulated thyroid remnant gets large enough, hyperthyroidism will recur (see "Lilian's Story" on pages 309–311). On the other hand, recurrence of hyperthyroidism after radioactive iodine treatment is uncommon.

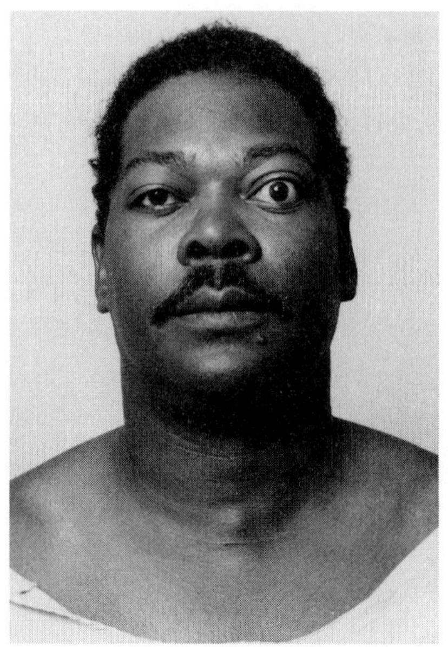

Figure 7.12. Patient with Graves' disease treated with both a thyroidectomy and radioactive iodine. Note the exophthalmos.

Prior to surgery, patients are treated with one or more of the following—beta-blockers, iodine, or antithyroid drugs. Without preoperative treatment, hyperthyroid patients could develop thyroid storm, a life-threatening thyroid crisis described at the end of this chapter.

Ordinarily, patients with thyroid disease are advised to avoid excess iodine. Therefore, it may seem paradoxical to give iodine to hyperthyroid patients prior to surgery. Although too much iodine can induce hyperthyroidism in susceptible individuals, a large amount of iodine, prescribed for no more than ten to fourteen days, blocks the release of thyroid hormone from the thyroid gland. For this reason, hyperthyroid patients undergoing surgery may be pretreated with iodine for seven to ten days.

Other Treatments for Hyperthyroid Patients

In unusual circumstances, drugs other than sedatives, beta-blockers, and antithyroid drugs are prescribed to treat patients with Graves' hyperthyroidism. These drugs include steroids, iodine, perchlorate, lithium, and iopanoic acid (an x-ray dye containing iodine). Calcium channel blockers may be used to control the heart rate in patients who cannot take beta-blockers. On rare occasions, excess thyroid hormone is removed by plasmapheresis (circulating blood through a machine).

Treatment of Patients with Graves' Eye Disease

The course of Graves' eye disease is unpredictable, variable, and often frustrating. Patients' frustration with their symptoms naturally leads to a desire to do something, anything, to relieve those symptoms. Watchful waiting, symptomatic treatment, steroids, and radiation, rather than definitive surgical treatment, are often the best options during the eighteen- to twenty-four-month period known as the active phase of Graves' eye disease.

A general rule in Grave's eye disease is that patients must be patient.

During the active phase, there is ongoing, fluctuating inflammation and swelling of many parts of the eye, especially the eyelids, the muscles that move the eye, and the fat behind the eyeball. For this reason, physicians are reluctant to operate on the eyes during the active phase, fearing that ongoing inflammation and swelling will cause the eyes to change again after surgery. Thus, most physicians advise patients to defer surgery for eighteen to twenty-four months until their eye disease goes into an inactive phase. Of course, if symptoms are severe, or if loss of vision is threatened, then all available treatments will be used at any time, even during the active phase.

When inflammation and swelling are relatively mild, symptoms are also relatively mild. When inflammation and swelling of the eye muscles and fat increase even a little, the eye condition may deteriorate rapidly. The reason for this rapid deterioration is that the eye, together with its fat and muscles, sits in a bony structure (orbit) that cannot expand. Therefore, if the eye becomes very inflamed, pressure builds up, and the eye has nowhere to go but out. If the inflammation and swelling create pressure on the optic nerve, vision may be threatened, and the pressure must be relieved.

Fortunately, most patients with Graves' hyperthyroidism have few, if any, eye symptoms, and, if they do have symptoms, they are usually mild. Nonetheless, ophthalmologists are ordinarily involved in the treatment of patients with Graves' eye disease. Since Graves' eye disease is unpredictable and can worsen rapidly, baseline measurements and an established relationship with an ophthalmologist are invaluable. Most thyroidologists and endocrinologists can recommend ophthalmologists experienced in the treatment of Graves' eye disease.

Patients requiring only symptomatic treatment during the active phase of Graves' eye disease may be advised to do one or more of the following:

- discontinue smoking
- avoid smoke-filled rooms
- use lubricating eye drops and ointments
- avoid decongestant eye drops
- cover eyes while sleeping
- wear wrap-around dark glasses outdoors during the day
- elevate the head of the bed to reduce overnight eye swelling
- wear prism glasses, or cover one eye with a patch, to relieve double vision
- use oral or topical nonsteroidal anti-inflammatory drugs
- turn ceiling fans off before going to bed
- avoid exposure to strong sunlight
- avoid or limit wearing contact lenses
- restrict salt intake
- take diuretics temporarily to relieve swelling around the eyes

When eye symptoms are severe, steroids, radiation therapy of the eye(s), or eye surgery may be advised, either individually or in combination (see "Debbie's Story" on pages 202–208). The choice of therapy and the timing of therapy require a great deal of thought on the part of the team caring for patients with Graves' eye disease. The list below summarizes medical and surgical treatment options for the small percentage of patients with severe Graves' eye disease:

- large doses of steroids to reduce inflammation
- radiation to the tissue behind the eye(s) to reduce inflammation
- surgical adjustment of eyelid placement, including lower eyelid implants
- plastic surgery for swelling around the eye(s)
- eye muscle surgery for realignment of the eye(s)
- orbital decompression
- orbital expansion
- orbital rim augmentation

Surgery can relieve certain signs and symptoms, such as lid retraction, swelling around the eyes, or double vision (diplopia). Ophthalmologists specializing in plastic surgery of the eye perform the surgery to relieve lid retraction and swelling around the eyes. Double

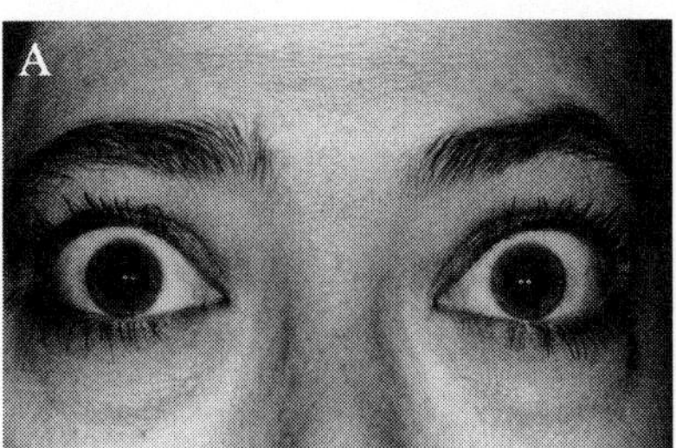

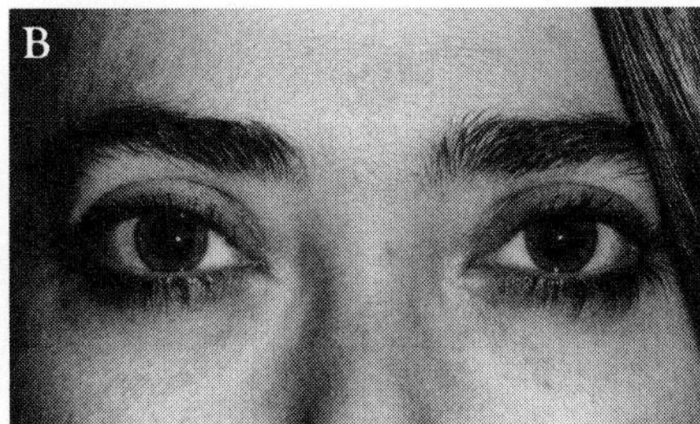

Photographs Courtesy of James R. Patrinely, M.D., Houston, Texas

Figure 7.13. Patient with eyelid retraction and mild exophthalmos. (A) Preoperative appearance. (B) Appearance following corrective eyelid surgery alone.

vision occurs when the muscles attached to the eye become stiff and do not work well together. If the six muscles attached to the eye do not move in unison, a patient will see double images. Ophthalmologists specializing in eye muscle diseases perform the operation(s) to relieve double vision.

Orbital decompression, orbital expansion, and orbital rim augmentation are three surgical procedures that may improve a patient's appearance, correct or protect a protruding eye, or relieve pressure on the optic nerve when the pressure threatens vision. During orbital decompression, an experienced ophthalmologist removes the inflamed and swollen tissue from the orbit to allow more space for the eye and surrounding tissue. In orbital expansion, the eye surgeon removes some of the bone around the orbit to provide more space. Finally, orbital rim augmentation may be necessary for some patients. In this procedure, the eye surgeon pulls the facial bones forward to make more room for the eye and its surrounding tissue. Unfortunately, each of these orbital operations may create or worsen double vision. When this occurs, additional surgery on the eye muscles may be necessary.

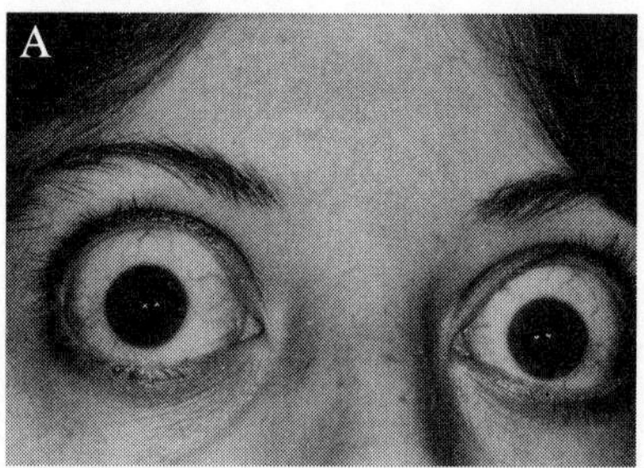

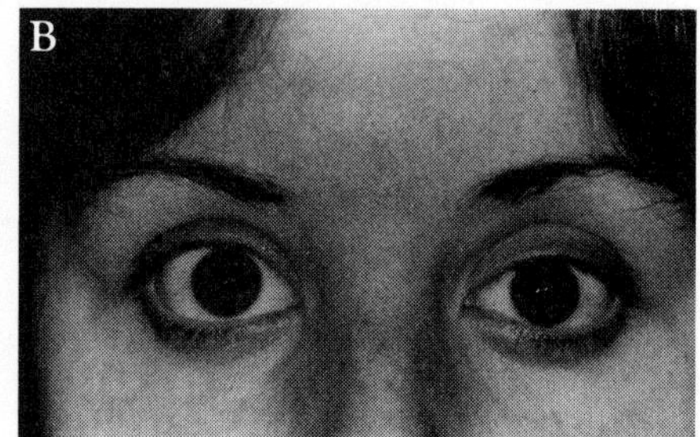

Photographs Courtesy of James R. Patrinely, M.D., Houston, Texas

Figure 7.14. Patient with marked exophthalmos. (A) Preoperative appearance. (B) Appearance following orbital decompression surgery performed on both sides.

It is understandable that many patients with significant Graves' eye disease are frustrated, anxious, and impatient. The psychological effects of Graves' eye disease may be profound. Some patients experience social withdrawal as a result of the changes in the appearance of their eyes. For example, one patient told her physician that she was unable to look people in the eye for years because of the "terrible stare in my eyes." Another patient recalled not dating for years because she was too embarrassed by her appearance; four months after reconstructive surgery, she became engaged.

In addition to experiencing social withdrawal, some patients cannot perform their jobs because their vision is too impaired. For example, a physical education teacher had to stop refereeing because he could not see what was happening during the games. In another case, a telephone repairman could not climb telephone poles because of his impaired vision. He also said that he "scared children into screaming." Fortunately, cosmetic surgery can improve the appearance of a patient's eyes, and corrective eye surgery and other treatments can improve vision.

Treatment of Hyperthyroid Patients with Graves' Dermatopathy

Graves' dermatopathy (skin disease) is both uncommon and difficult to treat. Steroids can be either injected or applied directly to the affected skin. The services of a dermatologist are invaluable in the treatment of Graves' dermatopathy.

Treatment of Patients with Toxic Autonomously Functioning Thyroid Nodules or Toxic Multinodular Goiters

When an autonomously functioning thyroid nodule produces sufficient thyroid hormone to cause hyperthyroidism, it is called a toxic autonomously functioning thyroid nodule (TAFTN). Sometimes, a patient with a large (greater than 3 centimeters) autonomously functioning thyroid nodule is treated in anticipation of the nodule becoming toxic. Occasionally, a toxic autonomously functioning thyroid nodule will spontaneously bleed and self-destruct, leaving the patient euthyroid and eliminating the need for any further treatment (see "Elaine's Story" on pages 287–288).

When a patient has more than one nodule, she has a multinodular goiter. If one or more of the nodules produces sufficient thyroid hormone to cause hyperthyroidism, the goiter is called a toxic multinodular goiter (TMNG).

The treatment of a patient with a toxic autonomously functioning thyroid nodule or a toxic multinodular goiter may involve one or more of the following:

- surgery
- radioactive iodine
- antithyroid drugs
- ethanol injections

Surgery

To reduce the risk of thyroid storm (see page 199), most patients will be treated before surgery with antithyroid drugs until they are euthyroid. Surgery for a toxic autonomously functioning thyroid nodule involves removal of the lobe containing the nodule while the remainder of the thyroid gland is left intact. When patients with toxic multinodular goiters are treated surgically, most of the thyroid gland is removed. Levothyroxine therapy is then started in patients with toxic multinodular goiters and in selected patients with toxic autonomously functioning thyroid nodules.

One advantage of surgery over radioactive iodine in the treatment of patients with either toxic autonomously functioning thyroid nodules or toxic multinodular goiters is that surgery reliably removes the nodules, whereas radioactive iodine usually only decreases the size of the nodules. Furthermore, patients whose toxic multinodular goiters are surgically removed are less likely to develop thyroid cancer than patients treated with radioactive iodine.

Radioactive Iodine

The dosage of radioactive iodine used to treat patients with toxic autonomously functioning thyroid nodules or toxic multinodular goiters is usually higher than that used to treat patients with Graves' disease.

(Treatment with radioactive iodine is described on pages 176–181.) Unlike the thyroid glands of patients affected by Graves' disease, the thyroid glands of patients with toxic autonomously functioning thyroid nodules or toxic multinodular goiters contain some tissue that is not hyperfunctioning. Indeed, this thyroid tissue is suppressed and will not take up any radioactive iodine. Nonetheless, the suppressed tissue is exposed to radiation because of its proximity to the toxic nodule or nodules that are avidly taking up radioactive iodine, and it may be destroyed along with the toxic nodule or nodules. Therefore, some patients treated with radioactive iodine will become permanently hypothyroid and require levothyroxine therapy, while others will not (see "Erendira's Story" on pages 289–292).

Pregnant or breastfeeding women should not take radioactive iodine.

Some patients with toxic autonomously functioning thyroid nodules or toxic multinodular goiters who are treated with radioactive iodine may become temporarily hypothyroid. In approximately 50% of patients, the previously suppressed thyroid tissue will recover its function. The recovery process may take eight weeks or more.

Antithyroid Drugs

Patients with toxic autonomously functioning thyroid nodules or toxic multinodular goiters are usually treated with either surgery or radioactive iodine. However, some patients are not good candidates for either of these treatments. In these situations, selected patients will be treated indefinitely with antithyroid drugs instead. (For a detailed discussion of antithyroid drugs, see pages 181–184.)

Patients with toxic autonomously functioning thyroid nodules or toxic multinodular goiters are treated with antithyroid drugs indefinitely. Unlike patients with Graves' disease, they cannot go into remission. In patients treated indefinitely with antithyroid drugs, levothyroxine may also be prescribed a few weeks or months after starting the antithyroid drugs (see the discussion of the block-replace method on pages 182–183).

Ethanol Injections

Although seldom used in the United States, ethanol (alcohol) injections may be given to some patients with toxic autonomously functioning thyroid nodules. Depending upon the size of the toxic nodule, three to six injections of ethanol are given directly into the nodule either weekly or twice a week for several weeks with the expectation that the nodule will be destroyed. Side effects are usually minor and may include mild burning during the injection, fever, or a temporary change in voice. Ethanol injections are used more often in Europe where toxic autonomously functioning thyroid nodules are a more common cause of hyperthyroidism.

Pregnancy

Since toxic autonomously functioning thyroid nodules and toxic multinodular goiters tend to occur in an older age group, they are relatively uncommon during pregnancy. When they do cause hyperthyroidism during pregnancy, the hyperthyroidism tends to be mild. Nonetheless, an occasional patient will require treatment during pregnancy.

Just as in pregnant patients with Graves' hyperthyroidism, the treatment options for pregnant patients with toxic autonomously functioning thyroid nodules or toxic multinodular goiters are limited to antithyroid drugs or to surgery. Usually, surgery is performed during the second trimester to reduce the possibility of a miscarriage during the first trimester or of premature labor during the third trimester. It is unknown if ethanol injections are safe for pregnant patients who have toxic autonomously functioning thyroid nodules.

Treatment of Patients with Subclinical Hyperthyroidism

The treatment of patients with subclinical hyperthyroidism is controversial. While most patients with subclinical hyperthyroidism do not progress to overt hyperthyroidism, some patients are at greater risk of complications than other patients are. Therefore, the treatment of patients with subclinical hyperthyroidism must be individualized. For example, physicians may be more likely to treat older women with osteoporosis and heart disease than younger, otherwise healthy women.

In fact, as previously mentioned, one study suggested that subclinically hyperthyroid patients over sixty years of age have an increased mortality rate during the ten years following the initial finding of a low TSH level. The primary cause of the increased number of deaths was heart disease. Nonetheless, there is no evidence yet that treatment of patients with subclinical hyperthyroidism prevents the increased mortality.

Once the decision to treat is made, subclinically hyperthyroid patients are generally treated in the same ways as overtly hyperthyroid patients. Subclinically hyperthyroid patients with Graves' disease, however, are more likely to be treated with antithyroid drugs than with either radioactive iodine or surgery. There are two reasons for this prudent approach. First, many patients with subclinical hyperthyroidism have small goiters, making remission more likely. Second, physicians are reluctant to destroy a thyroid gland that may be causing no symptoms when other treatments are available. Further research should clarify the natural history of subclinical hyperthyroidism and the identification of patients who need treatment.

Treatment of Patients with Hyperthyroidism from Unusual Causes

As mentioned earlier in this chapter, there are uncommon causes of hyperthyroidism, such as a pituitary tumor, struma ovarii, hydatidiform mole, choriocarcinoma, hyperemesis gravidarum, and factitious hyperthyroidism. Patients who have hyperthyroidism from these unusual causes are treated by unusual methods, and it is not practical to describe these treatments in detail in this book.

Children with Hyperthyroidism

Although hyperthyroidism is uncommon before puberty, it does occur, especially if there is a family history of thyroid disease. A child's doctor needs to know if either the mother or father has a hereditary autoimmune disease, such as Graves' disease or Hashimoto's thyroiditis. The doctor will then pay particular attention to the child's thyroid examination.

The two most common causes of childhood hyperthyroidism are neonatal hyperthyroidism and Graves' disease. Approximately one out of 100 babies born to mothers with Graves' disease develops transient neonatal hyperthyroidism. This hyperthyroidism is the result of thyroid-stimulating antibodies (TSAb or TSI) crossing the placenta and stimulating a newborn's thyroid gland (see "Karen's Story" on pages 211–217). Neonatal hyperthyroidism is temporary and lasts until the baby metabolizes, or uses up, its mother's TSAb or TSI.

The signs and symptoms of hyperthyroidism in children are similar to those seen in adults with hyperthyroidism. However, the first sign that children are hyperthyroid may be a decline in their grades. The treatment options for hyperthyroid children are also the same as those for adults.

Signs & Symptoms of Childhood Hyperthyroidism

- poor grades
- mood swings
- emotional outbursts
- hyperactivity
- inability to concentrate
- goiter
- rapid heart rate
- palpitations
- nervousness
- difficulty sleeping
- fatigue
- high blood pressure
- protruding eyes
- tremor
- increased appetite with a decrease in weight
- increased sweating
- feeling hot

Treating hyperthyroid children with antithyroid drugs before puberty is more complicated than treating hyperthyroid teens and adults for two reasons. First, children's growth and development are affected by their thyroid function and, therefore, must be closely monitored. Second, the normal ranges for TSH and free T_4 vary from age to age prior to adulthood; therefore, thyroid function tests must be done frequently. For these reasons, pediatric endocrinologists are usually consulted in the management of hyperthyroid children.

In the past, physicians were reluctant to use radioactive iodine to treat hyperthyroid children with Graves' disease; antithyroid drugs were the treatment of choice. However, this reluctance is giving way since several studies have demonstrated the long-term safety of radioactive iodine in children. In particular, there is no evidence of an increased risk of cancer or reduced fertility in adults who were treated with radioactive iodine when they were children. There is also no evidence of an increased risk of birth defects in the offspring of adults who were treated with radioactive iodine when they were children. There is, however, a small increased risk for the development of benign thyroid tumors following treatment with radioactive iodine in childhood.

Since hyperthyroidism is uncommon in children, and since the symptoms of hyperthyroidism can be confused with those of other disorders, it may be overlooked (see "James' Story" on pages 224–228). Once the correct diagnosis is made, the treatment of children with hyperthyroidism is very effective.

Heart Disease and Hyperthyroidism

Hyperthyroidism can complicate pre-existing heart disease and can cause heart problems in patients without known heart disease. Patients with stable heart disease who develop hyperthyroidism may experience angina pectoris (chest pain), atrial fibrillation (a serious heart rhythm disturbance), or congestive heart failure (failure of the heart to pump blood effectively, resulting in the accumulation of fluid in the lungs and legs).

Patients without a history of heart disease may also develop atrial fibrillation, just as former President George H. W. Bush did. Atrial fibrillation is a particularly worrisome complication since it predisposes hyperthyroid patients to strokes and blood clots. For these reasons, blood thinners, such as Coumadin, are prescribed at the same time as the hyperthyroidism and atrial fibrillation are treated.

Patients with known heart disease and untreated hyperthyroidism have an increased risk of worsening heart disease and thyroid storm during and after thyroid surgery and, possibly, after treatment with radioactive iodine. Therefore, prior to thyroid surgery, hyperthyroid heart patients take antithyroid drugs until they are euthyroid. Also, antithyroid drugs are sometimes prescribed prior to treatment of hyperthyroid heart patients with radioactive iodine. Some patients, depending on their age, the nature of their heart disease, and other individual factors, may elect to continue antithyroid drugs indefinitely rather than have either surgery or radioactive iodine. The treatment of patients must be individualized according to their particular situation.

Interestingly, amiodarone, an iodine-rich drug used to treat atrial fibrillation and other dangerous arrhythmias, can actually cause hyperthyroidism and further compromise heart function. In some patients with heart disease, amiodarone is the best, or the only, drug to control heart rhythm disturbances. Therefore, some patients cannot stop taking amiodarone, even if it makes them hyperthyroid.

Amiodarone-induced thyrotoxicosis (AIT), or amiodarone-induced hyperthyroidism, occurs in approximately 5% of patients taking amiodarone. Two types of amiodarone-induced thyrotoxicosis are recognized. Type I amiodarone-induced thyrotoxicosis occurs most often in patients with multinodular goiters; it is characterized by increased thyroid hormone production and secretion. Type II amiodarone-induced thyrotoxicosis often occurs in people with normal thyroid glands. It is characterized by a high interleukin-6 level and increased release of thyroid hormone from a disrupted, and sometimes tender, thyroid gland. Nonetheless, in practice, it is often difficult to distinguish between the two types.

Treatment of patients with amiodarone-induced thyrotoxicosis may be difficult for three reasons. First, as previously stated, many patients cannot discontinue taking amiodarone. Second, even when amiodarone is discontinued, residual iodine remains in the body for six months or more and continues to affect thyroid function. Finally, since the radioactive iodine uptake is often low in patients with amiodarone-induced thyrotoxicosis, treatment of Type I patients with radioactive iodine is not always possible.

Patients with Type I amiodarone-induced thyrotoxicosis are usually given antithyroid drugs, although they may also need uncommonly prescribed drugs such as perchlorate. Steroids in large doses are often helpful in patients with Type II amiodarone-induced thyrotoxicosis. Since it may be difficult to distinguish Type I from Type II amiodarone-induced thyrotoxicosis, hyperthyroid patients taking amiodarone may be given both antithyroid drugs and steroids. Finally, some physicians will recommend a thyroidectomy for some patients with amiodarone-induced thyrotoxicosis. For example, patients who cannot stop taking amiodarone and patients who are experiencing side effects from the medications used to treat their hyperthyroidism could be candidates for thyroidectomies (see "Jim's Story" on pages 88–90).

Nonthyroidal Surgery in Hyperthyroid Patients

Hyperthyroid patients who have been successfully treated and have normal thyroid function generally do well when they have nonthyroidal surgery. However, patients who are still hyperthyroid require special consideration before they undergo any surgery because they are at risk of developing thyroid storm. Therefore, hyperthyroid patients should postpone elective surgery until they are euthyroid. If hyperthyroid patients require emergency surgery, they may be given medications such as antithyroid drugs, iodine, iopanoic acid, beta-blockers, steroids, or a combination of two or more of these drugs.

Thyroid Storm

Thyroid storm is a severe and life-threatening form of hyperthyroidism; the mortality rate may be as high as 40%. Causes of thyroid storm include surgery, infection, or severe medical illness in hyperthyroid patients. Patients with thyroid storm may experience fever, nausea, vomiting, diarrhea, dehydration, altered mental status, and pulse rates of 150 or more beats per minute. This uncommon complication requires immediate treatment in the Intensive Care Unit, as well as larger and more frequent doses of the same drugs that are used to treat hyperthyroidism.

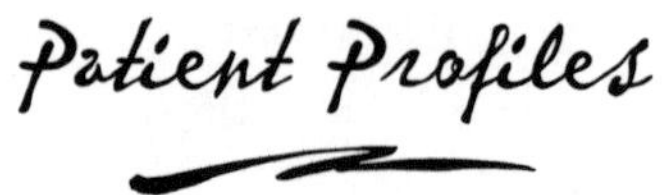

PATRICK'S STORY

"Patrick" is a sixty-year-old husband, father, physician, college professor, and author. He recounts his experiences—common and uncommon—when he had Graves' hyperthyroidism:

> I began experiencing symptoms in 1976. The first thing I noticed was the color of the signs on the freeway; they were more vivid than usual. The green and white were shimmering, but I liked it! Then I noticed a tremor in my hands when I was operating. A nurse asked me if I was nervous. I just thought I needed a vacation.
>
> I also noticed that my interest in women increased enormously. Every woman was so beautiful in every way. Any woman who came within my orbit was of interest. I started chasing anything with a skirt on and vice versa. I had sex with three different women a day for a year. I learned a lot about women during this time. I could read the signs if they were willing.
>
> I started losing weight—twenty-six pounds in eight months—despite a voracious appetite. For dinner, I would eat two steaks, four packages of frozen vegetables, and then clean up everybody's plate. My wife called me the human garbage disposal.
>
> After dinner when we went to bed, my sexual appetite was as voracious. Then my wife told me that she couldn't keep up with me any more. She said I could have other women as long as I was discreet.
>
> I was also losing muscle strength. I would measure my grip strength with a gripometer. My grip went from

146 to 86 pounds, so the decline was 60 pounds or 41%. I also had trouble climbing stairs and getting off the toilet. I was short of breath when I exercised, which was unusual; I used to referee.

I was always warm. All the ladies said, "You feel so warm." My wife said it was like sleeping next to a human furnace. I radiated heat.

I diagnosed myself as having ALS, Lou Gehrig's disease. I had all the same signs and symptoms. I thought I was just going to go out. I didn't believe in doctors!

One day in the faculty lunchroom, the head of endocrinology said, "Your eyes are too prominent." I even moved faster, and he commented that I was too revved up. Later, when he examined me, he said that I was hyperthyroid. My wife said, "No. It's just that you're too sexual."

We had to decide how to treat the hyperthyroidism. [My endocrinologist] presented my case at Grand Rounds. Everyone voted for radioactive iodine treatment. But my endocrinologist said I had a small thyroid gland, and he thought I would go into remission with antithyroid drugs.

Three months after I started taking antithyroid drugs, my strength came back, but the lights and colors were not as vibrant, and my orgasms were less intense. But I knew I had to take my medication.

I developed a rash—diffuse hives—and stopped taking methimazole [Tapazole]. I switched to PTU and took it for another three months. I was checked every week for a while and then every three months, six months, and now once a year. My thyroid levels have been normal since that time, and I don't need to take levothyroxine. The first doctor was right; I didn't need radioactive iodine.

> While I was hyperthyroid, I wrote eleven papers [for medical journals], but they were all rejected because the editors said they were too flamboyant. I revised them after I became euthyroid, and every one of them was accepted.
>
> Graves' disease is such an individual thing for each person. For me, there were pros and cons to having it, and some of it was fun. If it weren't for the muscle weakness, I would have preferred to be hyperthyroid. I'm not exactly proud of all the sex I had; it was an isolated incident.
>
> My thyroid gland still hasn't burned out and probably won't now. The unique aspect of my case is that I became euthyroid, not hypothyroid.

Although hypersexuality is an extremely uncommon complication, "Patrick's" story highlights the dramatic and personal changes that may occur in the life of someone who develops hyperthyroidism. While some patients might be uncomfortable talking to their doctors about their private lives, sharing this information is very helpful in both the diagnosis and treatment of thyroid disorders.■

DEBBIE'S STORY

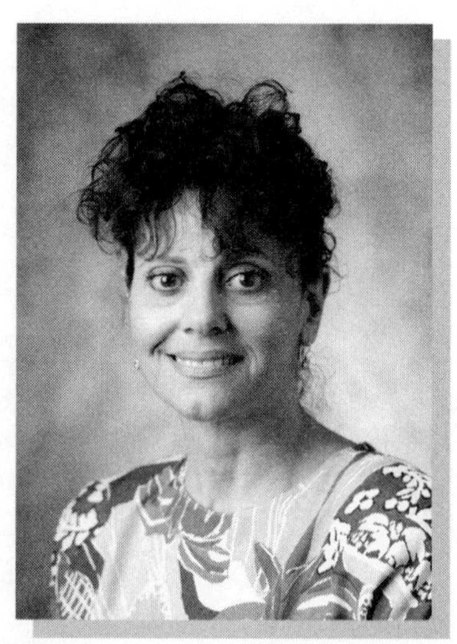

Forty-six-year-old Debbie remembers 1997 vividly. It was the year of El Niño—the year in which she bought a house, started working on her master's degree in business administration, and developed Graves' disease.

> In June of 1996, I had LASIK surgery done because I'm nearsighted. Everything seemed fine. About six months later, I noticed I was having night

sweats. I'd be watching television, and my heart would start racing. My hair was brittle, and I noticed I was more jittery, more on edge. But I've always been a hyper person. I was eating constantly—I'm talking mass quantities. I thought okay, I'm having night sweats because maybe I'm going through menopause; I'm anxious because of the stress at work; my hair is brittle because of the perm I had. I had excuses for everything.

I went to a [business] conference. I'm not much of a drinker, but when you're entertaining customers, you have to. I had one or two margaritas, and then we all went to a club. I had three Kamikazes! I went back to my room to go to sleep, and woke up at 6:00 A.M. for a golf outing. My eyes wouldn't open; they were swollen shut. I felt really funny, kind of dizzy. I got out of bed and dropped to my knees. I thought, "Is this what a hangover is like?"

I soaked a washcloth with cold water and put it over my eyes. Finally, I could open one eye. I was seeing double; my eyes were really swollen and tearing. I just laid down on the bed with my head elevated and kept the washcloth on my eyes for about thirty minutes. Finally, the double vision went away, so I rested until the afternoon activities. That night I didn't drink anything, but the next morning, the same thing happened for about an hour. It happened all week.

When I got back from the conference, I went to the surgeon who did my LASIK surgery to see if that might be the cause. He said it wasn't. He said it was because I had been drinking and was tired and gave me some antibiotic drops. I used them for a week, but the same thing happened every morning. My eyes were swollen, and I had double vision.

The following week, my eyes were red, dry, and tearing, so I made an appointment with an ophthalmologist.

She was mystified and said it was probably El Niño. Supposedly, the weather from El Niño created conditions that aggravated allergies. She thought it was an allergy causing my eyes to swell and gave me allergy drops.

So I take the allergy drops, but my eyes don't get better. It takes me two hours to get ready for work every morning. It's been three weeks, so I say, "Okay, I'll go to an allergist." He pokes me with every imaginable substance, and says I'm not allergic to anything, but he gave me Allegra. He also used the El Niño excuse.

By Easter, it feels like someone is putting burning coals in my eyes. My sister is an ob-gyn nurse, and she said, "You might want to check your thyroid." I said, "What's a thyroid and where is it?"

So the next week I went to my primary care physician and told her about my eyes. She couldn't explain what it was. I asked her how to test the thyroid, and she said, "You don't have any symptoms." So I said, "Just humor me; do the test." I had to talk her into it!

She called the next day and said, "I've made an appointment for you with an endocrinologist." I said, "What's that?" So I went to see him, and he takes one look at me and says, "It's Graves' disease." My TSH was low, and my thyroid hormone levels were off the charts. I'm thinking, what are they talking about? I don't know all these terms. He explained that it was an autoimmune response. He measured my eyes and said, "Your eyes are not closing at night." That's why they were drying out. I asked him what this had to do with my thyroid, and he explained that [Graves' eye disease] runs a parallel course [with Graves' hyperthyroidism].

After Debbie's physician explained the treatment options for Graves' hyperthyroidism, she chose antithyroid drugs. Unfortunately, she was one of the 6% of patients who develop an allergic reaction to antithyroid drugs.

> It was Memorial Day weekend; I had been to a party on a farm. I thought I had poison ivy. Then I thought it was the strawberries I had been eating a lot. I called the doctor, and he said to stop the medicine, but I said, "No, I think it's the strawberries." He said no, it was serious and I had to stop the medicine. It lasted a week. My joints hurt. It was the only time I took off from work even though I had had double vision for eight months.
>
> So I took the atomic cocktail [radioactive iodine] the first week in June and glowed in the dark for a week. Just kidding! It was just like drinking water. You're in an iron-clad room; they leave, and you drink it. I had to wait about half an hour to be sure I didn't get sick, and then I left.

Debbie's symptoms of hyperthyroidism began to disappear, but her eyes still bothered her.

> Because of the double vision, I would lean my head to drive. I was a danger to society on the road! The doctor explained that my eye muscles could not control my eye—it was like my eyeball was in Jell-O, just floating around.
>
> My vision would change every day. I was in school and couldn't take notes. I bought over-the-counter reading glasses, and an eye doctor who specialized in treating double vision placed a film in one lens to trick the other eye and clear up the double vision. I had to take my glasses off to look at the board and put them back on to read.

Meanwhile, a friend brought Debbie some literature about Graves' eye disease. That led her to the Internet, where she read about various treatment options she had been unaware of, including radiation treatments of the eyes. After a consultation with an ophthalmologist experienced in the treatment of patients with Graves' eye disease, Debbie began two weeks of daily radiation treatments.

> I went to three ophthalmologists before I found someone who could help me. It mystified me that there were these professionals you're paying who don't do anything or explain what your options are. It was very frustrating and discouraging. I'd been so healthy all my life. If I didn't have faith, family, and a support system, I would have never made it.
>
> By December, the double vision went away. I had also been on cortisone for three months and had chipmunk cheeks; it was hideous!

Debbie worked in the marketing division of her company. However, when her inflamed eyes changed her appearance, she believed that she had to make certain adjustments.

> I couldn't look my customers in the eye. I had been in marketing but asked to be taken out of sales. I didn't want to subject my customers to [my swollen, bulging eyes]. My employers didn't suggest it; I just felt that it was what I should do.

Although Debbie no longer suffered from double vision, she continued to have difficulties with her irritated, protruding eyes.

> In March, through the office grapevine, I heard about another woman who was seeing [an ophthalmologist specializing in plastic and reconstructive eye surgery.] I called her, and she told me about the doctor and the surgery. In December of 1999—that's how I brought in the millennium—I had orbital decompression. I was

out of work for six weeks. They did one eye the first day and the other one the next day. I stayed in the hospital overnight. It really wasn't very painful.

In March, I had eyelid surgery because my lids would freeze open. They wake you up at the end of surgery and tell you to open and close. Then snip, snip—you hear the scissors clipping and feel pressure, but no pain. It's a little weird, a little bizarre. I was out of work for one week with that surgery, but I orchestrated it around my school break.

In August, I did the under-eye thing [surgery to remove fat from lower lids]. You could say he rearranged the fat under my eyes.

My eyes still don't close at night. I sleep with a mask or headband. I've put goop in my eyes, and I've taped my eyes shut with Band-Aids, but my eyebrows and eyelashes got ripped out. I've put little sandbags, little bean bags on my eyes to keep them closed. I've put a cottonball or cosmetic patch and taped over it, top and bottom. Now I've learned to position the headband at night.

That's the miracle of being a human—you learn to cope. You just do it. After the surgeries, people came up to me and said, "You never complained." They said that they would look to me for strength because of how I had dealt with all of this. I didn't know. You don't know people are watching you. You don't know the impact you're having on people.

I would say when you notice symptoms, don't write them off. Don't make excuses. Check into it. I didn't recognize the symptoms, so I didn't think anything was wrong. It's easy to write off symptoms to other things. I think everybody should have a thyroid test regularly once a year.

> I have a twenty-three-year-old son, and I'm concerned about him. My mother, both sisters, and an aunt on my father's side had [hypothyroidism]. Nobody in the family had too much thyroid.

Debbie is one of the small percentage of patients with Graves' disease who develop severe eye disease. Furthermore, her Graves' hyperthyroidism and Graves' eye disease have run independent courses. Throughout her frustrating illness, Debbie has been patient and has taken one day at a time.■

KYM'S STORY

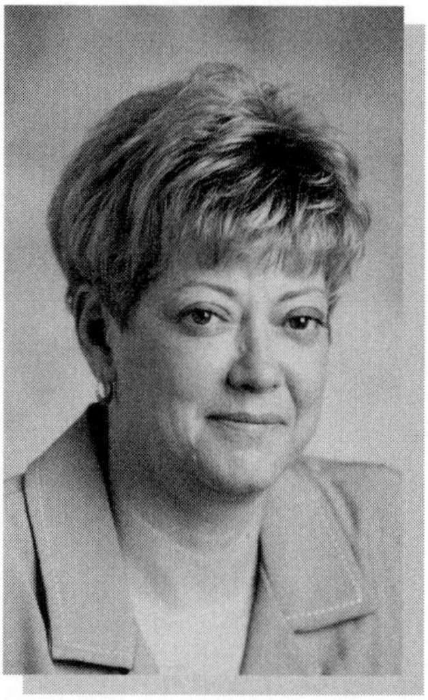

Kym believes that her thyroid problems began when she had her first child sixteen years ago; however, she did not do anything about it at the time.

> I think it probably started the summer after I had my son, but who's going to complain about losing weight?
>
> About five or six years ago, I started feeling worse. I was tired constantly, my eyes were red, my feet were swelling, and I gained thirty pounds in six months. The doctors kept giving me water pills and told me to exercise more. One internist put me on fen-phen, but my heart raced and my body felt really weird, so I stopped taking it after a month.
>
> He also put me on a low dose of [levothyroxine]. After six or seven months, I was still not better, so I went to see [an endocrinologist]. He bumped up the thyroid medicine and checked me every three months.

> I read the pamphlets [about hyperthyroidism and hypothyroidism] and felt like I had symptoms of both. Finally, [my endocrinologist] told me that I had Graves' disease. It had started as hyperthyroidism, then my thyroid burned out, and I became hypothyroid.

Unfortunately, Kym also had Graves' eye disease and Graves' dermatopathy. Frustrated with the progression of her disease, Kym sought the advice of another endocrinologist. He recommended that she consult an ophthalmologist and a dermatologist.

> My eyes had started to protrude and burn. They still feel tired all the time. I hate air blowing or fans. I would prefer to work in the dark! I used drops for a few months and wore a mask at night, but I thought it was too obnoxious. [My new endocrinologist] referred me to [an ophthalmologist specializing in plastic and reconstructive eye surgery]. He did my upper and lower eyelids, but it probably won't stop there. I might need to have decompression surgery.
>
> I had the surgery as an outpatient. There wasn't a lot of pain; it was just inconvenient. My kids freaked out when they saw me, but, after the surgery, I got quite a bit of relief. I couldn't get up too fast and had to have someone guide me at first. I also had to watch how much weight I picked up and how fast I moved.

Kym became equally frustrated with her Graves' dermatopathy. In particular, she had problems with extensive myxedema and acropachy, both of which are difficult to treat.

> My feet were swelling more. The lumps were getting harder and harder. It seems to bother other people, so I wear pants all the time. The left leg is worse than the right. It makes it awfully hard to shave my legs. The skin texture is different—like an orange peel on my feet.

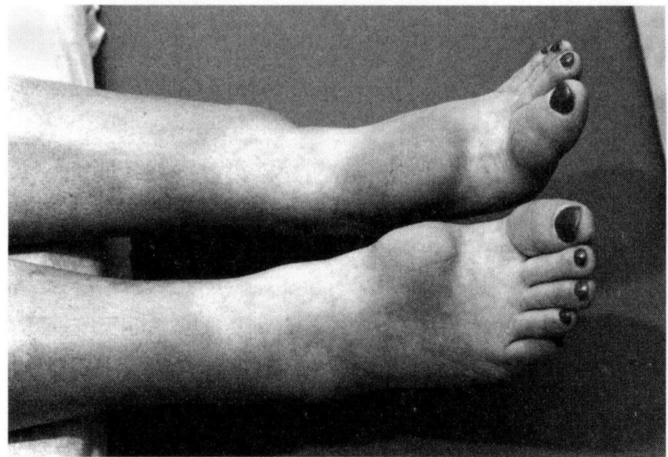

Kym's extensive myxedema

I also noticed changes in my hands. Both hands are affected equally. My ring size went from a 5 1/2 to an 8. I notice the thicker fingertips, but other people notice the curved nails more.

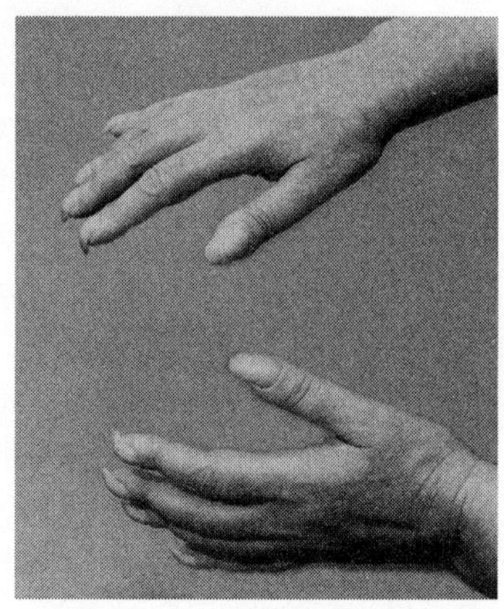

Kym's hands. Note the enlargement of her fingertips and the curve of her fingernails.

[My endocrinologist] sent me to a dermatologist who treated me with lots of creams with steroids, but it didn't help. I didn't want the [skin] biopsy he suggested. There's no pain in my hands or feet; I just don't have as much dexterity. We also tried wrapping my feet with Saran Wrap [and steroid cream], and that helped some at the time. I can't understand why they can't scrape it off, but they can't operate.

I tried an experimental drug [Octreotide] that [my endocrinologist] had read about. I had injections three times a day. My husband and daughter and a friend learned how to give me them to me in my leg and back of my arm. I just couldn't do it! But there was

> not one ounce of change—nothing. The doctors think that it's as bad as it'll get; I probably won't get any worse.
>
> My mother had Graves' disease, and my sister developed it after I was diagnosed, but they never talked about it. I asked [my endocrinologist] to look at my sixteen-year-old daughter to make sure she didn't have it. I was worried because she went from a size 9/10 to a size 5 without trying to lose weight.
>
> Sometimes I wonder if I let this get too far along before I got help. Could I have avoided or prevented some of this? My advice to others is don't just chalk up your symptoms like they're just something that happens.

Unfortunately, Kym experienced many of the most troubling aspects of Graves' disease. Her eye disease and skin disease were more difficult to treat, and caused more frustration, than her hyperthyroidism. Nonetheless, she remains optimistic and hopeful that additional research will lead to new and better treatments of Graves' eye disease and dermatopathy.■

KAREN'S STORY

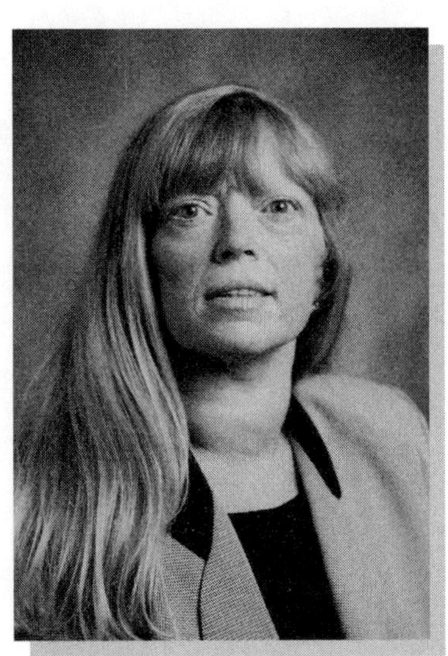

Forty-five-year-old Karen, a preschool teacher, discovered that she had Graves' disease in 1999.

> I didn't know what the thyroid was and how much in charge of our daily existence it was.
>
> I had been having trouble with sore throats and bronchitis. Something told me to go see my doctor about it. It had been ten months since my last

> appointment, and he immediately noticed my eyes. They've always been big, but they hadn't been sticking out so much. I also had a tremor in my right hand, and he found a goiter. Two days after I saw him, the test results came back, and he said I needed an endocrinologist.
>
> Looking back on it, I realized I had lost a lot of weight, but I was pleased about that. As far as diarrhea, I've always had colon and rectal problems, so I didn't think anything was unusual. And I was very emotional. It was all I could do to keep from crying. I was very nervous and had trouble sleeping. My heart was racing so much I felt like I could hear my heart beat.

Karen went to an endocrinologist who prescribed Tapazole and beta-blockers and asked her to return to his office every month. He increased her initial dosage of Tapazole when laboratory results showed no improvement in her thyroid hormone levels. He also suggested that she consult an ophthalmologist, who confirmed that she had Graves' eye disease.

> My vision is blurred. I have double vision and tearing. And it's painful; it feels as though someone is pressing down on my eyeballs. I have no peripheral vision, and it hurts to look up. [My ophthalmologist] plugged my tear ducts, but the plugs came out, and I'm still having eye problems.
>
> I was surprised when I found out I was pregnant even though my hyperthyroidism was still not under control. I have a thirteen-year-old daughter and had had a miscarriage in 1997. And then there was my age, but I really wanted this baby. It worried me that I might have another miscarriage.

Karen's case was unusual in several ways. First, hyperthyroid women sometimes have difficulty getting pregnant; however, Karen discovered she was pregnant while she was hyperthyroid. Second, for unknown reasons, pregnancy tends to lessen the symptoms of Graves' disease; however, Karen's thyroid hormone levels went up, and her symptoms became worse.

> I called my endocrinologist right away, and he called in a prescription of PTU for me. My obstetrician saw me right away because of my age and the Graves' disease. She wondered if I wanted to continue the pregnancy, but I did not want to terminate.
>
> I started reading all I could about thyroid disease. I began to wonder about my treatment and how all this was affecting my baby, especially when I read that pregnant women usually need about 200 mg of PTU. I was on much more. I decided to get a second opinion.

Karen visited another endocrinologist for a second opinion when she was twenty-seven weeks pregnant. She was taking 800 mg of PTU a day and, remarkably, was still hyperthyroid. Her endocrinologist referred her to an obstetrician specializing in high-risk pregnancies. An ultrasound revealed that the baby had a very large goiter. The baby's goiter was so large that it was preventing the baby from swallowing normally. Therefore, Karen's endocrinologist and obstetrician decided to inject thyroid hormone directly into the baby's muscle to reduce the size of the baby's goiter.

Ordinarily, thyroid hormone would be injected into the amniotic fluid, which the baby would then swallow, absorbing the injected thyroid hormone. However, since the baby's large goiter made swallowing difficult, levothyroxine was injected into its thigh. Within a few days of this intrauterine procedure, there was a 50% reduction in the size of the baby's goiter. Three weeks later, a second intrauterine injection of thyroid hormone was performed. This time, the obstetrician injected the levothyroxine into the amniotic fluid since the goiter was smaller and the baby was swallowing better.

> I panicked when they told me about the baby's goiter.

> But I believe in the power of prayer and that doctors are God's tools. I was relieved that now I had an obstetrician and an endocrinologist who were working together.
>
> Before, I felt that it was only me getting treated. Now both of us were being treated. I got hopeful knowing I was in better hands. Before this, I would sometimes have difficulty breathing when I was nervous. It was like I had hands around my neck. With the new information and the new doctors, it was like they removed those hands.

By the time Karen was thirty-four weeks pregnant, tests indicated that the baby's lungs were sufficiently developed for delivery. Since Karen's thyroid hormone levels remained elevated and since the baby's goiter continued to grow, her doctors decided to proceed with a Cesarean section.

A pediatric endocrinologist checked baby Savannah immediately after the delivery; her goiter was readily apparent. Savannah weighed 6 pounds 2 ounces even though she was six weeks early. Her doctor prescribed a combination of levothyroxine and PTU. She spent several days in the neonatal intensive care unit before being transferred to the premature nursery.

> About a week after Savannah was born, she had a thyroid storm and had to go back into [the neonatal intensive care unit]. Her temperature went up and her heart rate increased. I wasn't there; I was at home when it happened. It was so frustrating. I would go to the nursery every day, but I would try to be back home by the time my other daughter came home from school.

Savannah responded to treatment and continued to improve. When she was discharged from the hospital, her mother gave her PTU and levothyroxine until her thyroid hormone levels were normal.

> The PTU costs about $10 for a week's supply. It had

> to be refrigerated and was only good for seven days. Savannah was so good; she'd suck it right out of the syringe. I crushed up the levothyroxine, and she took it the same way. By the first of December, she was off all medication. Her goiter has completely disappeared. She really is doing so well.

On the other hand, Karen's thyroid hormones remained elevated after delivery, and she continued to suffer with symptoms of Graves' eye disease. She arranged to have radioactive iodine treatment before her baby came home from the hospital.

> After the baby's birth, my goiter got smaller, and my eyes didn't seem to protrude as much. I might have looked better physically, but I still had problems. My legs were so weak that I couldn't get up off the floor without help. I had to cover one eye just to walk down the hall in the morning. I still have to do that to see well. I can't drive and have to rely on my family and friends to drive me wherever I need to go.
>
> I knew before I had Savannah that I was going to have radioactive iodine, so I didn't breastfeed. I just wanted to get better as fast as I could. Just before I was scheduled for treatment, I woke up early one morning with a horrible headache. It was not like a normal headache; it was very intense. I had a temperature and my pulse was racing. My obstetrician said that I should go to the emergency room.
>
> My family took me to the emergency room by 7:00 A.M., and the doctor there wanted me to take iodine for a [CAT scan]. I remember asking him, "Sir, are you sure?" Somewhere in the back of my mind I thought I had read that I wasn't supposed to be taking anything with iodine. But he said he could get a clearer picture this way. The ER doctor authorized the iodine before he talked with my endocrinologist.

> It felt like I was burning up on the inside. I just couldn't stand it inside that [CAT scan] machine, so he stopped, injected me with something to calm me down, and put me back. I breathed through my nose as much as I could, but it was a horrible feeling; plus I was not at the height of my calmness. My thyroid was going ninety to nothing!
>
> I spent the day in the emergency room and went home around 5:00 that afternoon. I didn't get to see Savannah that day.

Because Karen was given iodinated dye for the CAT scan, her treatment with radioactive iodine had to be delayed.

> I finally had the treatment on December 14 [three and a half months after delivery], after Savannah had come home from the hospital. As of January 31, I was still a little hyperthyroid, but when I go back in April, I'm hoping that will be different. I feel a lot better; it's just my eyes that are bothering me now.
>
> I know that I'll eventually have to have surgery on my eyes, but I want to wait at least until this summer. I don't know what the surgery's called, but it has something to do with the muscle behind my eyeballs. I know [my endocrinologist] wants me to see someone who has done this surgery a lot.

Karen has this advice to pass on to others:

> If you have that gut feeling about your health, don't ignore it. My gut feelings got me to go to my general practitioner in the beginning and made me get a second opinion later on. Don't ignore that little voice inside; it's more powerful than you are.

Karen is now euthyroid on levothyroxine. Her patience and

persistence were rewarded with a beautiful, healthy baby.■

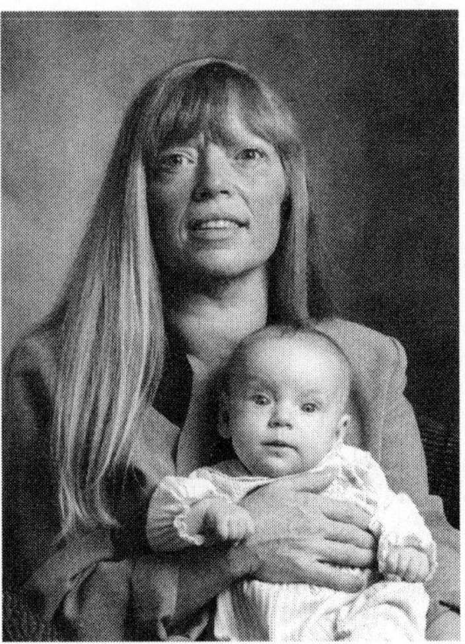

Karen and Savannah

JENNIFER'S STORY

Twenty-nine-year-old Jennifer went to her ear, nose, and throat doctor (ENT) when she noticed what she called "a bump" along her jawbone. When he said that he suspected she had an enlarged thyroid gland, she was taken by surprise.

> I didn't even know what a thyroid was! I wondered if I was going to die. My ENT suggested that I see an endocrinologist, and I chose one who was on my health plan. He was one of those chaotic professor types, and I wasn't really comfortable with him, so I changed doctors and went to someone not on the plan.

Records from the first endocrinologist indicated that Jennifer had both thyroid-stimulating immunoglobulins (TSI) and antithyroid antibodies. After ordering additional laboratory tests, Jennifer's new endocrinologist told her that she had subclinical hyperthyroidism (a low TSH level with normal free T_4 and T_3 levels). He discussed treatment options with her, and she chose to take PTU. However, forty-seven days later, her physician discontinued her PTU when he discovered that she had abnormal liver function test results.

> I didn't have any discomfort, but the lab work showed it, and the doctor told me to stop taking the [anti-thyroid] drugs.

Six months later, Jennifer was overtly hyperthyroid.

> I asked the doctor what the treatment options were. I still didn't have any symptoms, but I couldn't ignore the lab work. I researched on the Internet and asked lots of questions. My mother suggested that I look into alternative cures. I went to [an organic grocery store] to see what they had to offer, but I decided to rely on my doctor.
>
> I chose to go with radioactive iodine because it was the quickest fix. The word "radioactive" bothered me, but my doctor explained that just minimal amounts were used and that it would go straight to my thyroid.
>
> I really wanted to have a child, and I was worried about how this [hyperthyroidism] would interfere with conception. I discussed it with my doctor, and he advised me not to conceive until we got my thyroid condition under control.
>
> I took the radioactive iodine in the doctor's office. I had to sit there for half an hour in case I threw up. [Three] months after taking radioactive iodine, I experienced hypothyroid symptoms. I couldn't get enough sleep, but my work schedule was hectic. I was getting up at 5:30 every morning, so I just waited until my next doctor's visit to talk to the doctor about it. I gained about six or seven pounds without changing my diet.

> One of my biggest fears was developing Graves' eye disease. So far so good.

When Jennifer began taking levothyroxine, she became slightly hyperthyroid; therefore, her endocrinologist adjusted her dose. Three months later, Jennifer was euthyroid and had lost the weight that she had gained. She continues to be euthyroid and has shown no signs of Graves' eye disease.■

ED'S STORY

Forty-five-year-old "Ed" first noticed his heart racing in March 1999.

> I didn't know what to think. I thought that maybe I was going to have a heart attack. So what did I do? I started running! I figured if it was going to get me, that would do it. But exercise didn't affect it. It was strange; it only affected me at certain times—early in the morning and late afternoon.
>
> I went to see a cardiologist. He ordered a stress test and echocardiogram and also did some blood work. The thyroid panel came back and showed I had too much thyroid hormone.
>
> My sister works in the medical center in Houston, and she recommended that I see an endocrinologist there. So I've been making the six-hour drive to see him since then. [My endocrinologist] reordered the blood tests, and I had [a radioactive iodine] uptake [and] scan. He told me that I had some antibodies, and that it appeared highly likely that I had Graves' disease.

Treatment of "Ed's" Graves' disease was further complicated by the fact that he had lost an eye in a car accident in 1986. Although radioactive iodine is the treatment of choice for Graves' hyperthyroidism, some studies have indicated a possible increased incidence or worsening of Graves' eye disease among patients who have radioactive iodine treatment.

> We talked about the treatment options—antithyroid drugs, radiation, and surgery. Since eye disease may be more likely with radiation, I thought, "Why take a chance?" [My endocrinologist] recommended that I take antithyroid drugs for two years to see if I would go into remission. He explained that the odds were not great—that there was only a 30% chance of going into remission. But I have a small thyroid, and that increases the chances.
>
> I took Tapazole, and, two weeks to the day after I started, I had an allergic reaction. It looked like I had mosquito bites on my arms. I thought there were bed bugs in the hotel room I was staying in, so I changed rooms. But I woke up in the middle of the night because it was so painful and itched so bad.
>
> I stopped taking the Tapazole immediately. I kept off of it for two weeks and then started taking PTU twice a day. It took about a month before I started feeling good.
>
> [About five months after starting antithyroid drugs], I went from hyperthyroid to hypothyroid. My energy level was down, I was gaining weight, and my cholesterol went up. I've always loved the cold, but then I was too cold. I started on [levothyroxine] and started feeling better within a month or two. I got my energy back and stopped gaining weight. I'm losing the weight I gained now.
>
> It's been eighteen months since I was diagnosed. I never thought about the thyroid much before all this. Since I was diagnosed, I've found out that I know several people who also have Graves' disease—a friend

> from high school, a co-worker's niece, and another friend who had radioactive iodine. But there's no history of thyroid disease in my family.

"Ed" is now in remission—euthyroid without taking any medications—and has shown no signs of Graves' eye disease.■

JOE'S STORY

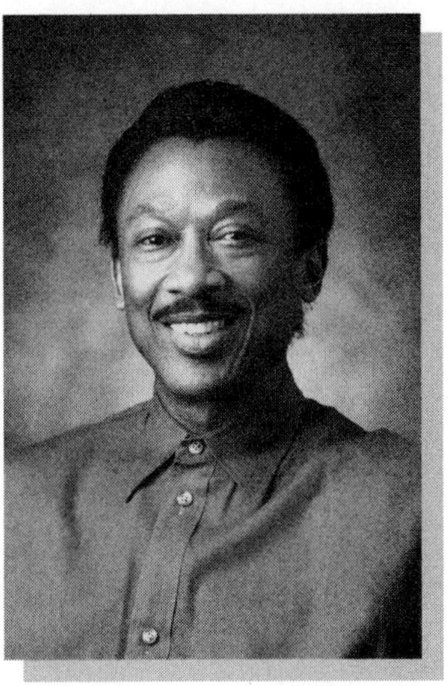

Fifty-six-year-old Joe is a teacher who has been taking antithyroid drugs for nine years to treat his Graves' hyperthyroidism.

> Shortly before my mother took ill, I started to lose weight. From time to time, I had noticed some nervousness, but I thought maybe it was work. At one point, I was so nervous, my hands were shaking so badly that I couldn't hold a pen. I had night sweats real bad; the bed linens would be wet in the morning. The other change was if I got angry or upset, I really had to sit down and calm myself. I'd be shaking so bad, it was noticeable; it was embarrassing. But I never had a problem sleeping.
>
> A friend at work said, "It might be your thyroid." I said, "Okay, come on, that's a woman's disease!" She gave me the name and address of [her endocrinologist] and said, "Just go and see him."

Joe followed his friend's advice and went to see the endocrinologist.

> In ten or fifteen minutes, he said, "You have a thyroid problem; you have hyperthyroidism, better known as

> Graves' disease." He told me what my options were. He said they could take it out, or I could have radioactive iodine—that it was painless. But I said, "Yeah, but you're talking about taking a major organ or destroying it. I don't want that." He explained that there were medicines, so that's the route I decided to go.

After reviewing the results of Joe's blood tests and thyroid scan, his endocrinologist prescribed PTU. However, when Joe's hives worsened, his endocrinologist recommended that he change from PTU to Tapazole.

Joe went to another endocrinologist for a second opinion. At that time, he had a goiter, a tremor of the hands, elevated free T_4 and free T_3 levels, a low TSH level, and positive TSI. Even though his new endocrinologist recommended radioactive iodine treatment, Joe chose to continue antithyroid medication. His physician prescribed Tapazole.

> We had to make four or five different adjustments. I started off taking one pill three times a day. It got to be a headache, so we tried to work out a system so that I could take it all at one time. I started taking three pills in the morning.
>
> Shortly after I started taking medication—about a month or two—I stopped losing weight; I couldn't fasten my shirt or pants! [The doctor's nurse] said, "You'll never be the same as when you first came in."
>
> Every time I came [back to the doctor's office], it seemed I gained three or five pounds. I was weighing 129, 130; now I was 150, 151. Exercise is what trimmed it down. I went from aerobics to lifting weights. Then I got into a swimming routine. Then I started running every other day. That was my routine. I also watched what I ate.

After seven months of treatment with Tapazole alone, his endocrinologist switched Joe to the block-replace method by adding levothyroxine.

> Then the weight got out of hand again. I was still taking three pills every morning, and the levothyroxine [my endocrinologist] had added. But it wasn't the pills. I was eating too late at night. I stopped eating so late and not so much. I lost ten to fifteen pounds after I stopped eating so late.

Two years after starting treatment for his Graves' disease, Joe stopped taking both drugs to see if he had gone into remission. Three months after discontinuing his medications, Joe was hyperthyroid again but chose not to take antithyroid drugs or have radioactive iodine therapy. Instead, he opted for a "natural alternative" and took various herbs and other over-the-counter preparations. When he returned for a follow-up visit four months later, he was still hyperthyroid and had lost ten pounds. Joe agreed to take Tapazole again and, four months later, he began taking levothyroxine as well. Joe has remained euthyroid on Tapazole and levothyroxine since that time, preferring not to stop his medications again.

> My visits [to the endocrinologist] were every three months up until very recently. Now I can go every six months. I still take three pills in the morning and drink lots of water. That's my own thing of always keeping myself flushed out.
>
> I didn't want to take [my thyroid gland] out; I didn't want to destroy it. I just wanted to calm it down. [My endocrinologist] has talked to me all along about taking the radioactive iodine pill. It's one thing I look forward to—how he'll try to get me to do it. But I just haven't wanted to go that route. This is working, and I do feel great! He said that I should be comfortable with whatever I choose. He's a great person; he listens and gives good advice.
>
> I would tell other people to make sure that they follow

> doctors' orders. Take medications as directed and take them every day. If there is any sign of some type of imbalance—either from the medication or the disease—call right away. Don't expect a miracle overnight; give it a chance.

Although many people do not like taking multiple pills every day and going to the doctor several times a year, some patients, like Joe, prefer this regimen to either radioactive iodine or surgery.■

JAMES' STORY

Fifteen-year-old James may be young, but he is an old hand at dealing with Graves' hyperthyroidism. His mother first noticed that something was different in his behavior when he was eight years old. She said:

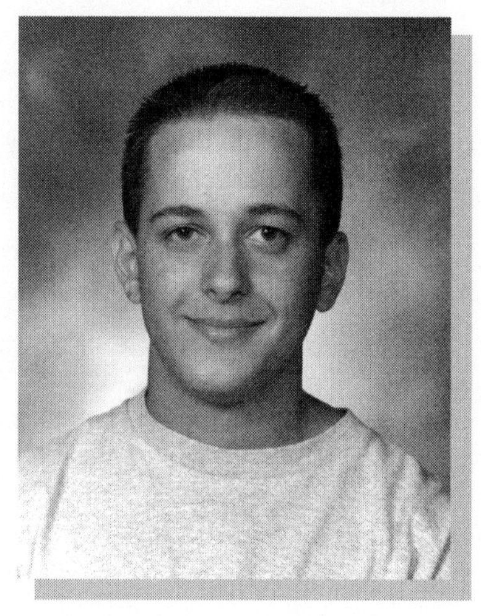

> Up until he started third grade, James was a normal boy. Then he got a stomach virus and lost eight pounds; he never gained it back. From that point on, things started going awry. Everything was affected. He had been a straight-A student; then he became a discipline problem. Things got worse and worse. It was a gradual process when he was eight, nine, and ten.
>
> I started talking to his pediatrician about six months into it, but he discounted it and said, "He's fine." After another six months, he said that maybe something was wrong and started to take it seriously. James was losing more weight, but he was getting taller. It got to where he was just bones. He had lots of diarrhea—constantly. In the fourth grade, he was real skinny, tired all the time, and had no energy. And he ate like a horse!

His father noticed the physical signs of James' illness: "He was weak; his legs would shake when he tried to get into the truck. His hands shook, and he couldn't perform athletically."

James missed participating in sports and explained, "I played baseball before, but I couldn't do it any more. I gave it up when I was nine. I couldn't run; I couldn't concentrate."

James' mother recalled that his behavioral problems became more evident when he was in the fourth and fifth grade:

> In the fourth grade, his teachers started calling. He couldn't do the work; he was just acting up, acting out. He couldn't understand directions. They wanted to put him on Ritalin. I about stood on my head!
>
> He had always been a loving, caring child. Then we were fighting all the time. He'd strike the wall, then start crying. He'd say, "I'm sorry; I don't know why I'm acting this way."
>
> His doctors did tests—a basic work-up. This was the first time they found elevated liver enzymes. Then they did a sweat test for [cystic fibrosis] and tested him for cancer. They even talked about doing a liver biopsy! Then they said that maybe he's lactose intolerant. So they took him off milk. That was really hard at this age. Finally, they told me, "You'll just have to come to the realization that he's a nervous child." I'm sure they thought I was neurotic, too.
>
> I think James was socially promoted when he finished the fifth grade. We decided to take him to a pediatric gastroenterologist. This was in June 1997, after three years. He did a bunch of blood work and talked about Crohn's disease and Wilson's disease.

James' mother knew that her grandmother and an aunt had thyroid disease and asked the pediatric gastroenterologist to check his thyroid:

> They said, "Oh yeah." It was just before the Fourth of July. His thyroid [hormone] levels were four times what high normal would be. The day before the Fourth, we saw a pediatric endocrinologist who explained that James had hyperthyroidism.
>
> They put him on beta-blockers to slow down his heart and on antithyroid drugs. He had to take PTU three times a day, every eight hours. We had to get up during the night to give it to him. We kept him on a rigid schedule.
>
> His eyes were getting kind of buggy, and he had every symptom on the list. We saw the [pediatric] endocrinologist every six weeks, and he kept adjusting [his antithyroid medication]. This was July, August, and September.
>
> His behavior started to improve; he started gaining weight; and his heart slowed down. Then one day I got a call from the school. They said, "Come get him; he's jaundiced." His eyes and tongue were yellow; his liver was very affected. His doctor said that his liver function was out of sight. He was having an adverse reaction to the medication that he was taking to correct his thyroid problem.
>
> They wanted to get him to the point—to get his thyroid to a level—to do [radioactive iodine therapy]. We waited about six weeks. When he was eleven years old, he had his first ablation [treatment with radioactive iodine]. It was the last of October.

James did not remember being concerned about what was happening. "I really didn't know what was going on. I didn't understand. It was just one more thing." Understandably, James' mother was anxious and looked forward to her son's health improving. She was pleased when James started to improve:

> Slowly things started to get better. We waited for six weeks to go by. The liver function was improving; the thyroid levels were coming down. Then by December, the doctor said [James] was where he was supposed to be.

James had a setback shortly after the Christmas holidays. His thyroid hormone levels began to rise again, and his mother was very concerned and somewhat surprised:

> The doctor had always intended to destroy [James' thyroid gland], and we knew he would have to take thyroid [hormone replacement]. His doctor said that [the radioactive iodine] should have killed his thyroid. That's when I got on the Internet and got [a book about thyroid disease]. I wanted as much information as I could get.

James' mother decided to take her son to another endocrinologist. After further evaluation, his new endocrinologist prescribed a second treatment with radioactive iodine. Within seven weeks, James was hypothyroid and began taking 112 mcg of levothyroxine daily.

James' parents are very pleased with his progress. According to his mother, James is back to normal:

> Basically, he lost three years of his life. But now he's getting straight A's again and playing golf and football and is on the weight-lifting team. His teachers comment about how good he is; he is really studious. His coaches couldn't believe his progress.

At the time of James' first radioactive iodine treatment, he weighed 110 pounds. While becoming euthyroid, he gained approximately seventy pounds, and his parents worried that he might gain too much weight. James' mother explained:

> During the years that he was hyperthyroid, he was able to eat anything he wanted and didn't gain a pound. After his thyroid problem was corrected, he continued

> to eat in the same fashion, as he had become accustomed. He was getting a little heavy and was becoming self-conscious. [In the last six months], James set out on a regimen of proper eating and exercise and has actually lost weight. He is down to about 145 pounds. He is really looking and feeling good. Now that he has lost some weight, his self image is much improved.
>
> My advice to others is don't take "no" for an answer. Even if you suspect something's wrong—even if you're wrong—it's worth looking into.

James' father echoes her sentiments and advises "If you think something's wrong, keep looking for the answer."

James' reaction? He sums up his feelings succinctly by saying, "I'm just glad it's over."■

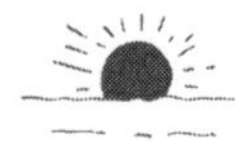

CHAPTER 8

WHAT IS THYROIDITIS?

Thyroiditis may be thought of as an inflammation of the thyroid gland. There are several different types of thyroiditis, and more than one type may occur in the same patient. For example, a patient with Hashimoto's thyroiditis, a common chronic type of thyroiditis, may also develop a transient type of thyroiditis, such as subacute thyroiditis.

One way of classifying the different types of thyroiditis is by their duration:

- chronic (permanent)
- transient (lasting less than a year)
- acute (rapid onset requiring immediate attention)

The table on page 230 shows a classification of the different types of thyroiditis.

CHRONIC THYROIDITIS: HASHIMOTO'S THYROIDITIS

In 1912, Dr. Hakaru Hashimoto first identified the chronic form of autoimmune thyroiditis that now bears his name—Hashimoto's thyroiditis. Other names for Hashimoto's thyroiditis are chronic autoimmune thyroiditis, chronic lymphocytic thyroiditis, and struma lymphomatosa.

Classification of Thyroiditis

CHRONIC	Hashimoto's thyroiditis Riedel's struma
TRANSIENT	subacute thyroiditis painless thyroiditis postpartum thyroiditis radiation-induced thyroiditis palpation-induced thyroiditis trauma-induced thyroiditis
ACUTE	suppurative thyroiditis

Autoimmune diseases are characterized by the presence of autoantibodies circulating in the bloodstream. Antibodies are proteins formed by the immune system to protect the body against foreign chemicals, bacteria, and viruses. In an autoimmune disease, antibodies are formed against the body's own chemicals. These antibodies, therefore, are technically called autoantibodies. Nonetheless, they are often simply referred to as antibodies. Although no one knows the exact cause of autoimmune diseases, studies indicate that they:

- tend to run in families
- affect women five to ten times more often than they affect men
- sometimes occur together

In patients with Hashimoto's thyroiditis, antibodies are formed against chemicals in the thyroid gland, such as thyroperoxidase and thyroglobulin. These antithyroid antibodies attack thyroid tissue, causing inflammation and a goiter (enlargement of the thyroid gland). The inflammation is almost always painless. Even though the thyroid gland may initially enlarge due to a combination of inflammation and compensatory growth of uninflamed thyroid tissue, its function is actually deteriorating. In some patients, the thyroid gland is smaller than normal (atrophic). At any stage of this autoimmune process, patients may become hypothyroid. Hashimoto's thyroiditis is the most common cause of hypothyroidism in the United States and in other iodine-sufficient areas of the world (see Chapter 5).

Since autoimmune diseases, such as Hashimoto's thyroiditis and Graves' disease, tend to run in families, it is not unusual for several generations of women to have thyroid disease (see "Jan and Suzanne's Story" on pages 245–248). The incidence of Hashimoto's thyroiditis increases with age, especially in women—from 15% at eighteen to twenty-four years of age to 24% at fifty-five to sixty-four years of age. By the time women are sixty-five years old, they have a one-in-four chance of developing Hashimoto's thyroiditis. Therefore, since Hashimoto's thyroiditis often causes hypothyroidism, it is not surprising that as women age, they are at increased risk of becoming hypothyroid. Women who have Hashimoto's thyroiditis should tell their mothers, daughters, sisters, aunts, and nieces about their condition so that their family members are aware that there is a hereditary disease in the family.

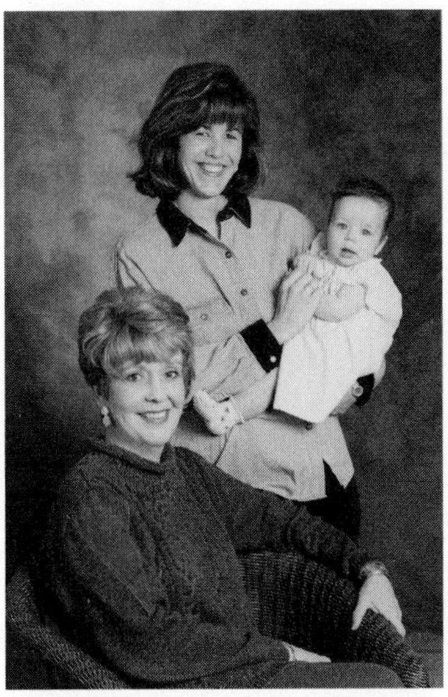

Figure 8.1. Grandmother and mother have Hashimoto's thyroiditis. Only time will tell if thyroid disease will appear in the next generation of this family.

Hashimoto's Thyroiditis and Other Diseases

Approximately 50% of patients with Graves' disease have the antibodies characteristic of Hashimoto's thyroiditis. Patients with Hashimoto's thyroiditis may also have other types of autoimmune diseases, such as vitiligo (a patchy loss of skin pigmentation) and prematurely gray hair. Women in their early thirties with gray hair and vitiligo very likely have Hashimoto's thyroiditis. When patients with Hashimoto's thyroiditis also have mitral valve prolapse, a common and benign heart valve disorder, they are more likely to have other autoantibodies, such as antinuclear antibodies (ANA). Finally, patients with Hashimoto's thyroiditis are slightly more likely than the general population to have serious autoimmune diseases, such as myasthenia gravis, rheumatoid arthritis, systemic lupus erythematosus, and Type 1 diabetes.

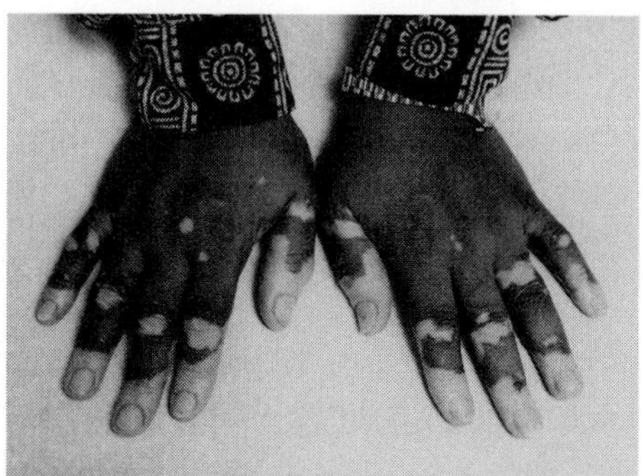

Figure 8.2. Vitiligo.

Similarly, patients with known autoimmune diseases, such as Type 1 diabetes, rheumatoid arthritis, and systemic lupus erythematosus, are more likely than the general population to have Hashimoto's thyroiditis. Premature menopause (failure of the ovaries before age forty) is also thought to be an autoimmune disease and is associated with a higher incidence of Hashimoto's thyroiditis. Patients with some non-autoimmune diseases, such as Turner's syndrome and Down's syndrome, also have a higher incidence of Hashimoto's thyroiditis.

Finally, patients with Hashimoto's thyroiditis may have other thyroid diseases besides Graves' disease. For example, a patient with Hashimoto's thyroiditis may also have a goiter, a thyroid nodule (lump), a multinodular goiter, or thyroid cancer. In other words, any thyroid disease can occur against a background of Hashimoto's thyroiditis, as demonstrated in Figure 8.3.

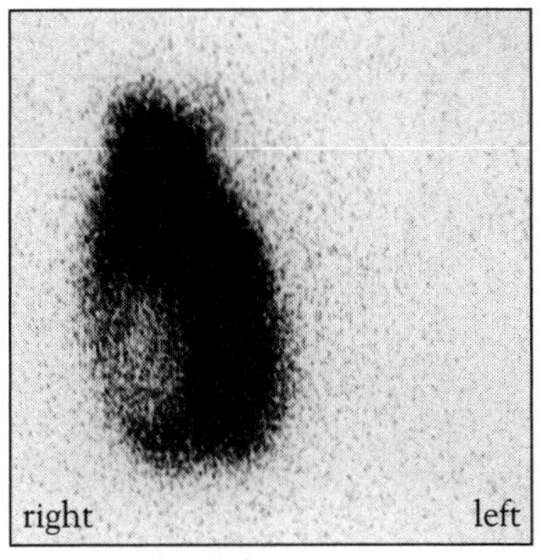

Figure 8.3. Thyroid image of patient with multiple thyroid diseases: congenital hemiagenesis with absence of left lobe and isthmus; thyroid cancer (light area) in right lobe; Hashimoto's thyroiditis was also found at surgery. The patient was euthyroid prior to surgery, hypothyroid after surgery, and temporarily hyperthyroid after levothyroxine treatment.

Hashimoto's Thyroiditis and Pregnancy

Women with Hashimoto's thyroiditis are predisposed to problems during pregnancy. For unknown reasons, women with Hashimoto's thyroiditis are at higher risk of miscarriage than women without it. In addition, patients who have had three or more spontaneous miscarriages have a higher than average incidence of Hashimoto's thyroiditis.

There are three theories explaining the association of Hashimoto's thyroiditis and pregnancy loss. The first theory suggests that a woman with Hashimoto's thyroiditis has a genetic predisposition to pregnancy loss. A second theory maintains that the pregnancy loss is due to mild hypothyroidism caused by Hashimoto's thyroiditis. The third theory proposes that the antithyroid antibodies found in a woman with Hashimoto's thyroiditis are the direct cause of the pregnancy loss. Additional studies are necessary to clarify the cause and treatment of pregnancy loss in women with Hashimoto's thyroiditis.

At least two-thirds of the women with postpartum thyroiditis, also called postpartum thyroid dysfunction (see pages 240–243), have Hashimoto's thyroiditis. Therefore, some physicians suggest screening all pregnant women for the presence of antithyroid antibodies to detect those women at greatest risk of developing postpartum thyroiditis. Other physicians recommend screening only the following pregnant patients:

- women with autoimmune diseases such as prematurely gray hair, vitiligo, Type 1 diabetes, systemic lupus erythematosus, and rheumatoid arthritis

- women with family histories of thyroid disease
- women with goiters
- women with recurrent miscarriages

Signs and Symptoms of Hashimoto's Thyroiditis

Some patients with Hashimoto's thyroiditis will not have any signs or symptoms—the only way to identify these patients is by the presence of antithyroid antibodies. Other patients will have goiters and no symptoms. The goiter caused by Hashimoto's thyroiditis often has a distinctive feel to it; it may be irregular and firm. Sometimes the goiter is very asymmetrical, with one side much larger than the other. Finally, many patients with Hashimoto's thyroiditis will have the signs and symptoms of hypothyroidism, with or without a goiter.

Tests for Hashimoto's Thyroiditis

The presence of thyroperoxidase antibodies (TPOAb) or thyroglobulin antibodies (TgAb) confirms the diagnosis of Hashimoto's thyroiditis. Almost all patients with Hashimoto's thyroiditis will have one or both of these antibodies. Since hypothyroidism is a common consequence of Hashimoto's thyroiditis, measurements of TSH (thyroid-stimulating hormone) and free T_4 are also indicated in patients with positive antibodies.

Physicians may use diagnostic ultrasound to evaluate patients with Hashimoto's thyroiditis and irregular goiters. A thyroid ultrasound can ordinarily distinguish a goiter caused by Hashimoto's thyroiditis from a goiter with one or more thyroid nodules. If the ultrasound demonstrates that only Hashimoto's thyroiditis is present, then further diagnostic studies to rule out cancer, such as thyroid imaging and needle biopsy, are not indicated.

Hashimoto's thyroiditis is sometimes discovered unexpectedly when doctors perform either a needle biopsy or thyroid surgery because of another thyroid problem. Experienced pathologists can diagnose Hashimoto's thyroiditis when they view thyroid tissue under a microscope.

Treatment Options for Patients with Hashimoto's Thyroiditis

Patient Status	Treatment
hypothyroid	levothyroxine
subclinically hypothyroid	levothyroxine
euthyroid with symptomatic goiter	levothyroxine
euthyroid with asymptomatic goiter	observation or levothyroxine
euthyroid without goiter	observation or levothyroxine

Treatment of Hashimoto's Thyroiditis

Treatment options for patients with Hashimoto's thyroiditis are shown in the table above. The choice of treatment depends upon which signs and symptoms are present.

A patient who has Hashimoto's thyroiditis and either hypothyroidism or subclinical hypothyroidism should take levothyroxine for the rest of her life. A patient with Hashimoto's thyroiditis and normal thyroid function (euthyroidism) who has a goiter that is causing symptoms should also take levothyroxine. Levothyroxine may decrease the size of the goiter and relieve the patient's symptoms. The last two groups of euthyroid patients shown in the table above can either be observed without treatment or be treated with levothyroxine. Patients in either of these two groups may choose to take levothyroxine in anticipation of the development of hypothyroidism, or they may choose to be observed on a yearly basis without treatment.

Chronic Thyroiditis: Riedel's Struma

Riedel's struma is an exceedingly rare form of thyroiditis, characterized by inflammation and scarring of the thyroid gland and, occasionally, of the tissue surrounding the thyroid gland. Dr. Riedel originally described it in 1896 as a "specific inflammation of mysterious nature producing an iron hard tumefaction of the thyroid." The cause of this condition remains unknown. The degree of scarring may be so extensive that it causes compression of the trachea, difficulty in breathing, and difficulty in swallowing. Surgery is the usual treatment for patients with Riedel's struma, although steroids and Tamoxifen, a drug used to treat patients with breast cancer, have also been tried.

There are several other uncommon diseases that could be confused with Riedel's struma. These diseases affect multiple organs, including the thyroid gland, and treatment is usually directed at the underlying disease process. Amyloidosis, hemochromatosis, sarcoidosis, cystinosis, scleroderma, and histiocytosis X are examples of these diseases. Hypothyroidism may occur with any of these diseases.

Transient Thyroiditis: General Considerations

While Hashimoto's thyroiditis is perhaps the most common thyroid disease in America, transient thyroiditis is relatively uncommon except for postpartum thyroiditis, which occurs after 5 to 9% of all pregnancies. Disruption of the thyroid gland and leakage of thyroid hormone from the gland characterize all forms of transient thyroiditis. Patients may have symptoms of hyperthyroidism for several weeks or months, followed by symptoms of hypothyroidism for weeks or months, before returning to normal thyroid function, as shown below.

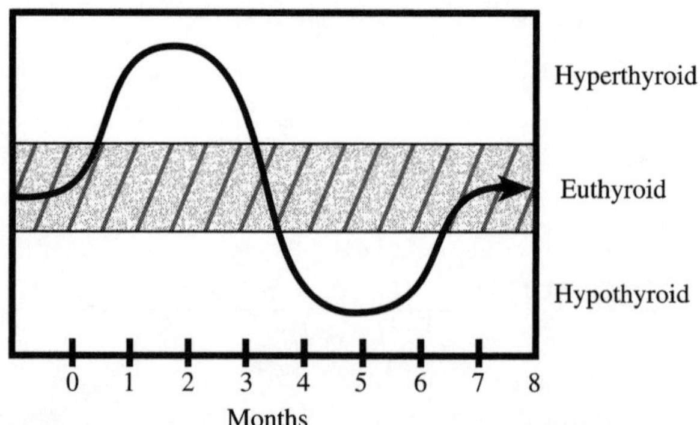

Figure 8.4. Diagram of the course of transient thyroiditis.

Hyperthyroidism in a patient with transient thyroiditis is caused by leakage of thyroid hormone from the damaged thyroid gland. The uncontrolled release of thyroid hormone will continue for several weeks or months until the stored thyroid hormone is depleted or until the thyroid gland recovers. During this hyperthyroid phase, beta-blockers may be prescribed for symptomatic patients.

Patients with asthma should not take certain beta-blockers since some beta-blockers can cause severe and, occasionally, fatal bouts of asthma.

If the damaged thyroid gland does not recover before thyroid hormone levels fall below normal, the patient may develop symptoms of hypothyroidism. This hypothyroid phase will continue for several weeks or months until the thyroid gland recovers. Levothyroxine may be prescribed during the hypothyroid phase, depending upon the severity of the symptoms. Most patients eventually return to a euthyroid state and will not require a lifetime of therapy with levothyroxine. However, some patients with transient thyroiditis will become permanently hypothyroid and require a lifetime of replacement therapy with levothyroxine.

The hallmark of transient thyroiditis is a low radioactive iodine uptake (see Chapter 4). The uptake is low because the thyroid gland is damaged and unable to take up iodine, an essential element for the production of thyroid hormone. Other features, described below, will distinguish one type of transient thyroiditis from another.

Transient Thyroiditis: Subacute Thyroiditis

Subacute thyroiditis (SAT)—also called de Quervain's thyroiditis, subacute granulomatous thyroiditis, giant cell thyroiditis, and subacute nonsuppurative thyroiditis—can be a very dramatic and enigmatic disease. As with most thyroid diseases, it occurs predominately in women—three to six times more often than in men. Subacute thyroiditis occurs more frequently in the summer months, and, in approximately 50% of patients, an upper respiratory viral infection precedes its development.

Typical signs and symptoms of subacute thyroiditis are pain and tenderness of an enlarged thyroid gland, malaise, fatigue, and fever (see "Iris' Story" on pages 249–251). The pain and tenderness in the thyroid gland may migrate from one side to the other, and the size of the thyroid gland may change rapidly over the course of several days. Sometimes only one side of the thyroid gland is involved (see "Joel's Story" on pages 251–252). Patients will usually have some of the signs and symptoms of hyperthyroidism as well.

Carotidynia (pain in the carotid artery) is sometimes confused with subacute thyroiditis. This harmless, but painful, inflammation of either of the two carotid arteries passing through the neck (literally a "pain in the neck") is almost always caused by stress. Patients with carotidynia usually have pain on the side of the neck, whereas patients with subacute thyroiditis usually have pain in the front of the neck. Carotidynia responds within a few days to treatment with nonsteroidal anti-inflammatory drugs, such as ibuprofen (Motrin and Advil).

The laboratory findings that confirm the diagnosis of subacute thyroiditis are:

- low radioactive iodine uptake
- sedimentation rate greater than 30 mm/hr (millimeters per hour)
- thyroid function test results compatible with hyperthyroidism

The treatment of choice for the early painful phase of subacute thyroiditis is an anti-inflammatory agent. These agents include:

- aspirin
- nonsteroidal anti-inflammatory drugs
- steroids

Aspirin or nonsteroidal anti-inflammatory drugs are usually very effective. (Acetaminophen, found in drugs such as Tylenol, is not a steroid, a nonsteroidal anti-inflammatory drug, or aspirin.) Treatment is continued until the neck pain and tenderness have completely resolved. In some patients, neither aspirin nor nonsteroidal anti-inflammatory drugs provide complete pain relief. Steroids, typically 30 to 40 mg (milligrams) of prednisone daily, may be prescribed for these patients. However, after discontinuing steroids, there may be a recurrence of symptoms. Symptoms do not usually occur after discontinuing aspirin or nonsteroidal anti-inflammatory drugs. In rare instances, surgery may be necessary to relieve the pain.

Most patients recover completely from subacute thyroiditis. Some patients may experience a recurrence within a few months of resolution of their initial symptoms. In the absence of any underlying thyroid disease, thyroid function almost always returns to normal.

Transient Thyroiditis: Painless Thyroiditis

Painless thyroiditis—also called subacute lymphocytic thyroiditis, silent thyroiditis, and lymphocytic thyroiditis with spontaneously resolving hyperthyroidism—is considered a variant of Hashimoto's thyroiditis. Antithyroid antibodies are present in many patients with the appropriately named painless thyroiditis. Furthermore, tissue specimens from the thyroid glands of patients with painless thyroiditis look similar to those obtained from patients with Hashimoto's thyroiditis.

The course of painless thyroiditis is similar to that of the other types of transient thyroiditis, with one major difference. Whereas most patients with transient thyroiditis recover after the hypothyroid phase, as many as 50% of patients with painless thyroiditis remain hypothyroid and require a lifetime of therapy with levothyroxine.

Certain drugs can cause painless thyroiditis. Amiodarone, a drug used to control serious heart rhythm disturbances, is one well-studied example of such a drug (see "Jim's Story" on pages 88–90). Interferon alpha (IFNa), a drug used to treat patients with hepatitis B or C and certain types of cancer, also causes painless thyroiditis. Approximately 1 to 5% of patients treated with IFNa for three months or longer will develop painless thyroiditis. Interestingly, they may also develop antithyroid antibodies or Graves' disease. The risk of any form of thyroid dysfunction is greatest in patients who have positive antithyroid antibodies prior to initiation of treatment with IFNa. As with other forms of painless thyroiditis, hypothyroidism may persist after IFNa is discontinued.

Transient Thyroiditis: Postpartum Thyroiditis

Dr. H. E. W. Robertson first pointed out the association between thyroid dysfunction and the postpartum period in a 1948 paper entitled *Lassitude, coldness, and hair changes following pregnancy, and their treatment with thyroid extract.* As the name suggests, postpartum thyroiditis occurs within the first year after the delivery of a baby. Many physicians consider postpartum thyroiditis a variant of Hashimoto's thyroiditis since at least two-thirds of all patients with postpartum thyroiditis have antithyroid antibodies. Postpartum thyroiditis is common, occurring after 5 to 9% of all pregnancies and after 25% of pregnancies in patients with Type 1 diabetes.

Women with one episode of postpartum thyroiditis will frequently experience another episode after each subsequent pregnancy. Hypothyroid patients taking levothyroxine who still have functioning thyroid tissue may also develop postpartum thyroiditis. Additionally, postpartum thyroiditis may occur after a miscarriage or premature delivery.

Postpartum thyroiditis may occur in three different patterns:

- transient hypothyroidism alone
- transient hyperthyroidism followed by transient hypothyroidism
- transient hyperthyroidism alone

The classic pattern of postpartum thyroiditis, which occurs in 20 to 30% of patients, is hyperthyroidism followed by transient hypothyroidism. In the hyperthyroid phase of postpartum thyroiditis, the thyroid gland is temporarily disrupted by inflammation, and stored thyroid hormones are released into the bloodstream. Too much thyroid hormone in the blood causes symptoms such as nervousness, irritability, insomnia, an inability to tolerate heat, tremor of the hands, weight loss despite an increased appetite, excessive sweating, hair loss, palpitations, fatigue, and muscle weakness (see Chapter 7). The symptoms of hyperthyroidism may last for several weeks or months.

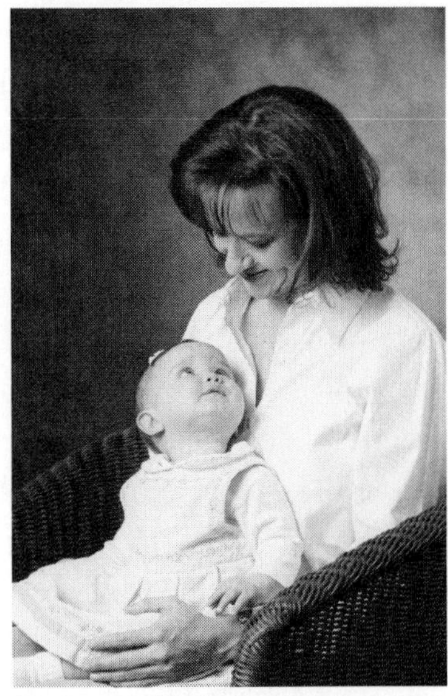

Figure 8.5. Young mother with postpartum thyroiditis.

As thyroid hormone is used up, there may be too little thyroid hormone in the blood if the inflamed thyroid gland has not fully recovered. A patient may then develop symptoms of hypothyroidism such as apathy, excessive sleeping, an inability to tolerate cold, difficulty in losing weight, fatigue, dry skin, hair loss, muscle cramps, and constipation. These symptoms may last for several weeks or months until the thyroid gland fully recovers and restores the amount of thyroid hormone in the blood to normal.

A patient with postpartum thyroiditis may experience wild swings in her symptoms and become very emotional. These symptoms may be incorrectly attributed to fatigue associated with the rigors of pregnancy and childbirth, changes in family relationships, sleep deprivation, postpartum depression, or other stresses in a mother's life. Furthermore, postpartum thyroiditis usually begins shortly after the routine six-week postpartum check-up (see "Laura's Story" on pages 252–255). Although a woman may feel well at that check-up, she may develop symptoms of postpartum thyroiditis later on and be unsure whether she should go back to her physician for another evaluation. She should.

Before the diagnosis of postpartum thyroiditis can be made, either the patient or her physician must suspect it. Once postpartum thyroiditis is suspected, the appropriate thyroid function tests will be performed. Blood tests done during the hyperthyroid phase will show a low TSH level and high free T_4 and free T_3 levels. Test results obtained during the hypothyroid phase will show a high TSH level and a low free T_4 level. A correct diagnosis will reassure the patient that her symptoms are not imaginary and that they are caused by an illness, which is not serious and is temporary.

In most patients with postpartum thyroiditis, thyroid function returns to normal after the disease has run its course, and no additional treatment is required. However, 20 to 30% of women with postpartum thyroiditis will develop permanent hypothyroidism, and they will require lifelong levothyroxine therapy. Studies have suggested that the following factors may predict whether hypothyroidism will be permanent:

- hypothyroid phase without a hyperthyroid phase
- high TPOAb (thyroperoxidase antibody) levels
- TSH greater than 20 mU/L (milliunits per liter)

Some physicians prefer to treat all women who have postpartum thyroiditis with levothyroxine indefinitely in an effort to minimize the effects of recurrent postpartum thyroiditis following subsequent pregnancies. They hope that levothyroxine will suppress thyroid hormone production so that there will be less stored thyroid hormone released during the destructive phase of subsequent episodes. However, other physicians are concerned that this treatment is not only ineffective, but could aggravate symptoms if the patients experience a hyperthyroid phase during their next episode of postpartum thyroiditis.

Graves' disease first detected in the postpartum period is sometimes confused with postpartum thyroiditis. Pregnancy can diminish the symptoms of Graves' hyperthyroidism to the point that they are not readily apparent, and the hyperthyroidism remains undiagnosed during pregnancy. Graves' disease may then flare up several months after the baby is delivered and be confused with postpartum thyroiditis. The distinction between Graves' disease and postpartum thyroiditis can usually be made by a radioactive iodine uptake—it is high in Graves' disease and low in postpartum thyroiditis.

Breastfeeding mothers should not have a radioactive iodine uptake unless they stop nursing for several days.

Postpartum thyroiditis and postpartum depression often overlap and may be confused with each other. Even though postpartum thyroiditis can aggravate postpartum depression, it does not appear to cause postpartum depression. In order to prescribe appropriate treatment, physicians must correctly diagnose each of these diseases.

Transient Thyroiditis: Radiation-Induced Thyroiditis

Radiation-induced thyroiditis may occur five to ten days after treatment with radioactive iodine; however, it is an uncommon occurrence. When it does happen, patients may experience neck pain and tenderness. Hyperthyroid patients may notice a transient worsening of their hyperthyroid symptoms. The treatment for patients with radiation-induced thyroiditis is the same as for patients with subacute thyroiditis (see pages 237–239). The symptoms ordinarily go away within one to three weeks.

Transient Thyroiditis: Palpation- and Trauma-Induced Thyroiditis

Palpation-induced and trauma-induced thyroiditis are both very uncommon. Vigorous palpation (manual examination) of the thyroid gland by the physician or by the patient may cause palpation-induced thyroiditis. Fine needle aspiration biopsy, especially of thyroid cysts, manipulation of the thyroid gland during surgery, and repetitive trauma to the thyroid gland from a seat belt are also causes of trauma-induced thyroiditis. Symptoms include mild neck pain and tenderness. Treatment of patients with either palpation- or trauma-induced thyroiditis is the same as for patients with subacute thyroiditis (see pages 237–239).

Acute Suppurative Thyroiditis

When the thyroid gland becomes infected with bacteria, the condition is called acute suppurative thyroiditis. This unusual thyroid disease affects both sexes equally and is more common among children than among adults. Children born with abnormal connections between the pyriform sinus (a structure above the vocal cord) and the thyroid gland are predisposed to acute suppurative thyroiditis. An upper respiratory infection usually precedes the onset of acute suppurative thyroiditis in children. Adults who get acute suppurative thyroiditis frequently have had chemotherapy or immunosuppressive drugs for cancer or AIDS.

Patients with suppurative thyroiditis usually have an acute onset of fever and a painful, tender thyroid gland. The skin over the thyroid gland may be red and hot. The diagnosis of acute suppurative thyroiditis often is made by a biopsy of the thyroid gland. Treatment requires hospitalization, intravenous antibiotics, and surgery on a relatively urgent basis.

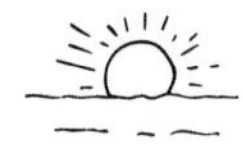

Patient Profiles

JAN AND SUZANNE'S STORY

Part I: Jan

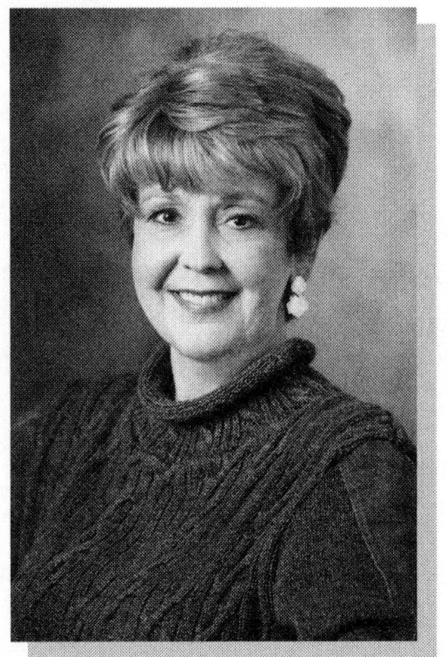

Jan is a fifty-seven-year-old homemaker who says she feels as though she has been hypothyroid all of her life.

> I was born tired; I've never had lots of energy. I've been cold most of my life. I've always loved wearing sweaters for fashion reasons, but I've also really needed them.

When she was twenty-seven years old and became pregnant, Jan described her symptoms to her obstetrician. He prescribed levothyroxine.

> I don't think he ran any tests; he just told me to take this pill.

Subsequently, Jan and her husband moved and changed pharmacies. When her levothyroxine ran out, she asked her physician for a new prescription, but he didn't remember prescribing it in the first place. This time he ordered blood tests to determine the level of thyroid hormones in her blood. According to Jan, the results were "low normal," and the doctor said that she didn't need to resume thyroid hormone replacement.

> But I was still so tired. I asked the doctor to put me back on the [levothyroxine], but he said, "You don't want to look bug-eyed, do you?" I kept complaining, and he just patted me on the hand and said, "Honey,

you'll be okay with a little nap."

Jan began to believe that it was just her nature to be tired all the time and that she would have to learn to live with it. She also struggled with heavy menstrual cycles and anemia.

> My periods were so messed up, and the iron I was taking for anemia was making my face break out. It's hard to describe how I was feeling. I just felt like I was floating away.

When she was thirty-nine years old, Jan changed doctors. Together they decided that a hysterectomy was necessary.

> We were hoping that once I had a hysterectomy, my energy level would improve.

As it turned out, the surgery provided only partial relief. Jan's ob-gyn referred her to an endocrinologist. Laboratory tests indicated that she was hypothyroid as a result of Hashimoto's thyroiditis. Once again, she began taking levothyroxine and started having more energy after several weeks of treatment.

> We had to do some fine-tuning of the dosage level, especially because of the estrogen I was taking, but I feel so good now. I'll never be without that tiny pill. What's the big deal about taking a pill every day when it makes your life better?
>
> I would tell all women to pay close attention to your body even if you're just tired. You don't need to suffer.

When Jan was diagnosed with Hashimoto's thyroiditis, she learned as much as she could about the disease and realized that it is a disease that can run in families.

> I've always known that my mother was hypothyroid,

> but I didn't know that meant I was more likely to have a thyroid condition.

Once Jan learned about the hereditary nature of Hashimoto's thyroiditis, she told her son and daughter about the disease and its symptoms. Jan's heightened awareness of thyroid disease helped her recognize that the symptoms her daughter Suzanne began to exhibit as a teenager required medical attention.

Part II: Suzanne

Suzanne is Jan's thirty-year-old married daughter.

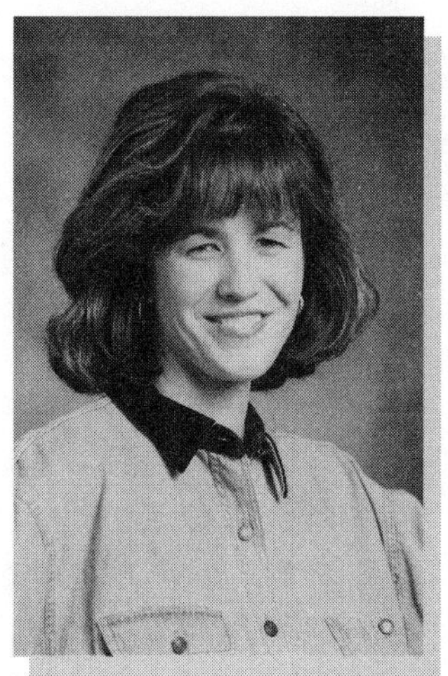

> I was vaguely aware of my mother's condition, but I really didn't remember much about it. Right before I left for college, Mom said she thought I might also have a thyroid problem. I thought she was just being motherly with all the usual warnings.

Jan noticed that during Suzanne's senior year of high school, it became more difficult to wake her up in the morning and that she seemed to be tired all the time. She said Suzanne had "nap attacks" and would sleep a lot. Since Suzanne was leaving for college soon, Jan took her to her endocrinologist. Laboratory tests confirmed Jan's suspicions—Suzanne also had hypothyroidism as a result of Hashimoto's thyroiditis. Suzanne explained:

> I was a little surprised when I found out. I thought, "Now what?" I knew Mom had the same condition so I was less concerned than I might have been.
>
> I didn't really notice a difference [in the way I was feeling] after I started taking [levothyroxine]. There was no dramatic effect—no miracle. Then I realized

> that I wasn't as tired.

Since beginning thyroid hormone replacement, Suzanne has made it part of her morning routine.

> It's no big deal. I just pop a little pill every morning. It's almost the first thing I do when I wake up. It's something you have to take care of. It just needs to be done. You are helping your body take care of itself.

Suzanne continued to see her endocrinologist once a year. When she married, he made sure that Suzanne knew the importance of telling him when she became pregnant. After she became pregnant, her endocrinologist made small increases in her levothyroxine dosage.

> I asked both [my obstetrician and endocrinologist] about the dangers of [levothyroxine] to the baby. I more or less figured that it was okay since the body needed [levothyroxine].

Suzanne gave birth to a beautiful little girl after an uneventful pregnancy. She plans on telling her daughter's pediatrician about the three generations of women who have thyroid disease so that this information will become part of her daughter's medical record.■

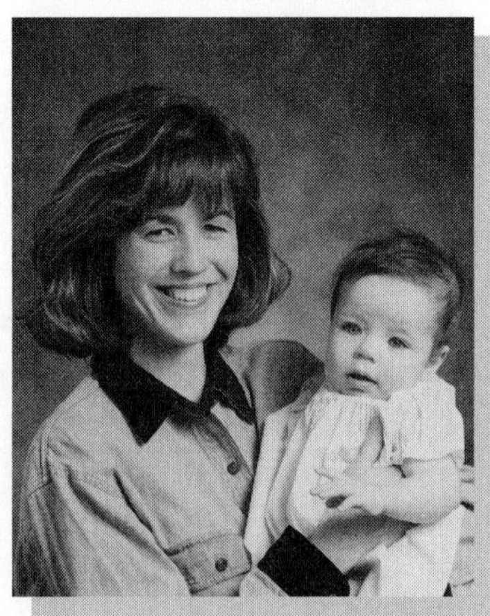

Suzanne and baby daughter

IRIS' STORY

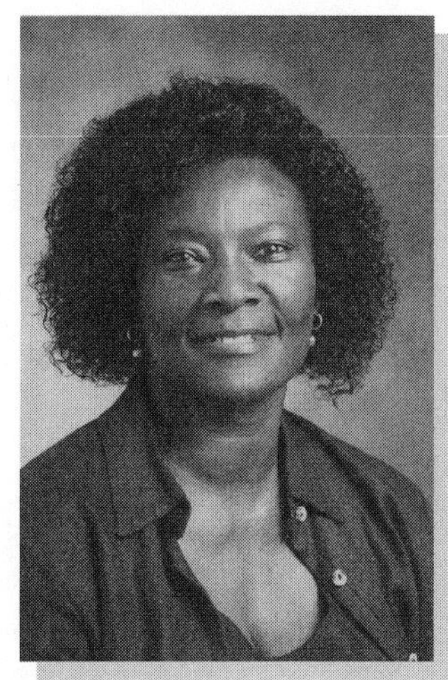

When forty-seven-year-old Iris began experiencing hot flashes, she attributed them to her age and menopause. Then she began to notice other symptoms.

> In December, after having a flu shot, I felt a little like I had a sore throat. It started on the left side and then moved to the right. It was weird. I had never felt this way before. The pain was lower than a typical sore throat. I kept looking in the mirror. I could see an outline of something swollen, and it hurt to touch. I was feeling very tired, my joints hurt, and my whole body ached. My memory was so bad! I thought it was a miracle that I got a job during this time. When I started working, it was hard getting up in the morning.
>
> I took Tylenol, but it didn't help. So I took ibuprofen. That helped some; it got me through the day. With the hot flashes and all these other symptoms, I thought, "This is terrible."
>
> In late February or early March, I went to my regular doctor. She knew what it was right away and said, "It's your thyroid." I already had high blood pressure, but now it went through the roof. It was 200/120! I thought the machine was broken. My doctor increased my blood pressure medication, and then she went on maternity leave.

Even though Iris was feeling tired, she continued to walk with a friend every morning.

> We walked in the neighborhood every morning and would talk while we were walking. Her oldest daughter

> had thyroid problems. She had a copy of [a book about thyroid disease] and gave it to me. When I read about subacute thyroiditis, I knew that was it. I made an appointment with [an endocrinologist], and he confirmed it.

Laboratory results showed that Iris had elevated thyroid hormone levels, a low TSH level, antithyroid antibodies, an elevated sedimentation rate, and a very low radioactive iodine uptake—all of which confirmed the diagnosis of subacute thyroiditis.

> I was hyperthyroid for about three to four months. I was eating a lot but losing weight. I lost about five pounds, which was unusual for me; my weight has always been steady. I kept taking ibuprofen but [at my endocrinologist's recommendation] increased it to three tablets, three times a day. I also had to increase my blood pressure medications again.
>
> For a brief period I felt okay, then I felt like I was bloating. I gained ten pounds even though I exercised regularly and watched what I ate. The hypothyroid phase lasted six weeks to two months. I didn't take anything for it because my symptoms were quite mild.
>
> The [throat] pain lasted a long time, even when I was in the hypothyroid phase. But I could live with the pain; it was localized. I've been pain-free since August. The hot flashes have stopped.
>
> I went to see [my endocrinologist] every six weeks. Now I see him every six months. I really go now because of my blood pressure. He told me a viral infection started the whole thing. He wouldn't say it was the flu shot. He told me it could happen again with other viral infections.

Iris went through a rocky course, experiencing both hyperthyroidism and hypothyroidism. Nonetheless, her thyroid function returned to normal four months after her endocrinologist confirmed that she had subacute thyroiditis.■

JOEL'S STORY

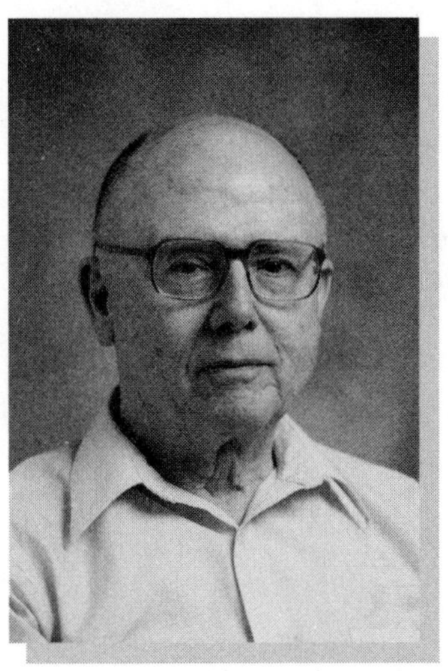

During a routine physical examination when Joel was fifty-eight years old, his internist discovered a lump in his thyroid gland.

> I wasn't too concerned, but I wanted it followed up.

Joel made an appointment with an endocrinologist who ordered thyroid function tests, a thyroid scan, a radioactive iodine uptake, and a fine needle aspiration biopsy. The thyroid function test results were normal. The scan revealed that Joel had a cold nodule in his right lobe, and his radioactive iodine uptake was 9%, a normal result. The pathology report from the fine needle aspiration biopsy was positive and highly suggestive of papillary thyroid cancer.

After consulting with his endocrinologist and an ear, nose, and throat doctor (ENT), Joel decided to have the suspicious nodule surgically removed. His ENT performed a right thyroid lobectomy.

> I knew all along that it might be cancer, but I had been told that [thyroid cancer] was slow-growing. The surgery went well; I had very, very little pain. The adhesive from the bandages caused the worst pain I had. In a matter of hours, I was up and walking.

The surprise came when the final pathology report indicated that the nodule was not cancerous; it showed that Joel had subacute thyroiditis.

> I trusted the doctors and knew I was in good hands. I understood the necessity of ruling out cancer. I believe that anyone in a similar situation should follow the same routine—have a needle biopsy and go ahead and have the surgery.

One month after surgery, Joel went to his endocrinologist complaining of a fever, neck tenderness, and pain with swallowing. The remaining lobe of his thyroid gland was tender, his skin was warm, and his reflexes were brisk. A 24-hour radioactive iodine was low at 1%, and both his free thyroxine index and sedimentation rate were elevated, indicating that Joel now had symptomatic subacute thyroiditis. His endocrinologist prescribed two aspirin every four hours, and the neck pain and tenderness resolved over the next two weeks. Six weeks later, Joel was hypothyroid, and levothyroxine was prescribed. Fifteen years later, Joel remembers to take his thyroid medication every day and still does not regret having the surgery.■

LAURA'S STORY

In May, thirty-two-year-old Laura had her first baby, a healthy little girl. After her six-week postpartum check-up, Laura noticed some unsettling changes.

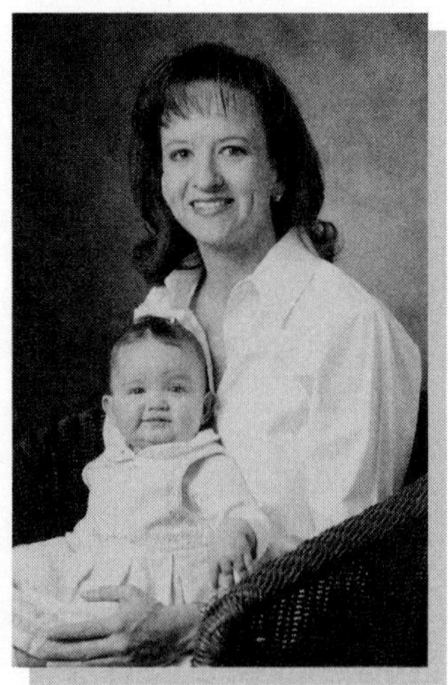

> Eight weeks after the baby was born, my hair started falling out. I had a ravenous appetite, but I didn't gain weight. I'd already lost the baby weight and maybe a little more. My husband noticed when I got out of the shower that I looked different.
>
> My legs were so weak that it was hard for me to get up

> off the floor. I attributed it to a lack of exercise; I was out of shape. My hips got sore when I sat. Chloe started sleeping through the night when she was two months old, but I couldn't!
>
> The other thing was the brain fog. That was just terrible! Not only could I not pay attention, I just couldn't retain anything. I wrote it off as sleep deprivation. My heart was racing, and my anxiety level was very high. Still, it was easy to write off every symptom. I had just gone back to work, I had a new baby, and I was worried about the hair loss.
>
> I called my [obstetrician], and she said right away, "Let's check your thyroid." My TSH was [less than] .01, and [my obstetrician] recommended I see [an endocrinologist]. My friends and co-workers also recommended the same doctor, so I went to him. I also started researching on the Internet.

Laura was experiencing the signs and symptoms of postpartum thyroiditis. When Laura's endocrinologist examined her, he noticed that she had a goiter, and an ultrasound revealed a small nodule in her right thyroid lobe. Laboratory test results showed that her free T_4 level and sedimentation rate were normal, but that her free T_3 level was elevated, her TSH level was low, and she had antithyroid antibodies.

Her endocrinologist recommended a radioactive iodine uptake to confirm the diagnosis of postpartum thyroiditis; a thyroid scan to determine whether the nodule was hot or cold; and a fine needle aspiration biopsy to rule out cancer.

> I had been put on birth control pills to try to help the hair loss, and [my breast milk] started drying up. But then I had to stop nursing for the radioactive [iodine] uptake, and that did it for nursing. I felt like it was ripped away from me. I freaked out!
>
> Then the cancer thing came into play. Everything

looked different. I started wishing I could have had longer with Chloe. I wanted a needle biopsy. We did it right away. It was painful, but it was a pressure pain, not very bad. There were no signs of cancer. It was such a relief!

Laura's endocrinologist explained that the hyperthyroid phase would eventually end without treatment and that she might also go through a hypothyroid phase.

> I went back to [my endocrinologist] a month after the biopsy, and the lump was still there, but my thyroid was getting smaller. My hair had stopped falling out by the end of November.
>
> My last check-up was in January. I'm still in the hyperthyroid phase, but I'm feeling better. I'm not looking forward to the weight gain and fatigue of the hypothyroid phase. Hopefully, I'll have more children, but I don't want to go through all of this again, especially the brain fog.
>
> I was still having problems with anxiety. I reacted to everything like the house was on fire, and I was quick to get angry. My emotions ran the gamut. I finally said yes to taking medicine to help it. [My endocrinologist] prescribed Xanax [for anxiety], and it has been really helpful. I've only taken it three or four times, mostly to help me sleep. It doesn't make me groggy. I highly recommend that anybody in my situation not resist trying something to take the edge off. Don't even think twice about taking something for anxiety.
>
> Most of my symptoms are better now, but if I'm under added stress, I feel it more. Just knowing what it is makes me feel better. I don't feel so weak, like why can't I control this? I feel sorry for any woman who has to go through this. There's enough to deal with having a new baby and all.

> Now that I have [thyroid disease], I know how common thyroid problems are. It's amazing how many of my friends and acquaintances have thyroid disease. I have three or four friends who had similar symptoms, but they were not diagnosed.
>
> My advice to other women is don't ignore the symptoms. Read about [postpartum thyroiditis] before you get pregnant and be aware of it.

One year after the onset of her postpartum thyroiditis, Laura's thyroid function is normal, and she does not require thyroid hormone replacement.■

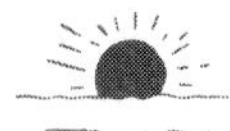

V

Could It Be My Thyroid?

Chapter 9

WHAT ARE GOITERS AND THYROID NODULES?

Any enlargement of the thyroid gland may be called a goiter. A goiter may be diffusely enlarged, irregular, lumpy and bumpy, symmetrical or asymmetrical, and may be associated either with hyperthyroidism, hypothyroidism, or normal thyroid function in various sequences and combinations. Enlargement caused by a solitary thyroid nodule (a lump in or on the thyroid gland) or multiple nodules is still called a goiter; a goiter with many nodules is called a multinodular goiter.

Some people become anxious when they find out that they have goiters with or without thyroid nodules. Their first thoughts may be that they will need surgery, that they have cancer, that their necks will become enormous, or all of the above. The following observations may provide perspective and alleviate undue concern:

- Thyroid surgery for a goiter is uncommon.
- Goiters that contain no thyroid nodules are very unlikely to be cancerous.
- The majority of thyroid cancers appear as a single thyroid lump (the solitary thyroid nodule).
- Approximately 90% of all solitary thyroid nodules are noncancerous.
- Enormous goiters are uncommon in iodine-sufficient areas, such as the United States.

Causes of Thyroid Gland Enlargement

Five general causes of thyroid gland enlargement are:

- tumors
- cysts
- inflammation/infection
- growth factors
- obscure or unknown (idiopathic) causes

Tumors

A thyroid tumor is an abnormal growth of thyroid cells. Although the exact cause of most thyroid tumors is unknown, certain types of radiation will promote their development. Unfortunately, the 1986 Chernobyl nuclear reactor explosion confirmed this effect of radiation. Children exposed to radiation from the Chernobyl explosion have developed more thyroid tumors, both benign (noncancerous) and malignant (cancerous), than unexposed children have.

Thyroid tumors are the most common cause of thyroid nodules. All tumors are nodules, but not all nodules are tumors—for example, nodules can also be cysts.

Cyst Formation

Cysts are fluid-filled nodules. Thyroid cysts most commonly result from degeneration of benign tumors into liquid, although malignant tumors can occasionally do the same thing. When the tumors degenerate, the residual nodules may be completely fluid-filled (cystic nodule) or partially fluid-filled (mixed nodule). Most nodules containing fluid are mixed nodules. Cystic nodules are less likely to be malignant than mixed and solid nodules are.

It is difficult for a doctor to determine from a physical examination whether a thyroid nodule is cystic, mixed, or solid. Ultrasound can readily distinguish between these different types of nodules. A nodule will sometimes degenerate by abruptly hemorrhaging, causing pain and swelling in the neck that may last a few days. An ultrasound cannot reliably distinguish between blood and other fluid in a cyst.

Inflammation/Infection

Inflammation of the thyroid gland with an accumulation of white blood cells is seen in many types of thyroiditis, as discussed in Chapter 8. The most common type of inflammation, and the most common cause of hypothyroidism in the United States, is Hashimoto's thyroiditis. Although very uncommon, infection of the thyroid gland also causes white blood cells to accumulate in the thyroid. Either inflammation or infection can cause the thyroid gland to enlarge.

Growth Factors

Three common growth factors cause thyroid gland enlargement. The most common cause is increased TSH (thyroid-stimulating hormone) production from the pituitary gland. When thyroid hormone is low, the pituitary gland secretes TSH, which stimulates growth of the thyroid gland and the release of more thyroid hormone. For example, since iodine is an essential component of thyroid hormones, iodine deficiency sets off a chain reaction that ultimately leads to thyroid enlargement. The sequence of events leading to goiter formation in these patients is:

iodine deficiency

↓

thyroid hormone deficiency

↓

increased TSH production

↓

goiter

Although iodine deficiency is very uncommon in the United States, there are approximately 655 million people worldwide with goiters caused by iodine deficiency. In iodine-sufficient areas, lithium, a drug used to treat patients with manic depressive illness, is a more common cause of elevated TSH and goiter formation.

A second growth factor is an antibody associated with Graves' disease that duplicates the function of TSH. This antibody is called thyroid-stimulating antibody (TSAb) or thyroid-stimulating immunoglobulin (TSI).

The third growth factor that will cause the thyroid gland to enlarge is a hormone called human chorionic gonadotropin (hCG). This hormone is produced during normal pregnancies and, ordinarily, does not cause any thyroid enlargement. In some uncommon cases, however, a pregnant woman may develop a growth in the uterus, such as a hydatidiform mole or a choriocarcinoma, which may lead to massive overproduction of hCG, a goiter, and hyperthyroidism.

Obscure or Unknown (Idiopathic) Causes

Sometimes a patient is frustrated and bewildered when there is no identifiable cause of a goiter. There could be an obscure or uncommon explanation for the goiter, but the process of identifying it may be too lengthy and costly to pursue. Identifying an obscure cause will not necessarily change the patient's treatment. At the end of the day, the cause of some goiters will remain unknown (idiopathic).

Evaluation of Patients with Thyroid Gland Enlargement

As mentioned above, any enlargement of the thyroid gland may be called a goiter, including enlargement caused by one or more thyroid nodules. Physicians distinguish between a goiter with and without nodules, since a goiter without nodules is very unlikely to be cancerous. Approximately 8 to 9% of goiters with a solitary thyroid nodule are cancerous. In general, patients with multinodular goiters have a lower risk of cancer than patients with solitary nodules do.

There may be advantages for patients with suspected thyroid nodules who consult endocrinologists as opposed to other physicians. According to a 1998 study in the *Journal of Clinical Endocrinology and*

Metabolism, "Early referral of patients with suspected thyroid nodules to an endocrinologist results in significant savings in both cost and patient's time as well as increased precision of diagnosis." For example, a patient with a suspected thyroid nodule may actually have only a goiter without any nodules, which essentially eliminates concern about thyroid cancer and additional, expensive testing.

Medical History

The first step in evaluating a patient with a goiter is the medical history. Important factors in the patient's medical history include:

- age
- size of the goiter
- symptoms
- history of radiation
- family history
- location of the goiter
- evidence of hypothyroidism or hyperthyroidism

The age of the patient and the size of the goiter are important, especially when considering treatment. For example, a young patient with many years to live and a very large goiter may request treatment because of the likelihood that the goiter will enlarge over the course of her lifetime. On the other hand, an older patient with a large goiter causing no symptoms may decide against treatment, particularly if that treatment involves some risk.

A patient with a very large goiter may experience certain unpleasant symptoms, such as difficulty in swallowing (dysphagia), difficulty in breathing (dyspnea), hoarseness, compression of the trachea, or redness of the face that is worsened by fully extending the arms upright along the side of the head (Pemberton's sign). These symptoms should not be confused with a feeling of something stuck in the throat. This sensation, called *globus hystericus*, is caused by tightening of the throat muscles in an anxious patient. Treatment of a goiter will not relieve globus hystericus.

Sometimes, a patient with a goiter experiences pain in the thyroid gland. This pain most often indicates either subacute thyroiditis or sudden bleeding in a thyroid nodule—not cancer. Occasionally, a patient with a goiter and pain in the neck may mistakenly believe that the pain is caused by the goiter. It is more likely that the pain is from carotidynia, a harmless, but painful, inflammation of either of the two carotid arteries passing through the neck (literally a "pain in the neck"). Carotidynia is almost always caused by stress.

Patients who have had radiation treatment or exposure are at an increased risk of developing both benign and malignant thyroid nodules. Therefore, patients should tell their doctors if they have had radiation treatment or exposure. Older patients may recall having radiation treatments as children for conditions, such as tonsillitis, acne, ringworm, or an enlarged thymus. Some patients may be unsure whether they had radiation treatments when they were very young. The answers to several questions could suggest whether they had such procedures.

- ***Were parents and medical personnel asked to leave the room during treatment?*** Parents and nonessential medical personnel were asked to leave the room when radiation was used. Nonpatients were not asked to leave the room when children were treated with purple ultraviolet or "UV" light, which does not use radiation and, therefore, does not cause thyroid dysfunction.

- ***Was the treating physician a dermatologist, and was the treatment for the scarring form of acne?*** If the answer is yes, it is likely that radiation was used.

- ***Were rods placed in the nose to shrink tonsils and adenoids?*** Radiation-tipped rods were sometimes inserted for this purpose. Fortunately, only a very small amount of radiation reached the thyroid gland with this type of treatment.

Patients treated with radiation for cancers, such as Hodgkin's disease, may also develop thyroid problems, particularly hypothyroidism. The dosages of radiation used to treat patients with Hodgkin's disease are much larger than those given to children with acne, tonsillitis, or ringworm. Although one might think that these larger doses of radiation would be more harmful to the thyroid gland than smaller doses, this is not the case. Smaller doses appear to stimulate development and growth of thyroid nodules and cancers, while larger doses tend to destroy the thyroid gland and cause hypothyroidism. Nonetheless, patients with Hodgkin's disease who receive radiation treatments do have a slightly increased risk of developing thyroid cancer.

Finally, some patients have been exposed to excessive environmental radiation that stimulates thyroid nodule formation. Included in this group are: people living near Hiroshima or Nagasaki when the atomic bombs were dropped in 1945; people living near certain nuclear bomb test sites; and people, especially children, living near the Chernobyl nuclear reactor explosion. Although radiation exposure and therapy increase the risk of a nodule being cancerous, they do not increase the risk sufficiently to proceed with surgery without additional diagnostic testing.

If there is a family history of Hashimoto's thyroiditis or goiter, it is more likely that the patient's thyroid enlargement is not cancerous. On the other hand, if a patient with a goiter has family members who have had medullary thyroid cancer, the patient is at increased risk of having a hereditary form of thyroid cancer, as discussed in Chapter 11.

Sometimes patients have goiters in unusual locations. For example, a patient may have a substernal goiter (an enlarged thyroid gland that grows behind the breastbone, or sternum). Because of its location, a substernal goiter is difficult to evaluate. A patient with a substernal goiter may require studies to determine whether nearby structures are involved. These studies might include thyroid imaging, chest x-ray, esophagram, and CAT scan or MRI of the neck and chest.

The physician will also ask the patient about a history of hypothyroidism or hyperthyroidism and symptoms suggestive of either. Knowledge of the patient's thyroid function may be helpful in determining the cause of a goiter. For example, a hypothyroid patient with a diffusely enlarged thyroid gland is likely to have Hashimoto's thyroiditis.

Physical Examination

Enlarged thyroid glands may be found during physical examinations in up to 10% of women and 2% of men. Thyroid nodules are found during physical examinations in more than 6% of women and in less than 2% of men. During a physical examination, a physician may also examine the patient for neck tenderness, enlarged lymph nodes, deviation of the trachea, and abnormal texture of the thyroid gland. In addition, the physician will look for signs of hypothyroidism or hyperthyroidism.

Diagnostic Tests

Based upon the medical history and physical examination, a physician will order the appropriate diagnostic tests. These tests may include blood work, thyroid ultrasound, thyroid imaging, x-ray procedures, and thyroid biopsy.

Thyroid function tests, such as a free T_4 and a TSH, are necessary to determine if a patient is hypothyroid, hyperthyroid, or euthyroid (normal thyroid function). When a patient has an enlarged thyroid gland, she often asks, "Does that mean I'm hypo or hyper?" The answer is, maybe or maybe not—having a goiter does not automatically mean that a patient is either "hypo" or "hyper."

A physician may also order a blood test for thyroid antibodies to determine if a patient has Hashimoto's thyroiditis. If a patient has a tender thyroid gland, the physician may order a sedimentation rate to rule out subacute thyroiditis.

Thyroid ultrasound is a diagnostic procedure that can readily distinguish among Hashimoto's thyroiditis, a multinodular goiter, and a solitary thyroid nodule. This procedure is particularly valuable in older patients or people with short necks in whom physical examinations are difficult or limited. Thyroid ultrasound can also accurately determine the size of a nodule. A series of ultrasound measurements can be compared to see if a nodule is getting larger or smaller. In addition, the components of a thyroid nodule can be accurately described by thyroid ultrasound; cystic structures have a different appearance than solid structures. Thyroid ultrasound can also demonstrate if the trachea is being pushed

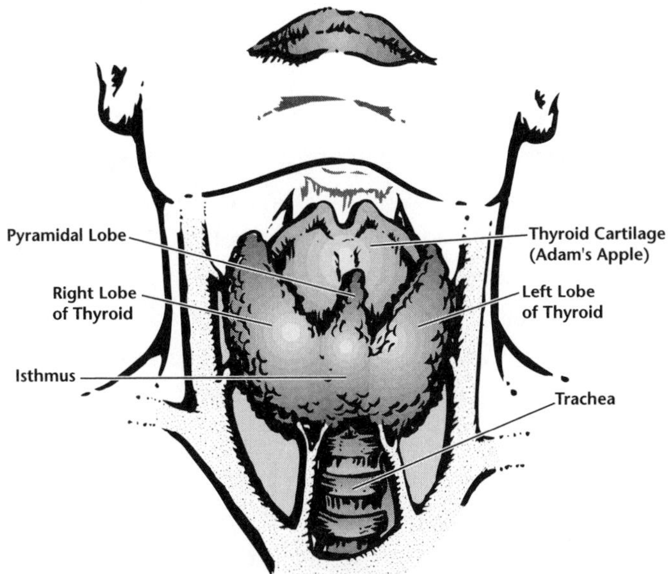

Figure 9.1. Front view of thyroid gland and neck, not drawn to scale.

Thyroid Self-Examination

You can actually examine your own thyroid gland if you can find your Adam's apple (thyroid cartilage). Begin by standing in front of a mirror with a cup of water. Then follow these steps:

- Locate your Adam's apple with your fingers.
- Drop down to the next tracheal ring of cartilage.
- Lift your head up and, while swallowing some water, look for the isthmus that lies over this ring of cartilage and for the thyroid gland that spreads out from the isthmus like a butterfly with its wings open.

Since the thyroid gland moves with swallowing, enlargement of your thyroid gland or lumps on your thyroid gland may become more apparent while swallowing.

out of its normal position (tracheal deviation) by an enlarged thyroid gland.

Thyroid ultrasound is most useful as a diagnostic tool when performed by a physician who is familiar with the anatomy of the thyroid gland and who wants to answer a specific question about a particular patient. It may eliminate the need for further diagnostic studies, such as thyroid imaging and thyroid biopsy. On the other hand, thyroid ultrasound is not a substitute for thyroid biopsy in determining whether a thyroid nodule is benign or malignant.

Thyroid imaging is sometimes used in patients with one or more thyroid nodules and almost always used in hyperthyroid patients with or without nodules. Thyroid biopsy is usually used only in patients with one or more thyroid nodules. Thyroid imaging and thyroid biopsy are discussed in greater detail later in this chapter.

Thyroid nodules are often found incidentally in diagnostic procedures examining other parts of the neck such as the carotid arteries or cervical spine. These nodules are, therefore, called thyroid incidentalomas. Physicians are finding incidentalomas more often for several reasons. Thyroid nodules occur more frequently in older patients, who are also more likely to have carotid artery disease and cervical spine disease than younger patients are. Since people are living longer, there is more need for diagnostic x-rays of the carotid arteries and cervical spine. Furthermore, diagnostic x-ray procedures are becoming less invasive and more sensitive. Therefore, physicians are ordering more diagnostic x-ray procedures and are frequently finding thyroid incidentalomas.

At the end of a thorough evaluation, a physician may classify a goiter as one or more of the following:

- simple goiter, or diffuse nontoxic goiter
- diffuse toxic goiter, or a goiter in a patient with Graves' hyperthyroidism
- goitrous Hashimoto's thyroiditis, or goiter caused by Hashimoto's thyroiditis
- goiter caused by transient thyroiditis

- goiter caused by infection
- solitary thyroid nodule (with or without a diffuse goiter)
- thyroid cyst
- substernal goiter
- autonomously functioning thyroid nodule
- toxic autonomously functioning thyroid nodule
- multinodular goiter
- toxic multinodular goiter
- thyroid cancer
- thyroid lymphoma
- Riedel's struma

Judging from this complicated list, it is no wonder that patients get confused. Therefore, to simplify matters and for the purposes of this book, patients with goiters will be divided into two basic categories—those with thyroid nodules and those without thyroid nodules. Patients with both goiters and thyroid nodules require further evaluation, as described on pages 270–278. Patients with goiters and no nodules require no further evaluation, and their treatment is described below.

Treatment of a Patient with a Goiter and no Nodules

The treatment of a patient with a goiter and no nodules depends upon the patient's thyroid function. When a patient is hypothyroid or hyperthyroid, or when a patient has transient thyroiditis, treatment is primarily oriented toward correcting the thyroid dysfunction. The treatment of a patient with these disorders is described in the following chapters:

- Chapter 5 – "What is Hypothyroidism?"
- Chapter 7 – "What is Hyperthyroidism?"
- Chapter 8 – "What is Thyroiditis?"

The treatment of euthyroid patients with goiters and no nodules is described below.

Euthyroid Patients with Goiters

There are four treatment options for a patient with a goiter, no nodules, and normal thyroid function. They are:

- observation
- levothyroxine
- surgery
- radioactive iodine

A patient who has no symptoms, a patient who has a small goiter, a patient who is not worried about the goiter growing, and a patient who does not like taking pills may choose observation without any treatment. Ordinarily, a patient who chooses this option will be re-examined every six to twelve months.

A second option is treatment with levothyroxine for an indefinite period of time. The theory underlying this approach is that levothyroxine will suppress TSH secretion from the pituitary gland, which, in turn, will prevent further stimulation of thyroid growth. Taking levothyroxine may reduce the size of the goiter or, at the very least, prevent it from growing. A euthyroid patient with Hashimoto's thyroiditis may choose to take levothyroxine for an additional reason. The patient wants to avoid hypothyroid symptoms that may eventually occur if the thyroid gland is sufficiently damaged by Hashimoto's thyroiditis.

A euthyroid patient with a very large goiter or one that is causing symptoms might consider surgery (thyroidectomy). Patients and doctors need to carefully weigh the risks and benefits of surgery. A younger patient who is a good surgical candidate may opt for surgery. An older patient with a higher surgical risk may be more hesitant. Once again, the size and location of the goiter, the degree to which the symptoms are affecting the patient, and the patient's overall health must be taken into account. Thyroidectomies are described in detail in Chapter 10.

Radioactive iodine (I^{131}) is a nonsurgical method of reducing the size of a large goiter. Although radioactive iodine has been used for more than fifty years to treat patients with hyperthyroidism or thyroid cancer, it has only recently been used to treat euthyroid patients with large goiters. The reduction in the size of the goiter following radioactive iodine treatment is less predictable than the reduction in size following surgery. However, radioactive iodine usually reduces the size of a goiter sufficiently to eliminate or greatly decrease the patient's symptoms (see "Johanna's Story" on pages 284–286).

Pregnant or breastfeeding women should not take radioactive iodine.

Goiters and Pregnancy

If a woman is already taking levothyroxine for a goiter diagnosed prior to pregnancy, she should continue taking it. Her thyroid function should be tested when she is six weeks pregnant and as often as necessary thereafter.

Goiters uncommonly arise during normal pregnancies in iodine-sufficient areas of the world. If a goiter is first detected during pregnancy and if the patient's thyroid function test results are normal, then no treatment is necessary. However, thyroid antibodies, characteristic of Hashimoto's thyroiditis, should be measured for four reasons.

First, since additional thyroid hormone is required during a normal pregnancy, a patient with a destructive autoimmune process like Hashimoto's thyroiditis may have trouble producing adequate amounts of thyroid hormone. Therefore, a woman with a goiter and positive thyroid antibodies should have thyroid function tests several times during her pregnancy. Frequent testing ensures prompt detection and treatment of mild thyroid failure, should it develop. Second, a patient who has thyroid antibodies is at a higher risk of developing post-partum thyroiditis. This patient will, therefore, be monitored more closely during the first year after delivery. Third, positive thyroid antibodies indicate that Hashimoto's thyroiditis is the likely cause of the goiter. Finally, a patient with Hashimoto's thyroiditis can alert her relatives to the presence of a hereditary autoimmune disease in the family.

Further Evaluation of a Patient with a Goiter and a Thyroid Nodule

As previously mentioned, the presence of a thyroid nodule raises concern about the possibility of cancer. Thyroid nodules are very common; on the other hand, thyroid cancers are very uncommon. Each year in the United States, more than 200,000 new thyroid nodules are discovered, of which about 17,000 are cancerous. Furthermore, death from thyroid cancer is uncommon, with only 1,300 patients dying from thyroid cancer each year. It is reassuring to know that most thyroid nodules are not cancerous and that thyroid cancers are usually cured.

A patient with a solitary thyroid nodule has approximately an 8 to 9% risk of the nodule being cancerous. In general, a patient with a multinodular goiter has a lower risk of thyroid cancer than a patient with a solitary nodules does. One way to understand the risk of cancer in a multinodular goiter versus a solitary thyroid nodule is to compare nodules on the thyroid gland to growths on the skin. If a person has many growths on the skin, it is unlikely that any of them are cancerous. On the other hand, if a single growth appears on the skin of a person with no other growths, then this solitary growth is more likely to be cancerous.

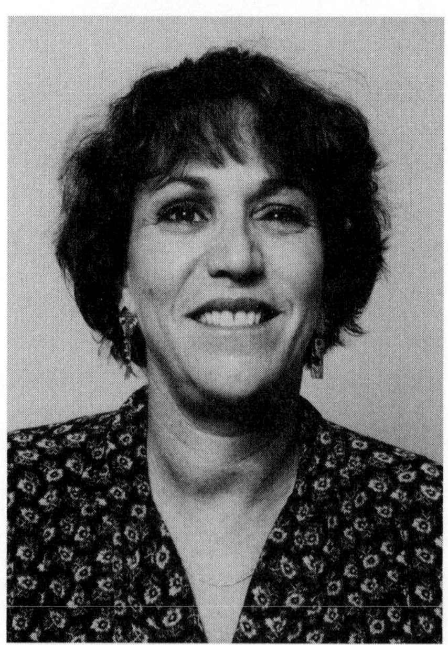

Figure 9.2. Patient with a solitary thyroid nodule in right lobe.

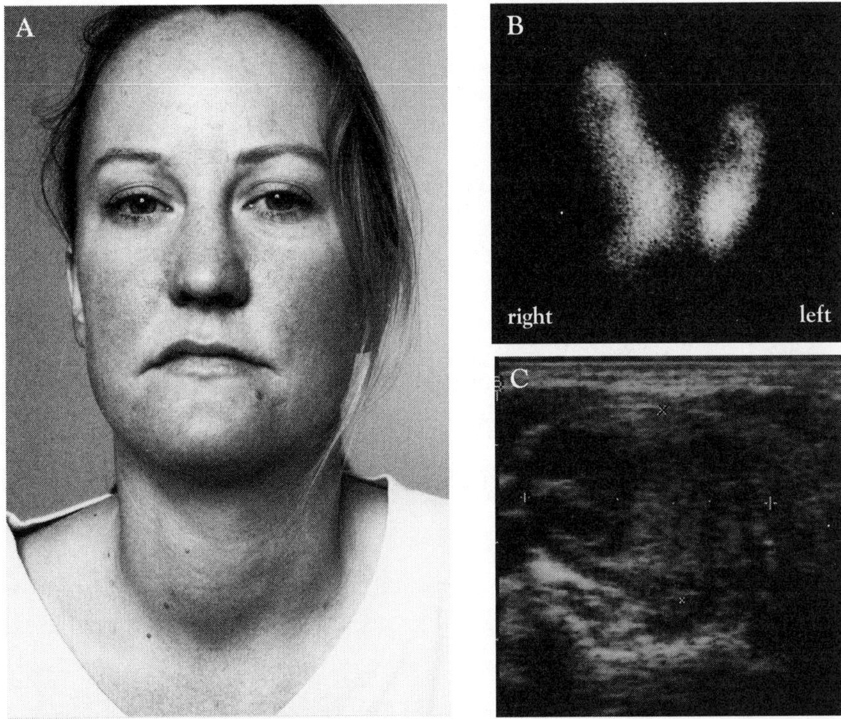

Figure 9.3. Dominant nodule in a multinodular goiter. (A) The patient. (B) Her thyroid image showing a dominant cold nodule in right lower lobe. (C) Her thyroid ultrasound.

In two situations, a patient may have more than one thyroid nodule and be treated the same as a patient with a solitary nodule. In the first situation, a patient may have only two or three large thyroid nodules. In the other situation, a patient may have multiple small nodules with one large nodule, the dominant nodule. In both situations, the large nodules are evaluated for cancer as if each were a solitary thyroid nodule. To better understand this point, compare again thyroid nodules to growths on the skin. If a large growth appears on the skin of a patient with multiple small growths, then this large growth is more likely to be cancerous.

Since a small percentage of patients with thyroid nodules have cancer, surgery is indicated only in those few patients who are likely to have thyroid cancer. Therefore, a careful evaluation of patients with nodules is necessary to identify those patients who are likely to have thyroid cancer and who are, therefore, candidates for surgery. The evaluation begins in the same way as the evaluation of a patient without a thyroid nodule. The physician asks about the medical history, performs a physical examination, and orders diagnostic tests. There will be, however, more extensive testing in order to classify nodules into those that suggest cancer and those that do not.

Sometimes a physician will advise a patient that an evaluation of nodules measuring less than 1.0 cm (centimeter) is unnecessary. First, these nodules have less than an 8% chance of being malignant. Second, even if they are cancerous, these small nodules are most often inconsequential and do not pose any threat to life. A papillary thyroid cancer (the most common type of thyroid cancer) measuring less than 1.0 cm is called an occult thyroid cancer. Pathologists have discovered occult thyroid cancers in up to 24% of autopsies done on patients who died of something other than thyroid disease. In other words, many people have small thyroid nodules that are unlikely to be cancerous. Even if the nodules are cancerous, they are unlikely to cause harm. Therefore, their physicians may recommend observation rather than a full diagnostic evaluation to determine if the nodules are cancerous.

Medical History

The age and the sex of the patient take on new significance when cancer is a consideration. Children and older individuals with new thyroid nodules are at greater risk of thyroid cancer than people of other ages are. Since thyroid disease is uncommon in children before puberty, the appearance of a thyroid nodule in a child is more suggestive of thyroid cancer than it is in an adult. Similarly, a new nodule in a seventy-five-year-old patient without a history of thyroid disease will raise suspicion that the nodule is cancerous.

Thyroid cancer is more common in women. However, solitary thyroid nodules in men are more likely to be cancerous because men are less likely than women are to develop thyroid nodules of any type.

Physical Examination

The size, firmness, and contour of a nodule are not particularly helpful in distinguishing benign from malignant disease. Benign and malignant thyroid nodules often feel the same.

A physical sign that is suggestive, but not diagnostic, of a cancer is involvement of the lymph nodes in the neck. Thyroid nodules and swollen lymph nodes from infection are both common, and they may be discovered simultaneously. The presence of enlarged lymph nodes in a patient with a thyroid nodule does not necessarily mean that the patient has thyroid cancer with lymph node involvement.

Diagnostic Tests

A physician may recommend measurement of calcitonin in addition to measurements of thyroid hormones, TSH, and thyroid antibodies. A calcitonin of more than 100 pg/mL (picograms per milliliter), or a rise in calcitonin to more than 100 pg/mL in response to a calcium infusion, is very suggestive of medullary thyroid cancer.

Diagnostic ultrasound can determine how many nodules are present. Interestingly, both ultrasound studies and autopsy studies show that up to 50% of patients have multiple thyroid nodules not previously detected. Therefore, ultrasound may reveal that a patient with a solitary thyroid nodule found during a physical examination actually has multiple thyroid nodules (a multinodular goiter). The presence of more than one nodule generally reduces the likelihood that any of the nodules are malignant. However, diagnostic ultrasound cannot reliably distinguish between benign and malignant disease.

Thyroid Imaging

Thyroid imaging using radioactive iodine (I^{123}) determines whether a nodule is hot or not. Nodules are classified as hot, warm, or cold. These are relative terms that describe how much radioactive material is taken up by the nodule as compared to the surrounding thyroid tissue. A nodule that takes up more radioactive material than the surrounding thyroid tissue is described as a hot nodule. Sometimes a nodule is so hot that it produces enough thyroid hormone to suppress the surrounding thyroid tissue. If this happens, the hot nodule will be the only thyroid tissue on the thyroid image. Hot nodules are rarely cancerous.

A nodule that takes up less radioactive material than the surrounding tissue is described as a cold nodule. While most cold nodules are not malignant, almost all malignancies are cold on thyroid imaging. Examples

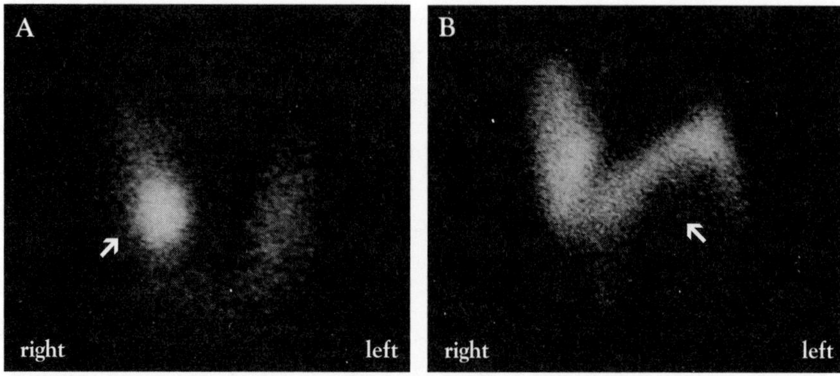

Figure 9.4. Thyroid images. (A) Hot nodule in right lobe. (B) Cold nodule in left lobe.

of hot and cold nodules are shown in Figure 9.4. A nodule that is neither hot nor cold is described as a warm nodule. While hot nodules are almost never malignant, warm nodules can be.

Pregnant or breastfeeding women should not take radioactive iodine.

Fine Needle Aspiration Biopsy

Fine needle aspiration biopsy (FNAB) is the most reliable and accurate method for distinguishing benign from malignant thyroid nodules. Therefore, virtually every patient with a cold or warm thyroid nodule, and some patients with hot nodules, should have a needle biopsy before consenting to surgery or to treatment with radioactive iodine.

There are almost no reasons to avoid a fine needle aspiration biopsy of the thyroid gland. The procedure is called a fine needle aspiration biopsy because the needle is very thin, much thinner than the needle used to draw blood. A needle biopsy may be performed safely even in patients taking blood thinners, such as Coumadin or heparin. The procedure is so safe that some doctors do not get a signed Informed Consent prior to the procedure.

Some patients may have been told that they should not have needle biopsies because they might spread thyroid cancer. Avoiding a needle biopsy for this reason is unwarranted. Only two cases of cancer spreading along a biopsy needle track have been reported among the hundreds of thousands of patients who have had thyroid biopsies. Furthermore, those two biopsies were not fine needle aspiration biopsies, and the patients already had widespread cancer at the time of the biopsies.

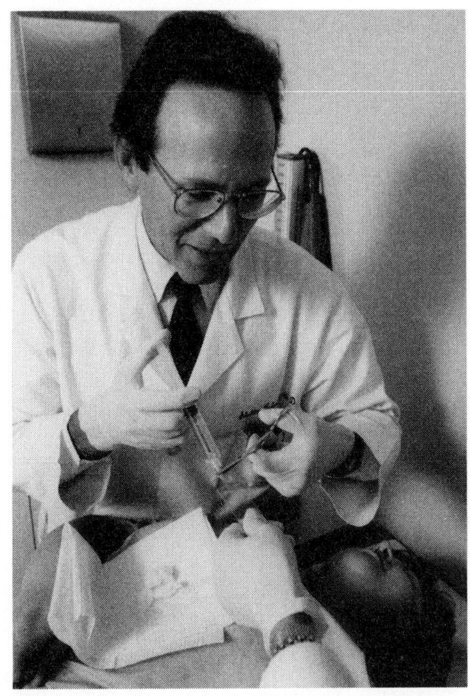

Figure 9.5. Doctor applying specimen to slide during fine needle aspiration biopsy.

During the needle biopsy, which takes about five minutes, a patient lies on her back with her neck extended over a pillow. The skin over the nodule is cleaned with alcohol swabs, and a local anesthetic may be injected into the skin. Either a thin needle attached to a syringe or only a needle is introduced through the skin and into the thyroid nodule. Most patients will be aware of a pressure sensation, but they usually experience minimal pain. After the needle is withdrawn, the biopsy sample obtained from the nodule is spread onto a slide, and the slide is sprayed with a fixative that prevents deterioration of the cells. Up to ten samples are obtained in this fashion, and the slides are then sent to a pathologist for processing, staining, and microscopic viewing.

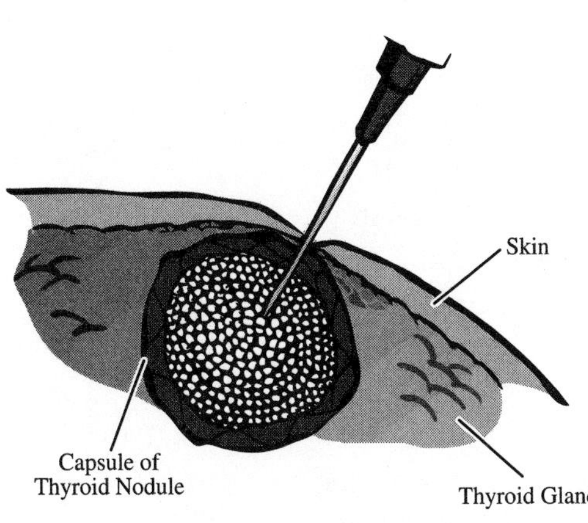

Figure 9.6. Fine needle aspiration biopsy.

Sometimes, a doctor will use ultrasound to guide

the placement of a biopsy needle. For example, if the nodule cannot be easily felt, or if the physician wants to biopsy the solid portion of a mixed nodule, he may do an ultrasound-guided biopsy.

Immediately after the last sample is obtained, pressure is applied and a Band-Aid is placed over the biopsy site. Sometimes, there is no evidence that a biopsy has been performed, and, at other times, there may be a bruise. A patient can go back to work or resume normal activities as soon as she leaves the doctor's office. Occasionally, a patient needs pain medications, such as aspirin or acetaminophen.

The choice of pathologist is very important. A pathologist with a great deal of experience in interpreting thyroid biopsies is invaluable. One of the main functions of a physician is to insure that the pathologist with whom he works is of the highest quality.

Biopsy results may be classified in several ways. One classification that has proven to be particularly useful includes four possible results from the pathologist:

1. *Benign* (or *negative*)—65 to 75% of patients receive this result. Enough cells are present, the cells appear benign, and there is nothing to suggest cancer.

2. *Non-diagnostic* (or *unsatisfactory*)—Approximately 10% of the time, the number of cells is inadequate for a pathologist to determine whether the nodule is benign or malignant. A small number of benign cells may be present, but not enough for the pathologist to call the nodule benign. If the specimen is non-diagnostic, a patient might be asked to return for a second or a third biopsy or even an ultrasound-guided biopsy.

3. *Malignant* (or *positive*)—In 5 to 10% of patients, the pathologist diagnoses cancer; sometimes he can specify the type of cancer.

4. *Suspicious* (or *inconclusive*)—In 10 to 15% of specimens, the cells have features suggestive of, but not diagnostic of, cancer. Inconclusive is not the same as a diagnosis of non-diagnostic or unsatisfactory.

Suspicious findings occur most often because cells from certain benign tumors (follicular adenomas) may look like cells from follicular cancers (see Figure 9.7). Also, if there are many Hürthle cells (a distinctive variant of follicular cells) present, suggestive of a Hürthle cell tumor, the biopsy result will be categorized as suspicious. At present, the only way to determine whether a follicular tumor or a Hürthle cell tumor is benign or malignant is by surgery. Hopefully, newer techniques for analyzing biopsy specimens will be able to distinguish between benign and malignant thyroid follicular cells without surgery.

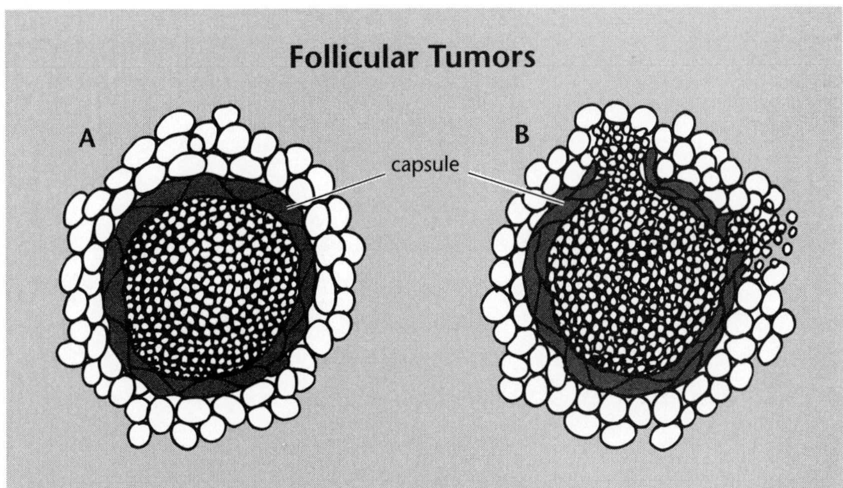

Figure 9.7. Follicular tumors. (A) Benign follicular adenoma. (B) Follicular cancer invading capsule.

Fine Needle Aspiration Biopsy during Pregnancy

Solitary thyroid nodules discovered during pregnancy are at least as likely to be malignant as nodules that develop in nonpregnant women. Nodules in pregnant women create diagnostic challenges. For example, a thyroid image cannot be done because pregnant women cannot take radioactive iodine. On the other hand, fine needle aspiration biopsy of the nodule can be performed safely during pregnancy. Some women, however, may wait until after delivery to have this procedure for the following reasons:

- Less than 10% of solitary thyroid nodules are malignant.

- If a thyroid nodule is malignant, it is likely to be slow-growing.

- In general, surgery during pregnancy should be avoided.

A study in the September 1997 *Journal of Clinical Endocrinology and Metabolism* comparing thyroid cancer in pregnant and nonpregnant women supports delaying surgery. It concludes that the outcome "of differentiated thyroid cancer is the same...and that the diagnosis and treatment of thyroid cancer during pregnancy can be delayed until after delivery in most patients."

Other women may elect to have a needle biopsy during pregnancy and then make a decision regarding surgery if the nodule is suspicious or malignant. If they choose surgery, the safest time to operate is during the second trimester.

Patients often ask me, "What would you do if I were your wife?" When responding to this question, I quote one of my favorite medical rules: *Don't order a test if you don't want to know the results*. In other words, patients should not have a needle biopsy if they are not prepared to deal with the results of the biopsy. Everyone wants a biopsy report indicating a benign nodule, for which surgery is not indicated. However, 15 to 25% of patients will have a result of either suspicious or malignant, for which surgery is indicated. These patients will then have to choose whether to have surgery during pregnancy.

The Decision to Operate

After the data from the medical history, physical examination, and diagnostic tests, including thyroid imaging and fine needle aspiration biopsy, are complete, a decision can be made regarding treatment. Surgery is not indicated for approximately 75 to 85% of patients with solitary thyroid nodules. Physicians will recommend surgery for the remaining

15 to 25% of patients to remove a cancer or a suspicious nodule.

Almost all patients whose biopsies are positive for cancer will have cancer at the time of surgery. In a small percentage of patients, the biopsy results show the characteristics of cancer, but the nodules are not cancerous (see "Joel's Story" on pages 251–252). Patients with suspicious results are less likely to have cancer, but there is no way of knowing which nodules are cancerous without surgery.

Treatment of Patients with Benign Thyroid Nodules, including Multinodular Goiters

After the data from the medical history, physical examination, and diagnostic tests are complete, most patients will be told they do not have cancer—they have benign solitary thyroid nodules or multiple benign nodules (multinodular goiters).

Hypothyroid Patients

Treatment of hypothyroid patients with benign nodules or multinodular goiters is relatively straightforward. Patients will take levothyroxine daily to restore the amount of thyroid hormone in their blood to normal. In addition, levothyroxine may reduce the size of the nodules in some patients. Hypothyroidism is discussed in Chapter 5, and treatment with levothyroxine is discussed in Chapter 6.

Hyperthyroid Patients

A patient who is hyperthyroid and has a benign solitary thyroid nodule may have either a toxic autonomously functioning thyroid nodule (TAFTN) or Graves' disease with a benign nodule. In the first case, the (toxic) nodule is producing too much thyroid hormone, causing the patient to be hyperthyroid. In the second case, the nodule is simply coexisting with Graves' hyperthyroidism. Similarly, a patient who is hyperthyroid and has multiple benign thyroid nodules may have either a toxic multinodular goiter (TMNG) or Graves' disease with multiple nodules (see "Erendira's Story" on pages 289–292).

A patient with Graves' hyperthyroidism, a toxic autonomously functioning thyroid nodule, or a toxic multinodular goiter has several

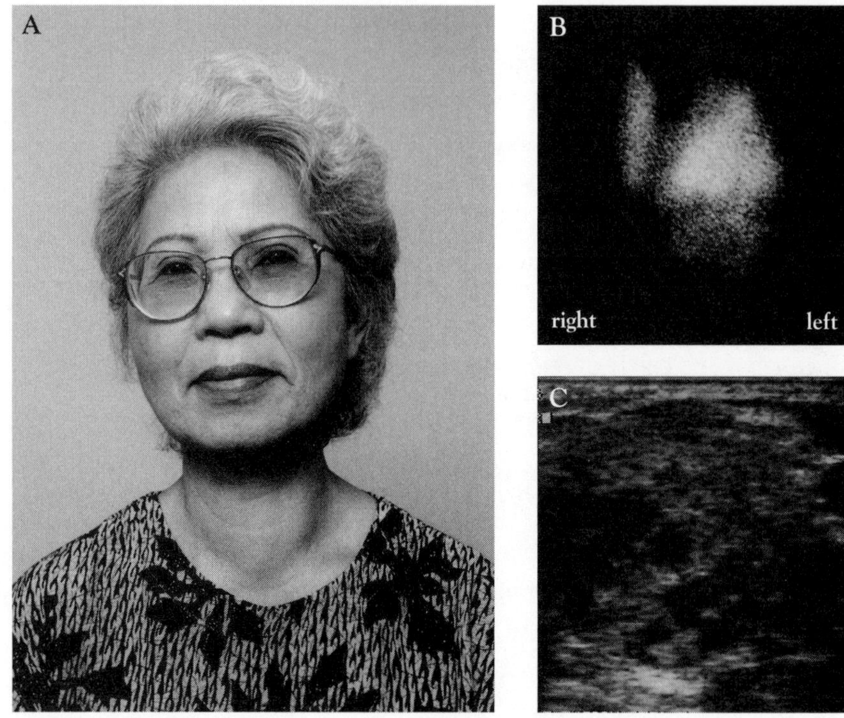

Figure 9.8. Multinodular goiter. (A) The patient. (B) Her thyroid image. (C) Her thyroid ultrasound.

treatment options. These options are discussed at length in Chapter 7.

Euthyroid Patients

The four treatment options for patients with one or more benign thyroid nodules and normal thyroid function are:

- observation
- levothyroxine
- surgery
- radioactive iodine

Patients without symptoms, patients with small nodules, patients who are not worried about their nodules growing, and patients who do not like taking pills may choose observation without any treatment.

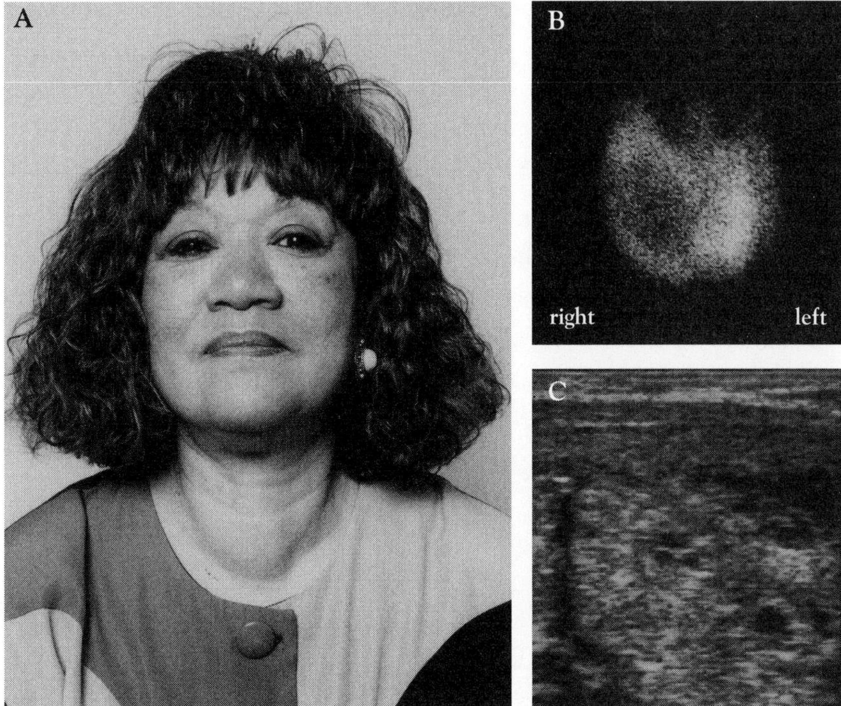

Figure 9.9. Multinodular goiter and Hashimoto's thyroiditis. (A) The patient. (B) Her thyroid image. (C) Her thyroid ultrasound.

Ordinarily, patients who choose this option will be re-examined every six to twelve months.

A second option is treatment with levothyroxine for an indefinite period of time. The theory underlying this approach is that levothyroxine will suppress TSH secretion from the pituitary gland, which, in turn, will prevent further stimulation of thyroid growth. Whether patients choose observation or levothyroxine therapy, some nodules will get smaller, and some will get larger, but most nodules will stay the same. Many physicians, however, believe that levothyroxine is more likely to prevent new nodule formation, to reduce the size of the existing nodules, or, at the very least, to prevent them from growing. Patients who choose to take levothyroxine will ordinarily be re-examined in about three months, in part to check their thyroid hormone levels.

Euthyroid patients with Hashimoto's thyroiditis may choose to take levothyroxine for an additional reason. Since Hashimoto's thyroiditis often causes hypothyroidism by destroying the thyroid gland, these patients hope to avoid the unpleasantness of hypothyroid symptoms.

Euthyroid patients with very large nodules or solitary nodules that are causing symptoms might consider surgery (thyroidectomy). The risks and benefits of surgery need to be carefully weighed. A younger patient who is a good surgical candidate may opt for surgery. An older patient with a higher surgical risk may be more hesitant. Once again, the size and location of the nodules, the degree to which the symptoms are affecting patients, and the overall health of the patients must be taken into account. Thyroidectomies are described in detail in Chapter 10.

Radioactive iodine (I^{131}) is a nonsurgical method of reducing the size of a large multinodular goiter. Although radioactive iodine has been used for more than fifty years in the treatment of patients with hyperthyroidism or thyroid cancer, it has only recently been used to treat euthyroid patients with large multinodular goiters. The reduction in the size of the goiter following radioactive iodine treatment is less predictable than the reduction in size following surgery. However, radioactive iodine usually reduces the size of the goiter sufficiently to eliminate or greatly decrease symptoms (see "Johanna's Story" on pages 284–286).

Pregnant or breastfeeding women should not take radioactive iodine.

Repeat Fine Needle Aspiration Biopsy

Benign nodules rarely become cancerous. Nonetheless, some thyroidologists recommend a second biopsy, even when the first result is benign and the nodule has not increased in size. Occasionally, a second biopsy yields a different result than the first biopsy. On the other hand, an informal survey of 1,000 patients rebiopsied one to two years after their first biopsy found that the diagnosis changed from benign to suspicious in only five (0.5%) patients, and to malignant in none. If the diagnosis of benign disease is confirmed by the second biopsy, then no more biopsies are performed unless the nodule enlarges significantly. If the nodule enlarges, a thyroid ultrasound may determine the cause of the enlargement and the need for a third biopsy.

Treatment of Patients with Thyroid Cysts

Sometimes a fine needle aspiration biopsy removes all of the fluid from a patient's cystic nodule, and it completely disappears without recurrence. Therefore, no additional diagnostic studies are necessary. In other cases, the cyst disappears after the biopsy, but then it recurs. If the cyst continues to recur after three needle biopsies, then further biopsies are very unlikely to cause the cyst to disappear.

If the result of the biopsy is benign, ultrasound-guided ethanol injection into the cyst might be considered for a patient with a recurrent thyroid cyst. Although ethanol injections can cause local pain and temporary paralysis of a recurrent laryngeal nerve, these injections are usually safe and effective. European physicians have more experience using ethanol injections since toxic autonomously functioning thyroid nodules—which may also be treated with ethanol injections—occur more commonly in Europe than in the United States. This procedure is seldom done in the United States.

The biopsy result from a cyst is often "unsatisfactory." A patient who has had three needle biopsies without either a diagnosis of benign disease or complete disappearance of the cystic nodule should consider surgery. Cystic nodules are malignant in less than 3% of patients, whereas mixed nodules are malignant in less than 10% of patients. The recommendation regarding surgery must be individualized.

Patient Profiles

JOHANNA'S STORY

Johanna is a seventy-seven-year-old great-grandmother who waited thirty-one years to treat her goiter.

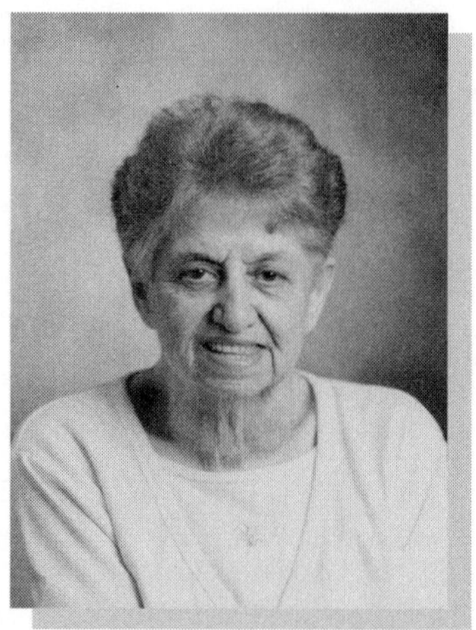

When I was a teenager, my face broke out, so I went to see a dermatologist. He told me to stay away from salt with iodine. I noticed that my neck started swelling some. I remember that the other people who went to the same dermatologist also had goiters. I've always thought that not eating iodized salt had something to do with this.

About thirty-one years ago, [my goiter] started getting really noticeable. I felt like I was choking sometimes. Every doctor I saw would ask about the goiter, but the only recommendation they ever gave me was to slice it out. Whenever they would mention a knife, that would end the conversation. They talked about how messy [the surgery] was, so I decided to take my chances and leave it there. I couldn't convince myself that I needed surgery. I thought I had a 50-50 chance, so I just let it go.

Cosmetically, it never really bothered me. Everybody else noticed it, but I really wasn't that self-conscious. You know, ladies have ways of hiding things. I wore a lot of scarves.

> A few years ago, I went to see my rheumatologist. When he saw my goiter, he sent me to [an endocrinologist]. He told me that I wouldn't have to say anything because [the endocrinologist] would know right away what was wrong with me.
>
> Until I saw [my rheumatologist], I wanted to let it go. But my daughter had been pressuring me to do something about it. My daughter and great-granddaughter literally pushed me in the door when we went to see [the endocrinologist].

When Johanna's endocrinologist first met her, he noticed that she had a raspy voice. Upon physical examination, he saw a massive multinodular goiter. It was compressing her trachea to the point that the trachea could not be identified on physical examination. When Johanna raised her arms over her head, her face turned bright red (Pemberton's sign). Her T_4 and T_3 were normal, but her TSH was low, indicating subclinical hyperthyroidism. A thyroid scan showed both hot and cold nodules, and a 6-hour radioactive iodine uptake was low at 2.8%. Biopsies of three of the largest nodules were negative.

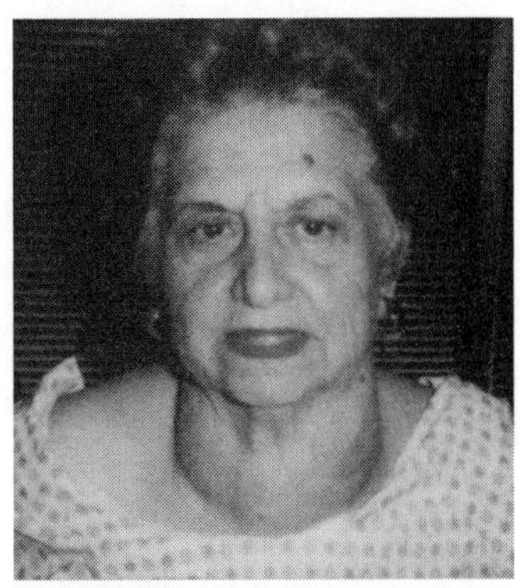

Johanna before treatment

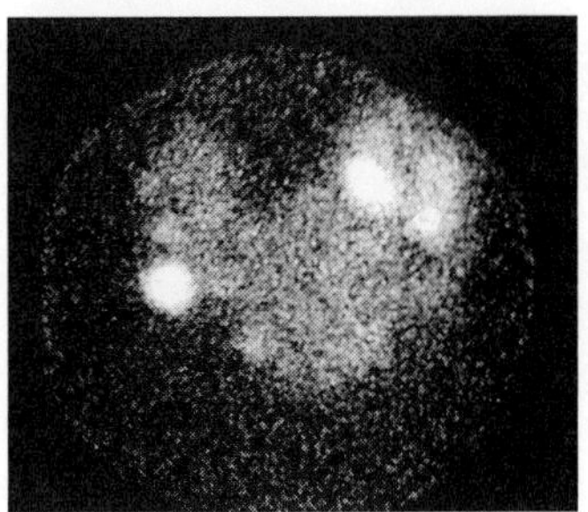

Johanna's thyroid image before treatment

Johanna told her endocrinologist that, because the goiter was choking her, she had to sleep with her head elevated. In addition, she tended to choke while eating, and, periodically, people would have to perform the Heimlich maneuver on her. She had even been in a situation where she had to "bang [her] back against the door to push air into [her] throat" when she was alone.

I didn't know there were specialists out there for this. [My endocrinologist] was the first to use the word "thyroid." He did a biopsy and scans. The tests showed a multinodular goiter. He recommended that I have radioactive iodine.

I had second, third, and fourth thoughts about [radioactive iodine]. It scared the heck out of me, but it scared me less than surgery. I did it pretty fast—about a month after the tests. I went to the hospital and spent the night. [My endocrinologist] told me how it was going to be. I was feeling frightened, but then he came by [my hospital room], and I felt better. I knew that he was watching over the process. Just seeing his face made a difference. I had a lot of confidence in him. He didn't lie to me about anything.

I took 100 millicuries of radioactive iodine. They told me to drink a lot of water. While I was in the hospital, I wrote down my experiences in a notebook—what it felt like to be cloistered and so forth. I was thinking maybe now this will be over. My thoughts as I left the hospital were ignited with thankfulness to God for a living family and to live in a country where you have the right to choose the doctor you want.

My advice to others is not to wait so long to get treatment. If you have a goiter problem, make your appointment as soon as possible to see an endocrinologist who specializes in goiter problems.

Over the next few months, Johanna's thyroid gland gradually became smaller. One and a half years after treatment, her thyroid gland remains very large, but it is half of its original size. Her TSH is normal.■

ELAINE'S STORY

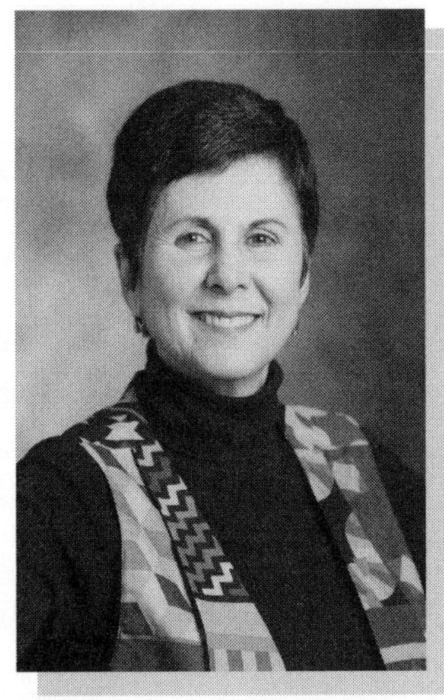

Ten years ago, fifty-four-year-old Elaine discovered a nodule in her thyroid gland.

> I thought it was a cyst at first. The doctor I went to ordered a scan and said I had a hot nodule. He said that we'd just watch it.
>
> I moved in 1994 and saw an ENT [ear, nose, and throat doctor] in 1997. It was not a positive experience. He ordered another scan, and it showed that I still had a hot nodule. He suggested a biopsy, but he only got liquid when he did it. He wanted to do a subtotal thyroidectomy just to make sure the nodule was benign, but I didn't want that. I had brain surgery in 1993 for an acoustic neuroma and lost the hearing in one ear. It left some scars, and I didn't want to be exposed to any unnecessary medical procedures.
>
> He put me on a low dose of [levothyroxine], but that made me hyper. My heart was racing, but I have ADHD [attention deficit and hyperactivity disorder] anyway and thought that I was just too wound up. My family doctor suggested that I see [an endocrinologist].

When Elaine arrived at the endocrinologist's office, she was taking 0.125 mg (milligrams) of levothyroxine daily. Her TSH level was low, and a thyroid scan showed that she still had a hot nodule that was not suppressed by levothyroxine. A fine needle aspiration biopsy was negative for thyroid cancer. Her endocrinologist told her that he did not believe surgery was indicated and advised her to stop taking levothyroxine.

> I was frustrated before I went to [the endocrinologist]. I felt negative. It was a rare thing for me to seek out another doctor, but when I got to him, I was reassured.

Elaine's nodule increased from 1.0 to 1.5 cm but eventually decreased to less than 1.0 cm. Two years after her initial visit to the endocrinologist, she returned for a check-up and told him that she was taking lithium prescribed by another physician for an unrelated problem. The hot nodule was no longer evident on the thyroid scan. In addition, she was now hypothyroid as a result of taking lithium. Since the nodule was no longer functioning autonomously, levothyroxine treatment was prescribed.

> I had not been quite as energetic but thought it was for other reasons. My skin was dry, and I was feeling cold. Then again, I've always been cold.
>
> My advice to others is to always get a second opinion—to try and find one of the top people. I didn't care what my insurance company said—it was worth it not to have needless surgery.

Hot nodules occasionally self-destruct, just as Elaine's did. She continues to take her levothyroxine daily and remains euthyroid.■

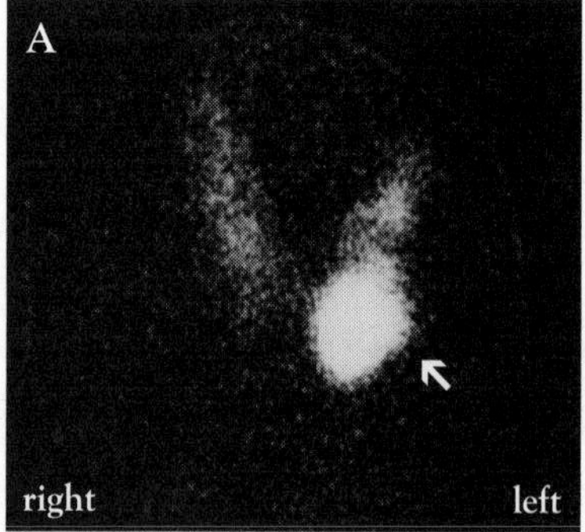

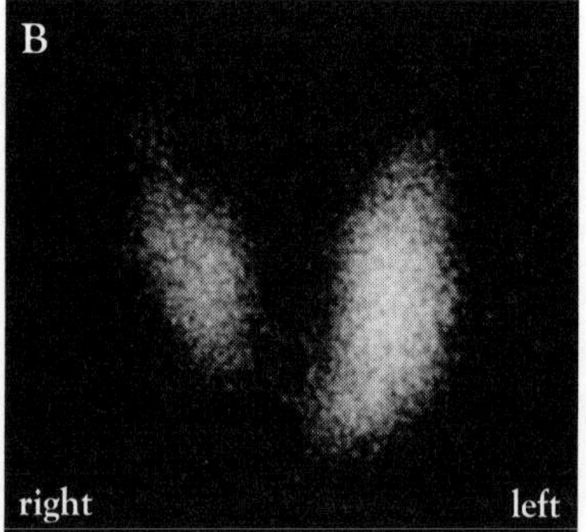

Elaine's thyroid scans. (A) Hot nodule in her left lobe. (B) After her nodule self-destructed, it was no longer visible on her thyroid scan.

ERENDIRA'S STORY

Even though she may not look it, Erendira is a fifty-four-year-old grandmother of five. Three years ago, during a routine examination by her gynecologist in Mexico City, she mentioned that she was nervous, losing weight, and becoming upset frequently. When he discovered that she also had a thyroid nodule, he referred her to a specialist.

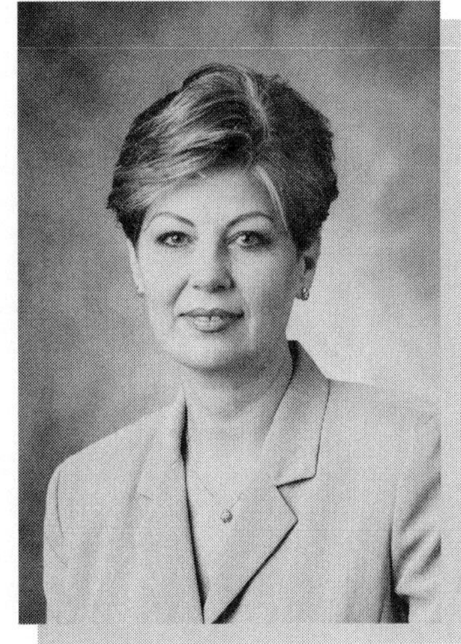

> He did an ultrasound that showed I had several nodules. He just said that I had a bad thyroid and prescribed [levothyroxine]. He said this medicine would stop the nodules from growing. He didn't draw any blood.
>
> I took the medicine for years, but it didn't help my symptoms. To the contrary—I had tachycardia [rapid heartbeat], shaky hands, and became angry with life because I didn't understand what was going on with my body.
>
> [Two years ago] I explained to the doctor that I was getting worse and that I was not happy. He told me I was a hysterical woman in front of my husband!
>
> Thirty years before, a doctor removed my sister's thyroid, but he didn't tell anybody what it was. To this day, I don't know why they removed her thyroid. Because of this history, I was concerned.
>
> For years, they did an ultrasound every six months, but they did not tell me what they saw. I would ask the technician if [the nodules] were growing, but she said she wasn't allowed to discuss it with me. I had to

> convince her to tell me, and she finally said, "You have a very large nodule and another behind that." I didn't know I had all these little ones. I had to ask the doctor to do lab work. Once he poked my neck four times to do a biopsy. A half hour later, he told me that it was not cancerous.
>
> I started smoking more and more and fighting with everyone. I'm sorry my life had to be like that. What a tragedy that you as a woman are supposed to understand your mate and children, but they can't understand when you are having trouble. My family just thought I was being bad.
>
> My sister is schizophrenic, and so I was terrified that it was happening to me, too. My husband left me for a while. He said I screamed too much. No one tried to understand me—that it was a disease.

When a friend told Erendira about an endocrinologist in the United States, she decided to fly from Mexico to see him. After examining her and reviewing the results of her lab work, ultrasound, and thyroid scan, he confirmed that she had a multinodular goiter with many hot nodules, and a suppressed TSH. Bilateral fine needle biopsies yielded benign cells.

> I was surprised he took so much time with me. The first day he did lab work, an ultrasound, and a scan. He told me that normally multiple nodules were not cancerous. He also told me to stop taking [levothyroxine] and to come back in [three months]. I noticed I was less hyper after a month. One definite change in my life was that I started gaining weight.

Three months after her first visit, Erendira returned to her endocrinologist for further evaluation. Even though she had stopped taking levothyroxine, her TSH was still low. Tests for Graves' disease were negative, and the thyroid scan and uptake were almost the same as when she was taking levothyroxine. Erendira's endocrinologist told her that she had subclinical hyperthyroidism from a toxic multinodular goiter.

> I had radioactive iodine May 1, 2000. I came back six weeks later and was still a little hyperthyroid. Then in November, [my TSH] was normal. I had started to feel swollen, and, in December, my thyroid hormone levels were quite low, but [my endocrinologist] wanted to see if it spiked back up before he started me on medication. It didn't, so now I can be treated for hypothyroidism.
>
> I'm very hypothyroid now. I'm sleepy all the time, and my eyes are puffy. My joints hurt. Yesterday I fell; my knees just gave out. I felt depressed and sad after the radioactive iodine. My hair even started falling out. I'm battling menopause, too, so I'm freezing then burning up. My skin is very dry and itchy. It looks like powder when I scratch it. My nails used to grow, and now they don't. I wear false nails now.

Erendira initially became euthyroid within six months of treatment with radioactive iodine. However, six weeks later, she was mildly hypothyroid with a TSH of 7.8 mU/L. After three months of observation without medications, her TSH had risen to 19 mU/L. It was now apparent, after four-and-a-half months of hypothyroidism, that the tissue surrounding Erendira's hot nodules was not going to produce sufficient thyroid hormone. Therefore, she began taking levothyroxine and has continued to improve.

> I have tried to tell my family about this disease. I tried to explain what it can do. Still they don't relate my behavior to the disease. It has been very, very difficult in my family. They have always been accustomed to me preparing the meals, always looking good. They never help; I do everything. They still don't like that Mother can't do everything.

> I feel that by being honest about all of this, it will help others. I'm worried about all the other women going through this. People need to understand it's a physical problem. Now my husband comes with me when I come to see [my endocrinologist]. He's beginning to understand what I have been going through. He wants to help.
>
> At first, he didn't understand why I had to keep coming back. He took all the [medical records] to a relative who is a pediatrician. He studied in this country, and he told my husband that everything that was being done was correct. He said that it was a process and takes time. Then he asked my husband, "Do you want your wife to die of a stroke, or do you want her to get better?" So it took another doctor to make him understand, but I am grateful he understands now and comes with me [to the United States].

A patient with a toxic multinodular goiter (or a toxic autonomously functioning thyroid nodule) treated with radioactive iodine has a 50-50 chance that only the hot nodules will be destroyed. When only the hot nodules are destroyed, the patient may temporarily become hypothyroid. Once the suppressed tissue around the hot nodules recovers, the patient's thyroid function returns to normal. On the other hand, if the tissue surrounding the hot nodules is also destroyed, the patient becomes permanently hypothyroid and requires levothyroxine therapy, just as Erendira did.■

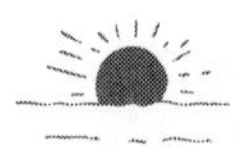

Chapter 10

WHAT IS A THYROIDECTOMY?

The reputations of many fine clinics in the United States, such as the Mayo, Cleveland, and Lahey Clinics, were built, in part, upon successful thyroid surgery in the first half of the twentieth century. However, starting in the 1930s and 1940s, other treatments diminished the need for thyroid surgery (thyroidectomy). For example, the iodination of table salt, pioneered by Dr. David Marine, virtually eliminated endemic goiter in the United States. Furthermore, once antithyroid drugs and radioactive iodine became widely used in the 1960s and 1970s, surgery on patients with Graves' disease was markedly reduced (see "Lilian's Story" on pages 309–311). In addition, fine needle aspiration biopsies have eliminated the need for surgery on many patients with thyroid nodules.

Since thyroid surgery is performed relatively infrequently today, few surgeons have accumulated extensive experience doing thyroidectomies; consequently, the choice of a surgeon must be considered carefully (see "Judy's Story" on pages 306–309). Many patients base their decision upon the opinion of an acquaintance who has had surgery. While trusted friends and relatives have the patient's best interests in mind, they cannot know the comparable experience and results of different surgeons (see "Stuart's Story" on pages 303–306). Therefore, it is prudent for patients to consult with their physicians to identify the most qualified thyroid surgeons in their area. Experience counts.

Thyroidectomy may mean any of the following:

- thyroid lobectomy—removal of one lobe with or without removal of part of the isthmus connecting the two thyroid lobes
- thyroid lobectomy and isthmusectomy—removal of one lobe and the isthmus
- subtotal, or near-total, thyroidectomy—removal of one lobe, the isthmus, and almost all of the other lobe
- total thyroidectomy—removal of the entire thyroid gland

Figure 10.1. Thyroidectomies.

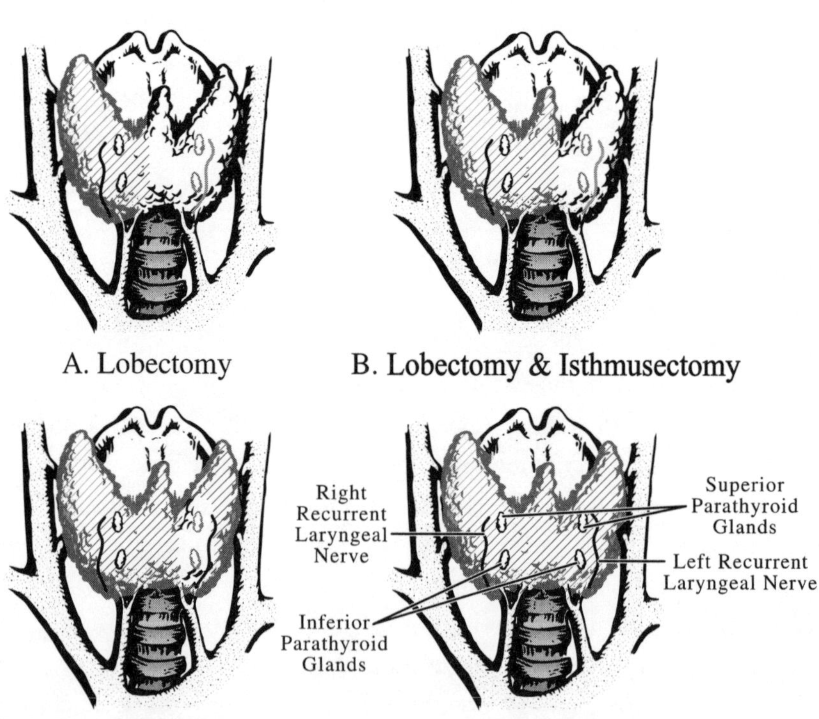

Regardless of which surgery is being performed, the procedure is almost always done under general anesthesia in a hospital and should be viewed as major surgery. In some unusual circumstances, however, surgeons may do thyroidectomies under local anesthesia. In fact, prior to 1920, local anesthesia was preferred for hyperthyroid patients since thyroid storm, a life-threatening thyroid crisis, occurred frequently after general anesthesia. Many physicians thought that thyroid storm could be avoided by using local anesthesia. With modern preoperative treatments, patients rarely experience thyroid storm after general anesthesia. Therefore, the primary indication for local anesthesia is fear of general anesthesia.

Indications for Thyroidectomy

Thyroidectomy is considered for the following:

- possible thyroid cancer
- known thyroid cancer
- large goiter, especially one causing symptoms
- toxic autonomously functioning thyroid nodule
- toxic multinodular goiter
- hyperthyroid children who cannot, or will not, take antithyroid drugs or radioactive iodine
- hyperthyroidism that cannot be controlled by either medications or radioactive iodine
- hyperthyroid adults who prefer surgery to either radioactive iodine or antithyroid drugs
- hyperthyroid pregnant women (preferably in their second trimester) who cannot tolerate antithyroid drugs
- patients with a family history of medullary thyroid cancer and a mutation of the RET proto-oncogene

The most common reasons for a thyroidectomy are possible and known thyroid cancer. There are other nonsurgical treatments for patients with goiters, toxic autonomously functioning thyroid nodules, toxic multinodular goiters, or hyperthyroidism. These alternative treatments are discussed in detail in the chapters dealing with each of those conditions.

Thyroidectomies during pregnancy are uncommon. When surgeons perform thyroidectomies on pregnant patients with Graves' disease, they prefer to do so during the second trimester for two reasons. First, the chances of a miscarriage caused by surgery are slightly less during the second trimester than during the first trimester. Second, the chances of premature labor caused by surgery are slightly less during the second

Thyroidectomies

Surgical Procedure	For a Patient with
lobectomy	a toxic thyroid nodule
lobectomy & isthmusectomy	a suspicious nodule a papillary cancer less than 1.5 cm
subtotal thyroidectomy	a typical papillary or follicular cancer a large goiter a toxic multinodular goiter Graves' disease
total thyroidectomy	an aggressive papillary or follicular cancer a Hürthle cell cancer a medullary cancer a small undifferentiated cancer

trimester than during the third trimester.

Patients may sometimes need diagnostic x-rays prior to surgery. Those patients who might have papillary or follicular thyroid cancer should avoid preoperative CAT scans or other diagnostic x-rays using iodinated dyes, if possible (see "Stuart's Story" on pages 303–306). The large amount of iodine given for these x-rays dilutes the small amount of radioactive iodine given for treatment of some patients with confirmed thyroid cancer. Treatment with radioactive iodine will, therefore, be delayed for six to twelve weeks until the body eliminates the excess iodine.

The Hospital Stay

Third parties in medicine (insurance companies, Medicare, Medicaid, HMOs, and PPOs) have shortened the hospital stay for thyroid surgery. Most patients are admitted to the hospital the morning of surgery rather than the night before. They are asked not to eat or drink anything starting the night before. Depending on the hospital's policies, preoperative tests are done either before or on the day of admission. An anesthesiologist, and possibly a medical student, intern, or resident will perform a physical examination. The patient will then go to the operating room, the recovery room, a hospital room, and finally home. The entire hospital stay may be as short as twenty-three to seventy-two hours.

What Happens During Surgery

After the patient is put to sleep, a three- to five-inch horizontal incision is made in the lower portion of the neck. A part or all of the thyroid gland is removed. This surgery may take from two to four hours.

A patient with a toxic autonomously functioning nodule who has chosen surgery usually has a lobectomy. A patient with a suspicious nodule typically has a lobectomy and isthmusectomy. Generally, a patient with a differentiated (papillary or follicular) thyroid cancer, Graves' hyperthyroidism, a toxic multinodular goiter, or a large goiter will have a subtotal, or near-total, thyroidectomy. For a low-risk patient with a papillary cancer less than 1.5 cm (centimeters) in diameter, the surgeon may choose to perform only a lobectomy or a lobectomy and isthmusectomy. The surgeon will ordinarily recommend a total thyroidectomy for a patient with medullary thyroid cancer, Hürthle cell cancer, or a small undifferentiated cancer.

If a thyroid cancer is found during surgery, the surgeon will look for and remove enlarged lymph nodes in the neck. Infrequently, the neck incision needs to be extended up toward one or both ears if there is extensive lymph node involvement. Years ago, surgeons performed radical neck dissections on patients with differentiated thyroid cancers that had spread to the lymph nodes. In this disfiguring operation, the surgeon removed neck muscles, veins, and nerves as well as enlarged lymph nodes. Today, modified radical neck dissection (thyroidectomy combined with the removal of only suspicious lymph nodes) is not disfiguring, and the outcome is as good as the outcome with a radical neck dissection.

Since surgery is the only treatment for medullary thyroid cancer, the initial surgery is more aggressive than the surgery for most papillary and follicular thyroid cancers. Surgery on a patient with medullary thyroid cancer includes removal of the lymph nodes in the nearby "central compartment" of the neck as well as a total thyroidectomy (see page 338). These lymph nodes are removed—even if they do not appear to be involved—since many patients with medullary thyroid cancer have undetected, microscopic lymph node involvement.

Frozen and Permanent Sections

During surgery on a patient with possible thyroid cancer, the suspicious nodule is sent to a pathologist for a frozen section. The specimen is frozen rapidly, sliced (sectioned), and prepared for viewing under the microscope while the surgeon (and the anesthetized patient) awaits the pathologist's report. Once the pathologist calls with his diagnosis, the surgeon decides upon the extent of surgery necessary for an optimal outcome.

After the surgery, the removed tissue can be sectioned and analyzed in a more meticulous fashion. It may take twenty-four to forty-eight hours to get a final report on these permanent sections. The permanent sections are more detailed and comprehensive than frozen sections and, occasionally, disclose a differentiated thyroid cancer—usually a follicular cancer—which was called benign or inconclusive on frozen section.

Papillary thyroid cancer, the most common thyroid cancer, is easily diagnosed because it appears so different from normal tissue. However, follicular cancer is sometimes difficult to diagnose. Cells from a follicular cancer are similar in appearance to those of a benign follicular tumor (adenoma) on fine needle aspiration biopsy. The distinction between a follicular cancer and a benign follicular adenoma may ultimately depend upon identification of invasion of either the blood vessels or the capsule of the thyroid nodule. Invasion indicates that the tumor is cancerous.

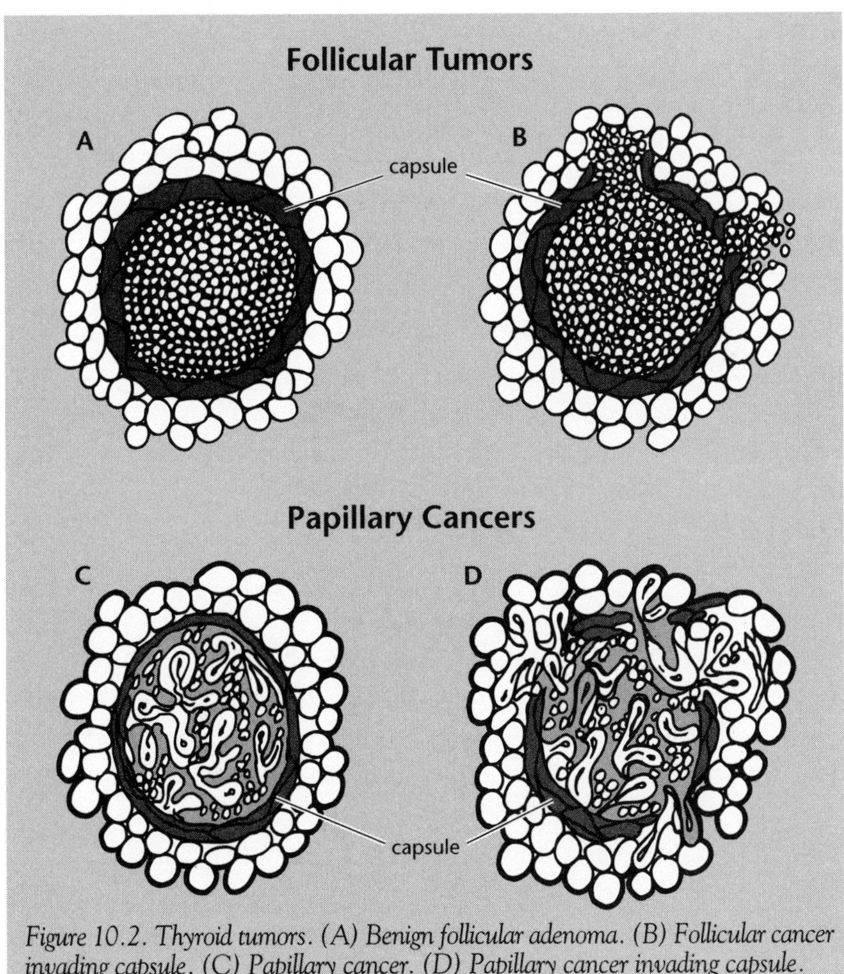

Figure 10.2. Thyroid tumors. (A) Benign follicular adenoma. (B) Follicular cancer invading capsule. (C) Papillary cancer. (D) Papillary cancer invading capsule.

Even when the pathologist examines the entire nodule on a frozen section, it may be difficult to identify invasion of either the blood vessels or the capsule of the nodule. Therefore, the pathologist may sometimes defer making a definitive diagnosis at the time of the frozen section. The surgeon, without the benefit of a frozen section diagnosis, then has to make a decision. Should he perform a subtotal thyroidectomy without a definitive diagnosis of cancer, or should he perform only a lobectomy and risk a second operation a few days later? Different surgeons will reach different conclusions at different times on different patients.

As previously mentioned, permanent sections are more revealing than frozen sections; therefore, permanent sections are more likely to identify invasion. When a thyroid cancer is diagnosed one to two days after the original operation, a patient who has had only a lobectomy may be advised to have a completion thyroidectomy. During a completion thyroidectomy, all or nearly all of the remaining thyroid tissue is removed.

After Surgery

Once the incision is closed, the patient is sent to the recovery room for observation until she wakes up. After she arrives in her hospital room, she may be served a meal. Most patients can get out of bed and have visitors the same day. A drain is often left in the operative site so that fluid does not accumulate under the skin; it is usually removed twenty-four to seventy-two hours after the surgery. If a subtotal or total thyroidectomy has been performed, a blood test for calcium may be done every six to twelve hours to be sure that there has been no damage to the parathyroid glands. (Parathyroid glands produce parathyroid hormone that controls the amount of calcium in the blood.) At the time of discharge, the patient is usually given pain medications, antibiotics, instructions about doctor appointments, and, when indicated, a prescription for levothyroxine.

The surgeon will recommend when a patient can return to work. Recovery time varies from patient to patient. A patient with a desk job usually can return to work one to two weeks after surgery; a patient with a physically demanding job may need to wait three or more weeks.

Complications of Thyroid Surgery

Infection or death rarely occurs as a complication of a thyroidectomy. A patient having a thyroidectomy does not usually require blood transfusions, so there is no need to worry about the transmission of AIDS or hepatitis.

A temporary drop in calcium (hypocalcemia) occurs frequently following a subtotal or total thyroidectomy. Hypocalcemia is due to reduced parathyroid hormone production (hypoparathyroidism) from injured parathyroid glands. A patient with mild hypocalcemia may experience numbness or tingling in the lips, arms, or legs. If the calcium level gets lower, a life-threatening spasm of the larynx can occur. Therefore, the patient is ordinarily given calcium by mouth or intravenously when numbness or tingling occurs. If the hypocalcemia persists for more than forty-eight to seventy-two hours, the patient may also be given Rocaltrol, a vitamin D preparation.

Hypocalcemia usually resolves in days or weeks. In less than 1% of patients, all four parathyroid glands are inadvertently removed or permanently damaged at the time of surgery. Some surgeons, in an effort to prevent permanent hypoparathyroidism, identify a parathyroid gland and transplant it into the patient's forearm at the time of the thyroidectomy. Untreated hypoparathyroidism can cause muscle spasms, convulsions, and cataracts. A lifetime of treatment with calcium and vitamin D is necessary in a patient with permanent hypoparathyroidism (see "Dick's Story" on pages 354–357).

The nerves that control the vocal cords (recurrent laryngeal nerves) are also near the thyroid gland. If one nerve is injured during a thyroidectomy, then the patient may have a hoarse and breathy voice, either temporarily or permanently (see "Estelita's Story" on pages 91–94). Permanent injury of one recurrent laryngeal nerve occurs in approximately 1% of patients. Permanent injury of both recurrent laryngeal nerves rarely occurs, but, when it does, the patient becomes hoarse and unable to breathe without a tracheostomy. Surgical treatment is available to patients with permanent injury to their recurrent laryngeal nerves, but it may be a difficult problem to correct.

Some patients worry about the appearance of the thyroidectomy scar. It is impossible to predict what the scar will look like, and it may take months for the redness to disappear and for the scar to heal completely. One patient made the following observation: "The scar is shown in its best light behind expensive jewelry, such as a necklace of pearls at least 13 millimeters in size, ideally purchased by a loving partner."

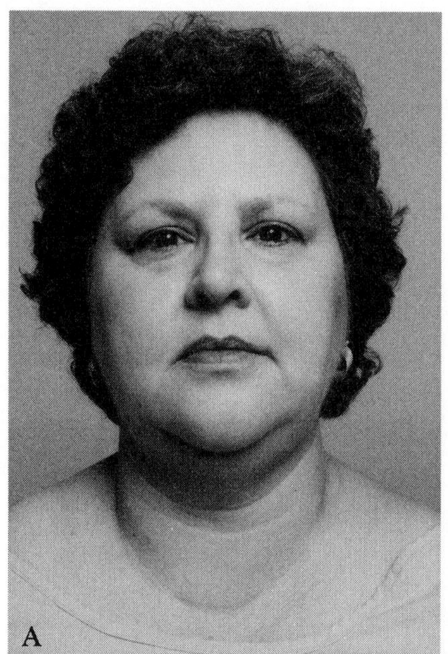

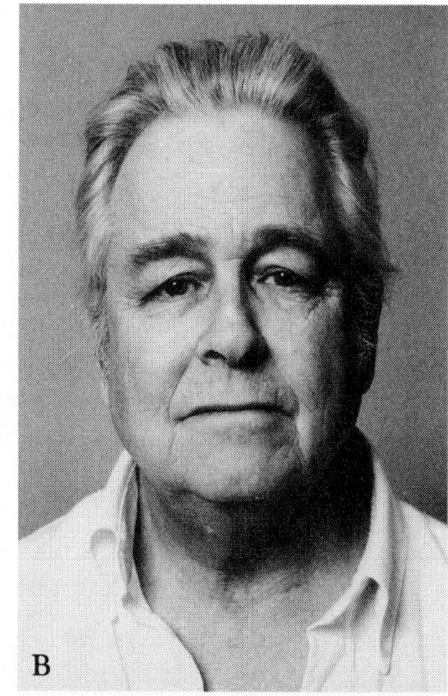

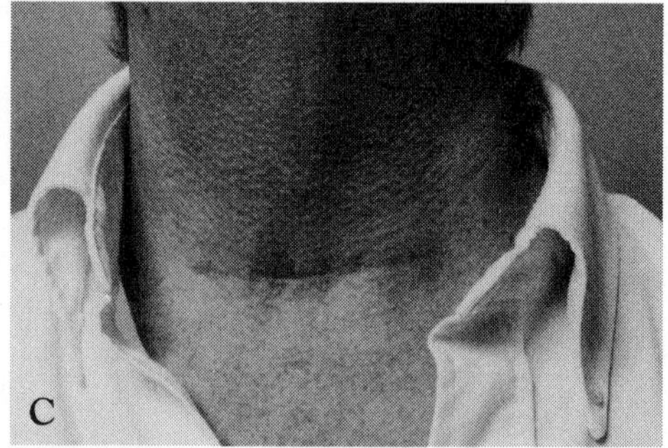

Figure 10.3. Thyroidectomy scars. (A) Patient with a sixteen-year-old scar. (B) Patient with a seven-week-old scar. (C) Close-up of the seven-week-old scar.

Postoperative Levothyroxine Treatment

Physicians will ordinarily recommend a lifetime of therapy with levothyroxine for patients who have had thyroidectomies for thyroid cancer. Many patients who have had thyroidectomies for other conditions will also take levothyroxine for one or more reasons. First, there may be too little thyroid tissue remaining to produce enough thyroid hormone. Second, levothyroxine may prevent the residual thyroid tissue from either enlarging or developing new nodules. The details of levothyroxine therapy are discussed in Chapter 6.

Patient Profiles

STUART'S STORY

In 1998, fifty-two-year-old Stuart was in a car accident and went to a neurosurgeon to treat the resulting neck pain. During the physical examination, his physician noticed that Stuart's thyroid gland was enlarged.

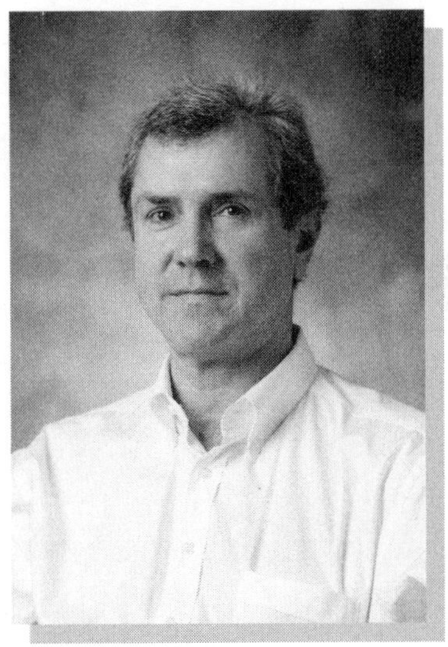

> I went to an [endocrinologist] who did a needle biopsy and put me on [levothyroxine]. The results of the biopsy were negative. He didn't really explain anything about nodules to me, and so I never really worried about it.
>
> I do have a niece who had thyroid cancer ten years ago, but she's doing fine. She has had two children since [she was diagnosed and treated]. I don't know what kind she had. No one else in the family has thyroid disease.

> Then [two years ago], my regular doctor stopped seeing patients, and I had to find another doctor. A friend of mine who has had thyroid cancer was seeing [an endocrinologist] and recommended him. So I went to him in November 2000.

When Stuart went to see the endocrinologist, he was taking 0.1 mg (milligrams) of levothyroxine once daily, as well as Dilantin, which had been prescribed to prevent seizures following a head injury. He was also taking a great deal of kelp. Both Dilantin and kelp can affect the results of thyroid function tests.

> [The endocrinologist] asked me to come back for [a scan and] an uptake in January, and he rebiopsied the nodule. The pathologist said that the results were suspicious.

The thyroid scan verified that Stuart had a large cold nodule, which was 7.5 cm long on an ultrasound. His endocrinologist recommended surgery.

> The same friend who referred me to [the endocrinologist] suggested I see his surgeon. I went to see him, and he said [the nodule] should be removed. The surgeon also ordered a CAT scan to better identify what was there.

Previously, Stuart's endocrinologist had advised him that a CAT scan was not a good idea, especially if his nodule turned out to be cancerous. The large amounts of iodinated dye used in a CAT scan could delay radioactive iodine treatment of differentiated thyroid cancer.

> I was not comfortable with this surgeon, so I kept an appointment I had already made with [another surgeon]. He had awards and pictures of famous people on his walls. I was more comfortable with him. I could tell he had more experience. We scheduled my surgery for March 15.

On March 15, Stuart's surgeon performed a lobectomy because a frozen section done during surgery showed only a "follicular lesion."

> The surgery went fine. I was a little uncomfortable, but that was mostly because I had to wait in the recovery room for about four hours before a room was available. I was released the next day because they thought the nodule was benign, but [my surgeon] explained that he wouldn't know for sure until the permanent sections came back.

The permanent section showed a minimally invasive follicular cancer and an occult 1.0-millimeter papillary cancer of the thyroid. His surgeon recommended a completion thyroidectomy.

> I got a call from my surgeon, and he said that he was sorry, but I would have to come back because he had to take out the other lobe. I went back within a few days for the second surgery. This experience was better than the first—I knew what to expect. I was more familiar with everything; I knew all the folks. I even recognized the anesthesiologist! I was in a private room quicker, and I wasn't as uncomfortable. I was released the next day.
>
> I went back a few days later for [my surgeon] to remove the bandage and then a few days after that for him to take out the drainage tube. Around the first of May, I had a [whole] body scan and then was put in isolation in the hospital for the radioactive iodine treatment. I stayed just one night. I drank plenty of water, and, by the next afternoon, the Geiger counter reading said that they could release me.

Fortunately, as it turned out, the large amount of iodinated dye given during the CAT scan in early January did not delay Stuart's radioactive iodine treatment. During the four months between the CAT scan and his radioactive iodine treatment, the excess iodine was eliminated from his body.

> I started taking 0.2 mg of [levothyroxine]. There was a gradual return of energy. My weight has stayed the same. Now, for the last three months, I've been going to the pool doing water aerobics for an hour, three times a week. I'm also getting back into yoga. All of this has helped my stamina.
>
> My wife even said that my schedule is better now that I'm taking levothyroxine regularly. I get up every morning and take it at 7:00 because I have to wait to take my Dilantin two hours later.
>
> [My surgeon] has been a jewel of a guy. I see him about every three months, and he feels around my neck. I will have another check-up with [my endocrinologist] in a couple of months and another [whole] body scan.
>
> I would tell people who have nodules that they should see a specialist as soon as possible. Friends' advice may be well intentioned, but it's not necessarily the best. It's good to get a second opinion. If you have any doubts whatsoever, seek another opinion and go no matter where it is—if it's the best. Go where you have the most confidence.

Stuart has done quite well since his surgeries and radioactive iodine therapy. In a few months, he will have a repeat whole body scan, which he hopes will be negative.■

JUDY'S STORY

Judy is a fifty-one-year-old thyroid cancer survivor and avid proponent of patient involvement. Unfortunately, she learned the importance of patient advocacy the hard way.

> My saga began in 1985, when I found a nodule in my thyroid. I was working with oncology patients at that time, so I was very alert to nodules.
>
> I had heard about [an endocrinologist] who was pioneering fine needle aspiration biopsy. It was considered advanced technology at the time. He did the biopsy, and the results showed cancerous cells. He referred me to a surgeon.
>
> At the time, I was married to a physician, and he preferred a friend of his, who was a general surgeon. I went to him, and he operated, but he didn't see anything, so he closed me back up. He didn't follow [my endocrinologist's] recommendation to rotate my thyroid to look for the nodule. I spent two or three days in the hospital.

Following surgery, Judy's surgeon wrote her endocrinologist and said, "The nodule in question was in fact a benign and normal lymph node." The surgeon also stated that he had biopsied two other small nodules in the area—one was normal fat, and the other was part of a healthy parathyroid gland.

> Later [my endocrinologist] talked to my husband and said I needed another operation. He was certain that I had cancer. I was so angry! Nobody believed him since fine needle biopsies were so new, and my surgeon didn't even look. I feel it was a good ole boy network in those days. They felt that they knew it all, but they didn't. They didn't listen to their patients.
>
> Six months after my first surgery, you could feel the nodule again, and I had another biopsy. This time I went to my endocrinologist's surgeon.

Although Judy's endocrinologist could feel the nodule again, the nodule was now above the isthmus of the thyroid gland, whereas it was below the isthmus when it first appeared. Her endocrinologist did another biopsy. The cells of the new nodule looked very similar to the cells from the first biopsy—suspicious.

While Judy was in surgery, the surgeon called her endocrinologist from the operating room to say that he could not find the nodule either. After the endocrinologist assured him that the nodule was there, the surgeon split her isthmus, and there it was, growing on a stalk from the back of her isthmus. Apparently, Judy had a "swinging" nodule—it was below the isthmus in the endocrinologist's office, behind the isthmus during the first surgery, above the isthmus when it reappeared, and behind the isthmus during the second surgery.

> This surgeon found it, and I had a complete thyroidectomy. I had papillary cancer mixed with follicular. I recovered from the surgery pretty fast. A month later, I had radioactive iodine treatment.
>
> The following year I went back for a scan, and they found remnant tissue. I had another radioactive iodine treatment. The worst part was going off thyroid medication before the scans. It is not fun. I had no energy—no reserve. I could work, but it took everything I had. But I knew it had a purpose and had an end, so I could handle it.
>
> I moved three years ago, and [my endocrinologist] referred me to an endocrinologist out here, but I had to go with [an HMO doctor]. My primary doctor didn't know anything about thyroid cancer, so I threw a fit. Now I'm allowed to see a specialist.
>
> Both my daughters now have enlarged thyroids. Both of them are on [levothyroxine]. My family history is sketchy, but I believe [thyroid disease] is genetic.

When asked if she had any advice for people in a similar situation, Judy had this to say:

> Go to a specialist. Trust your gut. Be your own best advocate. Tune into your body. Managed care pressures give doctors less time to spend with their patients. Don't give up until you get answers.

Despite Judy's unusual surgical history, she has done quite well and has remained free of cancer for more than fifteen years since her original diagnosis.■

LILIAN'S STORY

In 1953, Lilian had just given birth to her first son and was working as a nurse. When she started to lose weight, she assumed it was because she was busy trying to manage a career and family. She did not think anything was wrong until she returned from a vacation. A fellow nurse picked her up at the airport and commented on her appearance.

> She took one look at me and said, "You need to go to the doctor." I had lost weight, and my eyes were bulging. Looking back on it, I had all the symptoms. My throat was quite prominent, my pulse was very rapid, my hands were shaky, and I was very nervous. I ached constantly. I weighed about ninety-two pounds, but I was eating a lot. I should have put two and two together, but I didn't. I was just too busy.
>
> I realized that I probably had Graves' disease, so I went to a surgeon I knew. In those days, you went to surgery for Graves' disease. He did the surgery right away. I was in the hospital about a week. I did fine; the surgery went very well. I didn't have to take any [thyroid] medication at all; he left a very small amount of thyroid. I started gaining weight—back to where I had been before surgery. Gradually the symptoms went away; it wasn't overnight. I was just fine afterwards.

Forty-seven years later, Lilian went to see an internist for a complete physical.

> My children had been real worried; they kept after me to go to the doctor. Because my hands were shaking, my daughter thought I had Parkinson's disease.
>
> I knew something was wrong. I wasn't real sure, but I thought it was my thyroid. I had all the symptoms again. Right away [the internist] noticed how I looked. My eyes were just beginning to be prominent; my hands were shaky. I was eating like crazy but losing weight. I lost about twelve pounds; I went down to ninety-four pounds.
>
> [My internist] made the appointment for me with [an endocrinologist]. [The endocrinologist] did all the blood work, thyroid tests, ultrasound, and uptake.

The results of Lilian's diagnostic tests confirmed that she was hyperthyroid again—her thyroid gland, including her pyramidal lobe, had grown back during the forty-seven years since her thyroidectomy. Her endocrinologist recommended that she take radioactive iodine.

> He explained all the options to me and gave me [a book] to read. I had no hesitation; I followed his recommendation. I went to his office, and he gave me a capsule. When they brought it in, it was in a concrete canister. [The nurse] dropped it directly in my mouth. I thought I was going to glow in the dark! I didn't have any side effects from that at all. I didn't have to take any special precautions.

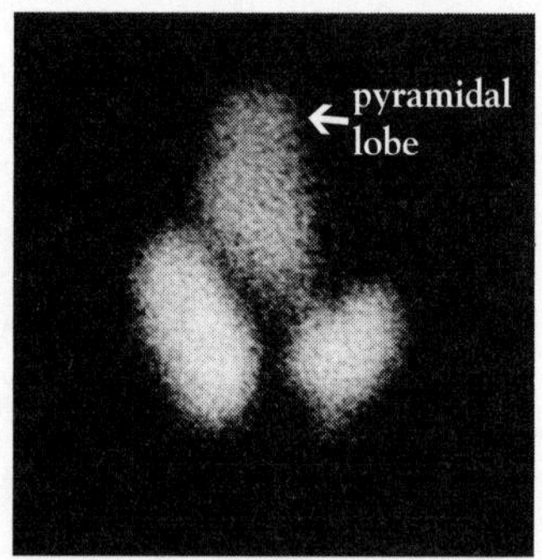

Lilian's thyroid scan showing that her thyroid gland, including her pyramidal lobe, had grown back since her thyroidectomy in 1953.

> I'd say it took about six weeks to stop shaking and for my goiter to start going down. I started to gain weight. It was just a few pounds at first, but now I'm up to 114 pounds, and I'm five feet tall! I'm going to have to buy an all new wardrobe. I wore a size six to eight for a while. Now I can't get into them. I'm an eight in some things; it just depends on how it's made.
>
> [My endocrinologist] put me on [levothyroxine] about a month after [the radioactive iodine]. It was a small dose. Then I didn't have to go back for three months. It was during that time when I gained the weight. I'm still hungry like I was before I was diagnosed. My appetite hasn't changed, so I'm gaining weight.
>
> The doctor suggested that I take up jogging, but I broke my leg three years ago, and they removed two inches out of my femur. I'm not in any pain; I just don't walk as well. I'm inclined to limp a little bit. I'm cutting down on what I eat. I just need to cut down on the calories I'm taking in. I don't want to get to the point I'm uncomfortable with my weight.

Lilian's experience demonstrates one complication of surgery for Graves' hyperthyroidism—recurrence. Since Lilian was still hypothyroid at her last check-up, her endocrinologist increased her levothyroxine dosage. She is expected to do well, without any more recurrences of her hyperthyroidism.■

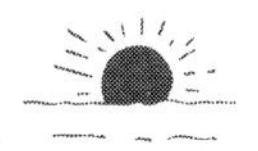

CHAPTER 11

WHAT IS THYROID CANCER?

Cancer is a scary word. Few words can evoke the sense of fear and panic that *cancer* does. Simply hearing the word can cause patients to react emotionally without evaluating the facts. Once patients learn the facts about thyroid cancer, they may be able to approach the diagnosis without undue fear and apprehension. Indeed, the outlook for most patients with thyroid cancer is excellent.

Each year more than 200,000 thyroid nodules—potential cancers—are discovered; however, only about 17,000 are actually cancerous. There are approximately 1,300 deaths per year from thyroid cancer, as compared to an estimated 40,000 from breast cancer and 31,000 from prostate cancer. It may be reassuring to know that most thyroid nodules are not cancerous and that patients with thyroid cancer are usually cured.

THYROID CANCER TERMINOLOGY

A thyroid nodule or growth that is noncancerous is described as benign; a cancerous growth is described as malignant. Another name for thyroid cancer arising from follicular or C cells (parafollicular cells) is thyroid carcinoma. Many thyroid cancers are contained within their capsules, the membranes around thyroid nodules. Some thyroid cancers break through their capsules but are contained within the thyroid gland. A thyroid cancer may also break through the thyroid gland and invade directly into surrounding structures, such as the windpipe (trachea) and esophagus.

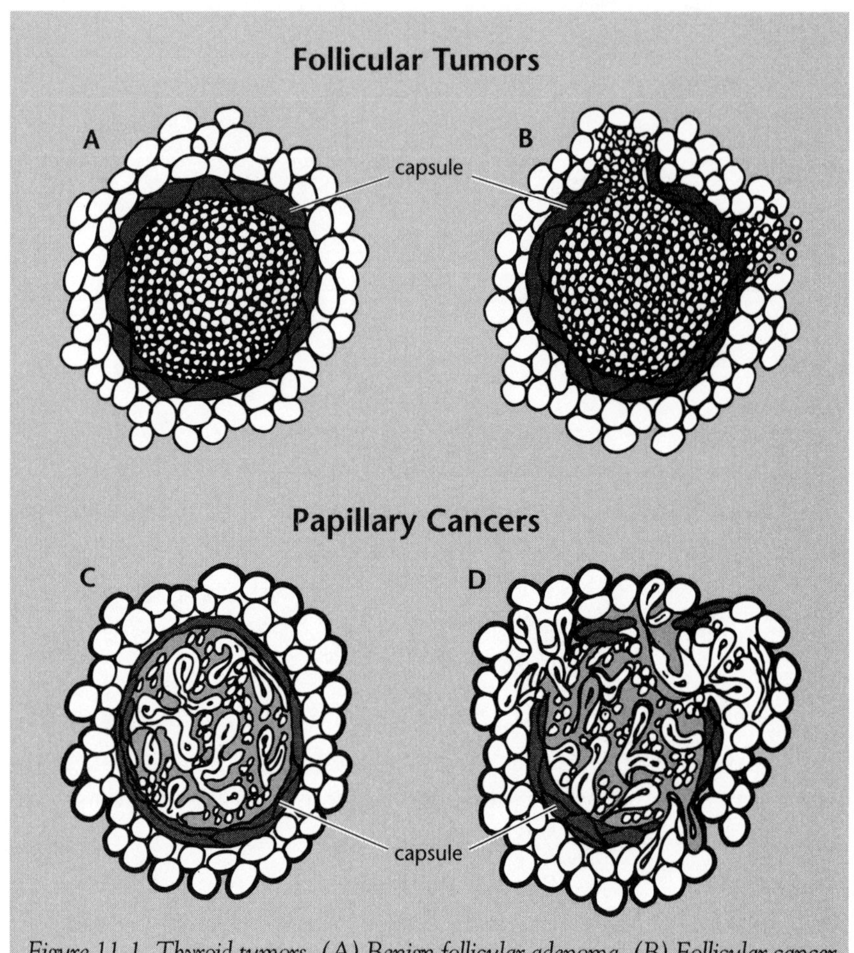

Figure 11.1. Thyroid tumors. (A) Benign follicular adenoma. (B) Follicular cancer invading capsule. (C) Papillary cancer. (D) Papillary cancer invading capsule.

Spread of thyroid cancer beyond the confines of the thyroid gland is called metastasis. One of the body's defenses against the spread of cancer is the lymphatic system, a collection of lymph nodes connected by vessels called lymphatics. Lymph nodes are glandular structures containing specialized white blood cells (lymphocytes) that are used to fight both cancer and infection. Thyroid cancer that spreads (metastasizes) through lymphatic channels is blocked from further spread by lymph nodes. In certain thyroid cancers, lymph node metastases in the neck indicate a less favorable outcome, or prognosis. In other thyroid cancers, the presence of lymph node metastases in the neck does not alter the prognosis. Cancers can also spread through the bloodstream to sites far away from the thyroid gland (distant metastases), such as the spine or the lungs. Distant metastases usually mean a less favorable prognosis.

When cells from a thyroid cancer look similar to normal thyroid follicular cells, the cancer is described as differentiated. The two types of differentiated thyroid cancers are papillary and follicular. When the cells from a thyroid cancer appear completely different from normal thyroid follicular cells, the cancer is referred to as undifferentiated (anaplastic). A differentiated thyroid cancer whose cells are recognizable as follicular cells, but barely so, may be described as poorly differentiated. Thyroid cancer arising from C cells is called medullary thyroid cancer (MTC).

Tumor markers are useful either for diagnosing cancer or for following patients with cancer. A tumor marker is a substance, usually a protein, that is ordinarily made only by the specific type of cell from which the cancer originates. For example, thyroglobulin is a protein made only by thyroid follicular cells and, therefore, it can be used as a tumor marker in patients with differentiated thyroid cancers. Once the cancerous thyroid gland has been removed, thyroglobulin should no longer be present. If it is, it could indicate recurrent cancer. Similarly, calcitonin, which is made by C cells, can be used as a tumor marker in patients with medullary thyroid cancer.

Types of Thyroid Cancer

The overwhelming majority of thyroid cancers are papillary cancers; the prognosis for patients with this type of thyroid cancer is usually excellent (see "Jerri Lynn's Story" on pages 341–345). Follicular cancer, the other type of differentiated thyroid cancer, occurs less commonly and may be somewhat more difficult to cure than papillary cancer. The names given to differentiated thyroid cancers by pathologists are sometimes confusing. For example, papillary-follicular cancer (also called follicular variant of papillary cancer) has elements that look like both papillary and follicular cancers. Fortunately, papillary-follicular cancer behaves the same as papillary cancer, which means it has a better prognosis

Thyroid Cancer in the United States	
Type of Thyroid Cancer	**% of All Thyroid Cancers**
papillary	70 – 80%
follicular, including Hürthle cell	10 – 15%
medullary	3 – 5%
undifferentiated (anaplastic)	2 – 5%
lymphoma	1 – 2%

than pure follicular cancer. "Pure" papillary cancers are uncommon; most thyroid cancers called "papillary" are actually papillary-follicular cancers. Hürthle cell cancer has a distinctive appearance under the microscope and is considered a somewhat more aggressive type of follicular cancer.

Medullary thyroid cancer makes hormones, such as calcitonin, by which it can sometimes be identified (see "Estelita's Story" on pages 91–94). Unlike papillary and follicular thyroid cancers, which are rarely familial (hereditary), medullary thyroid cancers sometimes run in families (see "Dick's Story" on pages 354–357).

Undifferentiated (anaplastic) thyroid cancers account for only a very small percentage of all thyroid cancers, and, fortunately, they are occurring less often than they did in the past. Anaplastic thyroid cancers appear most commonly during the seventh decade of life, more often in women than in men, and are almost always fatal.

The thyroid gland has lymphocytes and other cells found in all tissues in the body; cancers may arise in any of these cells. The most common of these uncommon cancers is lymphoma, cancer of the lymphocytes. Oncologists (cancer specialists) typically manage the treatment of patients with these rare forms of cancer. Since these cancers have very little in common with thyroid cancers, they will not be discussed further in this book.

People often assume that oncologists treat all patients with cancer. In fact, thyroidologists or endocrinologists, in conjunction with surgeons and nuclear medicine physicians, treat most patients with thyroid cancer.

Prognosis of Patients with Papillary or Follicular Thyroid Cancer

The outlook for patients with papillary or follicular thyroid cancer is very good. In general, patients with papillary cancer, the most common type of thyroid cancer, have a better prognosis than patients with follicular cancer have. With the appropriate treatment, more than 90% of all patients will be cured.

While cure rates have been determined for groups of patients with papillary or follicular thyroid cancer, it is nearly impossible to predict the outcome for an *individual* patient. Each person is unique (see "Melanie's Story" on pages 349–354). Nonetheless, medical scientists have made several attempts either to predict the prognosis of patients with differentiated thyroid cancers or to classify these patients into low- or high-risk categories.

A patient's prognosis is determined by multiple factors. The most important patient factor is age, although gender is also important. The most important characteristics of the cancer are size, type, extent of local invasion, and distant metastasis, although the number of tumors in the thyroid gland also influences the patient's prognosis. For example, the risk of a thirty-five-year-old woman dying from a papillary cancer smaller than 1.0 centimeter (occult thyroid cancer, or microcarcinoma) is very low. On the other hand, the risk of death is increased for a sixty-five-year-old male with a 5-cm (centimeter) follicular cancer that has extended beyond the thyroid gland.

A patient's prognosis determines, in large part, the extent of surgery and the follow-up treatment. For example, a thirty-five-year-old woman with a papillary cancer smaller than 1.5 cm may have only a lobectomy and isthmusectomy as opposed to a subtotal or total thyroidectomy since the prognosis for such a patient is excellent. On the other hand, a

Favorable Prognostic Factors for Patients with Differentiated Thyroid Cancers

age less than 45

tumor size less than or equal to 4 cm

papillary cancer, including follicular variant, with well-defined capsule

follicular cancer with minimal invasion of the capsule

absence of local invasion

absence of blood vessel invasion

absence of lymph node metatasis

absence of distant metastasis

single thyroid cancer

female gender

presence of Hashimoto's thyroiditis

sixty-five-year-old man with a 5-cm follicular cancer will have either a subtotal or total thyroidectomy followed by radioactive iodine. Once again, each patient must be treated individually, taking into account both the prognosis and the patient's personal preferences.

Although it would be ideal to classify a patient into either a low-risk or a high-risk category for the purposes of determining an accurate prognosis and the proper treatment, it is not always possible to do so. A low-risk patient with a high-risk cancer (for example, a thirty-five-year-old woman with a 5-cm follicular cancer and distant metastases) or a high-risk patient with a low-risk cancer (for example, a fifty-five-year-old man with a 3-cm papillary cancer without distant metastases) may fall into an intermediate-risk group. The outcome of this group is less favorable than the low-risk group but better than the high-risk group. When it is possible, classifying a patient into a risk group is useful in deciding how aggressive to be with surgery and other treatments.

Less Favorable Prognostic Factors for Patients with Differentiated Thyroid Cancers

- age 45 or greater
- tumor size greater than 4 cm
- papillary cancer with anaplastic transformation
- poorly differentiated follicular cancer
- tall-cell, columnar, or diffuse sclerosing variants of papillary cancer
- Hürthle cell type
- distant metastasis
- local invasion
- lymph node metastasis
- blood vessel invasion
- multiple papillary cancers (multifocal papillary cancer)
- insufficient surgery
- delay in therapy
- no levothyroxine therapy
- no radioactive iodine treatment in some patients
- male gender
- presence of Graves' disease

Treatment of Patients with Papillary or Follicular Thyroid Cancer

General Considerations

Some controversy exists in almost all areas of treatment of patients with differentiated thyroid cancers, but, hopefully, results from ongoing research will resolve many of these controversies. Patients with papillary or follicular thyroid cancer may receive the following treatments:

- surgery
- radioactive iodine (I^{131})
- levothyroxine
- external-beam radiation

Typical Treatment of a Patient with Differentiated Thyroid Cancer *	
Step 1	subtotal thyroidectomy treatment of transient hypocalcemia preparations for whole body scan
Step 2 *6 weeks after surgery*	physical examination blood tests for TSH, free T_4, and thyroglobulin thyroid ultrasound
Step 3 *1 or more days after Step 2*	whole body scan radioactive iodine (I^{131}) ablation thyroid hormone replacement with levothyroxine
Step 4 *5 to 7 days after I^{131} ablation*	post-treatment whole body scan
Step 5 *6 to 12 weeks after starting levothyroxine*	physical examination blood tests for TSH, free T_4, and thyroglobulin
Step 6 *8 to 12 months after I^{131} ablation*	follow-up tests additional treatment, if necessary

** does not apply to a patient treated with only a lobectomy*

The selection and the sequence of different treatments and follow-up tests may be confusing. Therefore, an overview of events following the diagnosis of papillary or follicular thyroid cancer may be helpful. The table on page 320 illustrates the steps in the typical treatment of a patient with differentiated thyroid cancer. It does not apply, however, to a patient treated with a lobectomy alone or to a patient with extensive local tumor invasion who requires external-beam radiation.

Surgery

Thyroidectomy, as discussed in Chapter 10, is the primary treatment for a patient with papillary or follicular thyroid cancer. The extent of thyroid surgery is determined by the characteristics of the patient and the cancer. For example, a thirty-five-year-old woman with a papillary cancer smaller than 1.5 cm may be treated with only a lobectomy and isthmusectomy. However, the same patient with a small papillary cancer that has spread to the lymph nodes in the neck will require a subtotal or total thyroidectomy. Subtotal or total thyroidectomy is also indicated for:

- a patient whose thyroid gland contains more than one papillary cancer (multifocal papillary cancer)
- a patient with a papillary cancer larger than 1.5 cm
- almost all patients with follicular cancer

In most patients with differentiated thyroid cancers, a subtotal rather than a total thyroidectomy is performed to avoid damaging all four parathyroid glands and both recurrent laryngeal nerves. The small amount of residual thyroid tissue can then be eliminated with radioactive iodine. A total thyroidectomy is generally reserved for a patient who has an aggressive follicular cancer, such as a Hürthle cell cancer, or an aggressive papillary cancer.

When cancer has spread to the lymph nodes in the neck, all apparently involved lymph nodes are removed. Adequate removal of a large number of involved lymph nodes sometimes requires extending the usual horizontal incision up toward one or both ears. In very unusual cases of extensive local invasion by an aggressive cancer, surgery may also include removal of part or all of the voice box (laryngectomy), creation of an opening in the windpipe (tracheostomy), removal of part of the esophagus, and reconstructive surgery. Fortunately, such extensive surgery is rarely necessary.

If the parathyroid glands are damaged during surgery, a patient may have low calcium (hypocalcemia). When this injury occurs, the patient may be treated with either oral or intravenous calcium, Rocaltrol (vitamin D), or both. The physician will see the patient within a week of discharge and as often as necessary until the patient's calcium level returns to normal.

Radioactive Iodine

Both a patient whose differentiated cancer has spread beyond the thyroid gland and a patient with multifocal papillary cancer are candidates for radioactive iodine (I^{131}) treatment. Many physicians believe that a patient who has had either a subtotal or a total thyroidectomy and whose cancer does not appear to have spread beyond the thyroid gland is also a candidate for radioactive iodine treatment. It is thought that radioactive iodine further reduces cancer recurrence in such a patient by destroying microscopic cancer within the thyroid remnant (the thyroid tissue remaining after a subtotal thyroidectomy).

While Hürthle cell cancers arise from follicular cells, they do not all share the characteristics of typical differentiated thyroid cancers. For example, 50 to 65% of Hürthle cell cancers do not take up radioactive iodine. Therefore, only 35 to 50% of patients with Hürthle cell cancer are candidates for radioactive iodine treatment.

Pregnant or breastfeeding women should not take radioactive iodine.

A patient who is a candidate for radioactive iodine treatment will have a whole body scan, usually six weeks after surgery. A whole body scan is obtained after administering a scanning dose of radioactive iodine. This scan consists of images of the "thyroid bed" (the area from which the thyroid gland was removed) and other parts of the body to which cancerous thyroid cells may have spread, such as the lungs, lymph

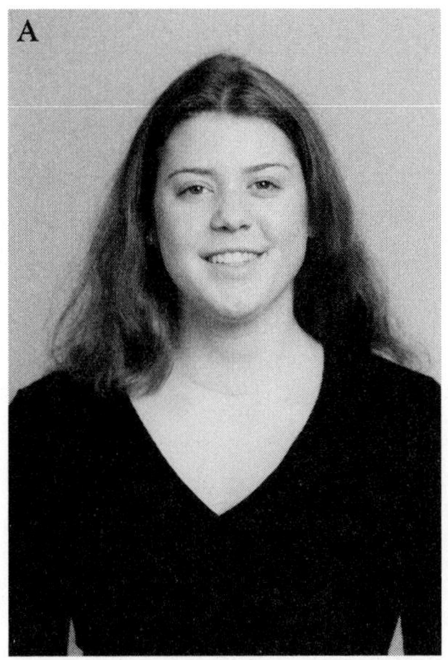

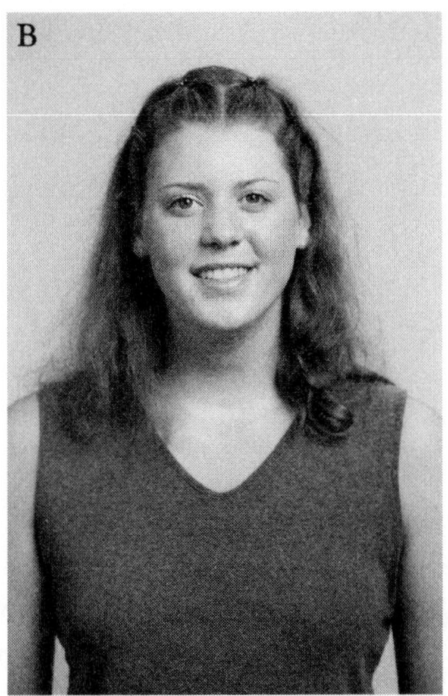

Figure 11.2. Thyroid cancer patient. (A) Hypothyroid six weeks after her thyroidectomy and the day after radioactive iodine therapy. Note the puffiness in her face. (B) Euthyroid after taking levothyroxine.

nodes in the neck, and bones.

A patient who will have a whole body scan is sent home after surgery without levothyroxine in order to elevate her TSH (thyroid-stimulating hormone). An elevated TSH is necessary for the uptake of radioactive iodine by any residual normal or cancerous thyroid tissue. The sequence of events leading to radioactive iodine uptake is:

surgery

↓

thyroid hormone deficiency

↓

increased TSH production

↓

stimulation of radioactive iodine uptake

Since most patients will become hypothyroid without levothyroxine during the six weeks between surgery and the whole body scan, they may take short-lived Cytomel (T_3) to reduce symptoms during the first four weeks. Eliminating Cytomel during the last two weeks allows the TSH to rise. The physician may also ask the patient to follow a low-iodine diet, consisting of a reduction of iodized salt, dairy products, eggs, and seafood for two to three weeks before the whole body scan. A low-iodine diet enhances radioactive iodine uptake by normal and cancerous thyroid tissue.

Six weeks after surgery, the physician will examine the patient and draw blood for TSH, free T_4, and thyroglobulin (Tg). The patient may also have a thyroid ultrasound to see if there are any abnormal lymph nodes in the neck and, sometimes, have a chest x-ray to look for spread of the cancer to the lungs. If any abnormalities are found, the patient may have additional x-ray studies, such as an MRI of the neck or chest, prior to the whole body scan to determine the extent of the spread of the cancer. Diagnostic x-ray procedures using iodinated dyes, such as CAT scans, should be avoided during this period. The large amount of iodine given for these x-ray procedure dilutes the small amount of radioactive iodine given for the whole body scan, making interpretation of the scan difficult.

If the TSH level is elevated to above 25 or 30 mU/L (milliunits per liter), the patient can proceed with a whole body scan. A patient having a whole body scan will take a scanning dose of one to five millicuries of radioactive iodine, go home, and return forty-eight to seventy-two hours later for the scan. The radioactive iodine will "light up" any residual normal or cancerous thyroid tissue so that it is visible on the whole body scan.

If any areas light up, the patient is usually admitted to the hospital for a treatment dose (ablative dose) of radioactive iodine large enough to destroy (ablate) any residual normal or cancerous thyroid tissue. Most patients are hospitalized in private rooms, and precautions are taken to protect hospital personnel, visitors, and future occupants of the room from radioactivity. For a patient perspective on radioactive iodine treatment, read "Rhonda's Story" on pages 31–34, "Jerri Lynn's Story" on pages 341–345, and "Lisa's Story" on pages 345–349.

There is no consensus on the correct ablative dose of radioactive

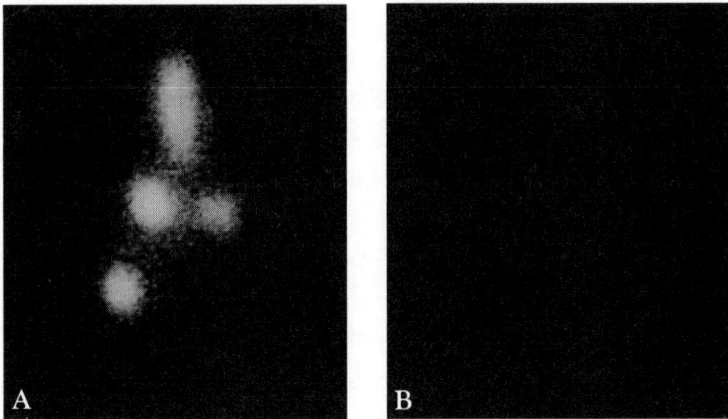

Figure 11.3. Images of patient with papillary thyroid cancer treated with surgery. (A) Before radioactive iodine treatment, residual tissue "lights up." (B) Eight months after radioactive iodine treatment, the repeat scan is negative—all residual tissue is gone.

iodine. Typically, an ablative dose is fixed at 100 to 200 millicuries of I^{131}. Some physicians advise selected low-risk patients to take doses as low as thirty millicuries, which may be administered on an outpatient basis in some states. Other physicians advocate the determination of the I^{131} dose based upon a calculation of the radiation delivered to cancer cells (dosimetry), especially in patients with distant metastases. However, dosimetry requires specialized equipment, technical support, and software.

Since radioactive iodine is eliminated primarily in the urine, drinking plenty of fluids helps to flush it out of the body. Once the level of radioactivity has been reduced to a safe range, usually within twenty-four to forty-eight hours, the patient is discharged from the hospital. Two to seven days after radioactive iodine treatment, the patient will have a post-treatment whole body scan in order to detect cancerous tissue that may become apparent only after the large treatment dose of radioactive iodine.

There are few side effects from a single ablative dose of radioactive iodine. Some patients, especially those receiving high doses of radioactive iodine, may need drugs to control nausea. A patient who has a large thyroid remnant may experience a brief period of pain and tenderness in the neck (radiation-induced thyroiditis) from inflammation of the residual thyroid tissue. Tongue pain or a decreased sense of taste may also occur briefly. In a few patients, radiation-induced salivary gland dysfunction may cause acute or chronic symptoms, such as pain or dry mouth. Chewing gum or sucking on hard, tart, lemon candies for several days may prevent these complications by stimulating salivary flow. A patient should begin these preventive measures shortly before taking radioactive iodine. If acute inflammation of either the neck or the salivary glands occurs, it usually responds to nonsteroidal anti-inflammatory drugs, such as Motrin or Advil.

Some patients have concerns about leukemia or other cancers, infertility, and genetic defects following radioactive iodine therapy. However, there is no conclusive evidence of an increased risk of any of these following a single dose of radioactive iodine. Nonetheless, after radioactive iodine treatment, it is prudent for a woman to avoid becoming pregnant until she is no longer hypothyroid—approximately six months.

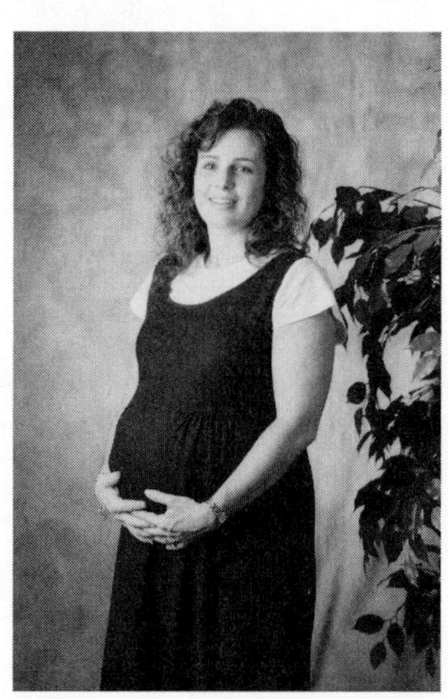

Figure 11.4. Successfully treated thyroid cancer patient, pregnant with her second baby since thyroid surgery and radioactive iodine treatment.

The miscarriage rate may be higher than expected in the first year after a thyroidectomy for cancer and even higher in a patient who is subsequently treated with more than 100 millicuries of radioactive iodine. A woman with thyroid cancer who is treated with radioactive iodine may experience menopause up to one-and-a-half years earlier than she would have without radioactive iodine treatment.

Nuclear medicine physicians often perform the whole body scans. In addition, they usually supervise the treatment of hospitalized patients receiving radioactive iodine. They can answer any additional questions that may arise about the specifics of this therapy.

Levothyroxine

Almost all patients with papillary or follicular thyroid cancer require a lifetime of levothyroxine therapy, which is discussed in Chapter 6. The physician will prescribe levothyroxine immediately after surgery for a patient who is not preparing for a whole body scan. A patient who has radioactive iodine treatment may start taking levothyroxine as early as a day after taking radioactive iodine. The dose of levothyroxine is relatively high for thyroid cancer patients compared to other hypothyroid patients because there is no residual thyroid gland function following a thyroidectomy and radioactive iodine treatment.

The physician will recommend the highest possible dose of levothyroxine that can be safely administered in order to suppress TSH secretion. Suppression of TSH is recommended because TSH stimulates growth of differentiated thyroid cancers. On the other hand, excessive levothyroxine therapy can cause complications, such as osteoporosis and heart rhythm disturbances. Therefore, before selecting a dosage, the prescribing physician will take into account the aggressiveness of the patient's thyroid cancer as well as the patient's risk factors for complications from excessive levothyroxine.

Ordinarily, a physician re-evaluates the patient approximately six to twelve weeks after starting treatment with levothyroxine. At this time, a patient will have a physical examination, blood work to measure TSH, free T_4, and thyroglobulin, and, possibly, a TRH (thyrotropin-releasing hormone) test to confirm adequate TSH suppression. If the dosage of levothyroxine needs adjustment, then the patient will return at six- to twelve-week intervals until the correct dosage is established.

External-Beam Radiation

External-beam radiation, radiotherapy from a source outside the body, is sometimes used in the initial treatment of patients with thyroid cancer. This type of radiation therapy is especially useful in two situations. First, when an aggressive cancer has invaded some structures next to the thyroid gland, external-beam radiation might prevent further spread of the cancer. Second, external-beam radiation can be useful to treat distant metastases to parts of the body from which the cancer cannot be completely removed by surgery. For example, external-beam radiation may prevent fractures and provide pain relief from bone metastases. Similarly, external-beam radiation can shrink brain metastases.

Goal of Treatment of Patients with Papillary or Follicular Thyroid Cancer

The goal of treatment of most patients with differentiated thyroid cancers is the elimination of all thyroid tissue, benign or malignant. (This goal is not applicable to patients who have been treated with lobectomy only.) Successful treatment can be characterized by the following results:

- no symptoms suggestive of recurrent thyroid cancer
- no evidence of thyroid cancer on the physical examination
- a thyroglobulin of less than 1 to 2 ng/ml (nanograms per milliliter) while the patient is taking enough levothyroxine to suppress TSH
- no rise of thyroglobulin in response to TSH stimulation
- no evidence of radioactive iodine uptake on a whole body scan
- no evidence of thyroid cancer on any diagnostic x-ray, ultrasound, or PET scan

Careful follow-up of patients with differentiated thyroid cancers is required to be certain that these results have been achieved.

Follow-Up of Patients with Papillary or Follicular Thyroid Cancer

General Considerations

Broadly speaking, the objectives of follow-up after the initial treatment of most patients with differentiated thyroid cancers are to confirm the absence of any residual thyroid tissue; to confirm the presence or absence of any recurrent thyroid cancer; and to treat recurrences, if necessary. Again, these objectives are not applicable to a patient who has been treated with only a lobectomy. The absence of all thyroid tissue increases a physician's ability to track the status of a thyroid cancer patient after the initial treatment. If there is any residual thyroid tissue in the thyroid bed after a subtotal thyroidectomy and radioactive iodine treatment, it may not be possible to distinguish between residual normal thyroid tissue and residual or recurrent thyroid cancer. On the other hand, if all normal thyroid tissue and all cancerous thyroid tissue have been eliminated from the thyroid bed, then anything that lights up on future scans is likely to be a recurrence.

Even though most recurrences of papillary and follicular cancers appear within the first five years after initial treatment, thyroid cancer sometimes recurs decades later (see "Joan's Story" on pages 360–364). Therefore, a patient must return regularly, over a long period of time, to the physician for follow-up visits. The physician identifies residual or recurrent cancer by the medical history, physical examination, blood tests such as thyroglobulin, whole body scans, and other diagnostic procedures, such as ultrasounds, MRIs, CAT scans, and PET scans.

After the initial postoperative evaluation, a patient who has had only a lobectomy will see the physician at yearly intervals. During these visits, the patient may have only a medical history, physical examination, blood work and, possibly, a thyroid ultrasound. On the other hand, the follow-up of a patient who has had a subtotal thyroidectomy and radioactive iodine treatment is more complicated. For example, not only will the patient require whole body scans, but the frequency and the type of whole body scan may depend upon whether the patient is classified as low-risk or high-risk. Using the criteria noted in the tables on pages 318 and 319, a patient with a favorable prognosis is classified as low-risk; a patient with a less favorable prognosis is classified as high-risk. In addition, a patient who has had a subtotal thyroidectomy and radioactive iodine treatment will have regular thyroglobulin measurements to detect cancer recurrence.

Thyroglobulin as a Tumor Marker

The relationship between thyroglobulin and differentiated thyroid cancer is an important one. Only thyroid cells produce thyroglobulin; therefore, an elevated thyroglobulin after a thyroidectomy and successful radioactive iodine ablation of all residual thyroid tissue may indicate recurrence of thyroid cancer. Therefore, thyroglobulin can serve as a tumor marker and may be helpful in making treatment decisions about a patient with papillary or follicular thyroid cancer.

Thyroglobulin can be measured either while a patient is taking enough levothyroxine to suppress TSH or while a patient has an elevated TSH level. After a thyroidectomy and successful radioactive iodine ablation of all residual thyroid tissue, a patient taking sufficient levothyroxine to suppress TSH should have a very low thyroglobulin, less than 1 to 2 ng/ml. A higher thyroglobulin level suggests the presence of recurrent thyroid cancer.

To prepare for a follow-up whole body scan, a patient taking levothyroxine who has a thyroglobulin of less than 2 ng/ml may be asked either to stop taking levothyroxine or to take synthetic TSH (Thyrogen). Either way, TSH will rise and stimulate thyroglobulin production. The TSH-stimulated thyroglobulin is a more sensitive indicator of recurrent thyroid cancer than a thyroglobulin measured while a patient's TSH is suppressed. If thyroglobulin rises from less than 2 ng/ml to more than 10 ng/ml after TSH stimulation, it is very suggestive of recurrent thyroid cancer.

There are, however, several problems that limit the usefulness of thyroglobulin measurements. First, there is no universal agreement among physicians regarding the interpretation of thyroglobulin measurements. Second, thyroglobulin cannot be measured in all patients with differentiated thyroid cancers. For example, a small percentage of papillary and follicular cancers fail to produce any thyroglobulin at all, and some papillary and follicular cancers that once made thyroglobulin will stop producing it.

Another problem with the measurement of thyroglobulin is the presence of thyroglobulin antibodies (TgAb). These antibodies, unfortunately, are present in up to 25% of patients with papillary or follicular cancer. Since thyroglobulin antibodies interfere with currently available tests for thyroglobulin, the usefulness of thyroglobulin in patients with TgAb is limited. Hopefully, either new methods of evaluating thyroglobulin or a thyroglobulin test that is independent of thyroglobulin antibodies will be available soon.

Not all laboratories provide a consistently reliable thyroglobulin measurement. Furthermore, when a patient moves or switches insurance plans, the new physician may use a different laboratory. Comparing thyroglobulin measurements from different laboratories may be more difficult than comparing thyroglobulin measurements from the same laboratory.

Withdrawal Scan

In order to evaluate the result of treatment with radioactive iodine, the physician will ask a patient to have another whole body scan eight to twelve months later. In most cases, the initial treatment with radioactive iodine will have destroyed all normal and cancerous thyroid tissue so that nothing lights up on the repeat scan. As mentioned above, the absence of all thyroid tissue increases a physician's ability to track the status of a thyroid cancer patient after the initial treatment. If all normal and cancerous thyroid tissue have been eliminated, then anything that lights up on future scans is likely to be a recurrence.

There are two ways to prepare for the second whole body scan—levothyroxine withdrawal and injections of synthetic TSH (Thyrogen). A patient preparing for a withdrawal scan will be asked to discontinue levothyroxine approximately six weeks before the scan. The physician may also ask the patient to follow a low-iodine diet, consisting of a reduction in the consumption of iodized salt, dairy products, eggs, and seafood for two to three weeks before the scan. A low-iodine diet enhances radioactive iodine uptake by normal and cancerous thyroid tissue. The physician will examine the patient, draw blood for TSH, free T_4, and thyroglobulin, and, possibly, perform a thyroid ultrasound the day before the scan is to begin.

The goal of preparation is to elevate the TSH above 25 or 30 mU/L. As noted above, TSH stimulates the growth of any residual normal or cancerous thyroid tissue so that it will be visible on the scan.

Because patients develop symptoms of hypothyroidism while preparing for withdrawal scans, they understandably dislike the process. Therefore, a patient is ordinarily given short-lived Cytomel (T_3) for the first four weeks after discontinuing levothyroxine. Nonetheless, the patient may become quite hypothyroid in the two weeks prior to the scan. Furthermore, the patient remains hypothyroid for several weeks after the scan, despite resuming levothyroxine therapy. Therefore, some physicians may give patients both Cytomel and levothyroxine for the first few weeks following the scan.

Thyrogen® Scan

As noted above, patients object to becoming hypothyroid while preparing for their withdrawal scans. Therefore, in the past, some physicians injected their patients with bovine (cow) TSH to increase their TSH rather than withdrawing their levothyroxine. While bovine TSH was effective in stimulating thyroid tissue, it frequently caused severe allergic reactions.

The development of synthetic TSH—also called thyrotropin-alfa, recombinant human TSH (rhTSH), or Thyrogen—has greatly improved the quality of life for many patients with differentiated thyroid cancers. The principle behind using Thyrogen is the same as that for using bovine TSH—elevating a patient's TSH without producing symptoms of hypothyroidism. Unlike bovine TSH, Thyrogen rarely causes allergic reactions and is now widely used in the follow-up of many patients with differentiated thyroid cancers. Although Thyrogen rarely causes allergic reactions, it can cause side effects. Studies indicate that 10% of patients experience nausea and 7% have headaches. Less common symptoms include weakness, vomiting, dizziness, numbness, chills, and fever.

After following a low-iodine diet, a patient is given an intramuscular injection of Thyrogen on two consecutive days, usually on a

Monday and Tuesday. The patient takes a scanning dose of radioactive iodine—preferably four millicuries of I^{131}—on Wednesday and has a whole body scan on Friday. Blood for TSH measurement is drawn on Tuesday or Wednesday and, sometimes, on Friday as well. On Friday, the physician will examine the patient, draw blood for thyroglobulin, and, possibly, perform a thyroid ultrasound before the patient completes the scan that day.

Withdrawal vs. Thyrogen® Scan

The advantage of Thyrogen scans is that the patient can remain on levothyroxine and, therefore, does not become hypothyroid. A disadvantage of Thyrogen scans is that a patient requiring radioactive iodine treatment cannot have it immediately following the scan because, as yet, there is no generally accepted and FDA-approved procedure (protocol) for this purpose. Therefore, if something lights up on the Thyrogen scan, the patient has to discontinue levothyroxine for six weeks before returning for radioactive iodine treatment. This disadvantage may be eliminated if current research leads to effective protocols for treating patients with radioactive iodine shortly after Thyrogen administration.

Understandably, patients prefer Thyrogen scans to withdrawal scans (see "Christine's Story" on pages 357–360). However, not all patients are candidates for Thyrogen scans. For example, a patient on levothyroxine with a suppressed TSH and a thyroglobulin above 5 ng/ml ordinarily is not a candidate for Thyrogen-stimulated diagnostic testing. Similarly, a patient with other evidence of recurrent thyroid cancer generally is not tested with Thyrogen. Both patients are likely to be retreated with radioactive iodine, which, as noted above, currently cannot be given immediately after Thyrogen administration.

Patients who will be considered for Thyrogen-stimulated diagnostic testing include those with:

- a reasonable expectation that all normal thyroid tissue has been ablated by surgery and radioactive iodine treatment
- a low risk of recurrent thyroid cancer

- a high risk of recurrent thyroid cancer and at least one negative withdrawal scan
- an inability to produce TSH because of pituitary or hypothalamic dysfunction
- thyroglobulin antibodies and one negative withdrawal scan
- an unwillingness to discontinue levothyroxine for a withdrawal scan
- the presence of medical conditions that could be seriously worsened by hypothyroidism

Regardless of the type of whole body scan performed, most patients will have a "negative" scan (a scan with no evidence of residual thyroid tissue or recurrent thyroid cancer) after a subtotal thyroidectomy and radioactive iodine treatment. Those patients who have "positive" scans (scans with evidence of residual thyroid tissue or recurrent thyroid cancer) will need additional treatment.

Treatment of Patients with Residual Thyroid Tissue or Recurrent Papillary or Follicular Thyroid Cancer

Hopefully, the results of all of the follow-up tests will confirm the absence of any residual thyroid tissue or recurrent thyroid cancer. If they do, then no further treatment is necessary other than resuming or continuing levothyroxine. However, a patient with evidence of residual thyroid tissue or recurrent thyroid cancer may need additional treatment.

A patient with residual thyroid tissue in the thyroid bed only or recurrent thyroid cancer confined to the thyroid bed, the neck, or the lungs on the whole body scan is admitted to the hospital for a second treatment with radioactive iodine (see "Rhonda's Story" on pages 31–34). On the other hand, a patient with other recurrences may require surgery or external-beam radiation as well as additional radioactive iodine treatment. For example, a patient with a palpable lymph node in her neck may have surgical removal of the lymph node followed by a withdrawal scan and, if necessary, another radioactive iodine treatment. If there is evidence of thyroid cancer metastases that may respond to external-beam radiation, such as metastases to the brain or bone, the physician will order this treatment as well (see "Melanie's Story" on pages 349–354).

Physicians have different opinions regarding the proper treatment dose of radioactive iodine for patients with residual thyroid tissue or recurrent papillary and follicular thyroid cancers. Some doctors advocate a fixed treatment dose of I^{131}, while others advocate the determination of the I^{131} dose based upon a calculation of the radiation delivered to cancer cells (dosimetry). Although dosimetry requires specialized equipment, technical support, and software, it may be particularly useful in patients with distant metastases.

Patients who have multiple radioactive iodine treatments for residual thyroid tissue or recurrent thyroid cancer may face additional risks. There may be a very small increased risk of leukemia, bladder or colon cancer, or infertility in both male and female patients who receive more than 500 millicuries of radioactive iodine during the course of multiple treatments. Therefore, if a physician anticipates that a young man may require high doses of radioactive iodine, he may suggest that the patient consider sperm banking. Scarring or fibrosis of the lungs may occur in patients who are given multiple large doses of radioactive iodine to treat thyroid cancer that has spread to the lungs. Finally, some patients may experience acute swelling or hemorrhage of metastases following treatment with a large dose of radioactive iodine. If the residual cancer is located in an area with very little room for enlargement of the tumor, such as the brain, spinal cord, or airway, serious complications may occur.

Follow-up of Patients with Residual Thyroid Tissue or Recurrent Papillary or Follicular Thyroid Cancer

If patients have had treatment of residual thyroid tissue or of recurrent differentiated thyroid cancers, their physicians may order additional whole body scans every eight to twelve months until one or two whole body scans are negative. Unfortunately, there is no consensus regarding the frequency of follow-up scans after one negative scan. In the past, physicians often refrained from frequent follow-up withdrawal scans because of low recurrence rates and because patients complained about being hypothyroid. However, since symptoms of hypothyroidism do not occur during Thyrogen scans, physicians and their patients may be inclined to do more frequent follow-up scans than they would have before Thyrogen became available.

While some follow-up scans are necessary to detect recurrences, too many scans can create problems. The recurrence rate for thyroid cancer in low-risk patients five years after surgery and radioactive iodine treatment is very low; the risk of false-positive scans and false-positive thyroglobulin elevations is also very low. However, the more Thyrogen scans patients have, the more likely they are to have false-positive results. Therefore, the risk of unwarranted patient anxiety and unnecessary tests increases with each additional Thyrogen scan.

Another controversy that sometimes arises is the proper treatment of patients with negative whole body scans and elevated thyroglobulin levels, with or without TSH stimulation. Hopefully, ongoing research will determine the best treatment for these patients, as well as how often thyroid cancer patients should have follow-up Thyrogen-stimulated diagnostic testing. Meanwhile, each patient's treatment must be individualized.

Chemotherapy

Occasionally, differentiated thyroid cancer, especially poorly differentiated thyroid cancer, progresses in spite of surgery, radioactive iodine treatment, and external-beam radiation. When progression occurs, a few patients may temporarily benefit from chemotherapy. Oncologists, or cancer specialists, usually supervise chemotherapy treatments.

Evaluation and Treatment of Patients with Medullary Thyroid Cancer

Medullary thyroid cancers account for less than 5% of all thyroid cancers. Medullary thyroid cancer arises from the C cells (parafollicular cells) of the thyroid gland, and is usually associated with excessive secretion of calcitonin. Calcitonin and, sometimes, carcinoembryonic antigen (CEA), can be used as tumor markers for medullary thyroid cancer, much as thyroglobulin is used as a tumor marker for differentiated thyroid cancer. Since medullary thyroid cancer arises from C cells, and not follicular cells, medullary thyroid cancer does not make thyroglobulin, take up radioactive iodine, or respond to changes in TSH.

Up to 25% of all medullary thyroid cancers are hereditary as opposed to sporadic (non-hereditary). When medullary thyroid cancers are hereditary, they may occur as part of three different types of multiple endocrine neoplasia type 2 (MEN 2)—MEN 2A, MEN 2B, or familial medullary thyroid cancer. MEN 2A, the more common form, is characterized by medullary thyroid cancer, one or more tumors of the adrenal glands called pheochromocytomas, and tumors of the parathyroid glands that can cause hyperparathyroidism, resulting in hypercalcemia. The less common MEN 2B is characterized by medullary thyroid cancer, one or more pheochromocytomas, and ganglioneuromatoses, which may include distinctive tumors located in the tongue, eyes, and gastrointestinal tract. Familial medullary thyroid cancer is considered a variation of MEN 2A (see "Dick's Story" on pages 354–357).

It is important to identify patients with hereditary medullary cancer since their evaluation and treatment will be more complicated than the evaluation and treatment of patients with sporadic medullary cancer. Physicians suspect that patients have MEN 2 when they have family histories of medullary thyroid cancer, pheochromocytoma, hyperparathyroidism, or ganglioneuromatoses. The diagnosis of MEN 2 is confirmed with a genetic test called the RET proto-oncogene and, in general, all patients with medullary thyroid cancer will have this test.

The treatment of a patient with medullary thyroid cancer is surgery, but the preoperative evaluation differs for a patient with a sporadic medullary thyroid cancer as compared to a patient with MEN 2. Both sporadic and hereditary medullary thyroid cancers often spread to the lymph nodes, chest, and liver. Therefore, the preoperative evaluation of all patients with medullary thyroid cancer might include an ultrasound or CAT scan of the neck as well as a chest x-ray or CAT scan of the chest and upper abdomen. A patient with MEN 2 will have additional tests for both pheochromocytoma and hyperparathyroidism. The preoperative identification of a patient with MEN 2 who also has a pheochromocytoma is important because it is dangerous to operate on a patient with an untreated pheochromocytoma. The preoperative identification of a patient with MEN 2 who has parathyroid tumors is also important since these tumors can be removed at the same time as the thyroid gland.

The initial surgery on a patient with medullary thyroid cancer is more extensive than on a patient with differentiated thyroid cancer. The reasons for more aggressive surgery are:

- surgery is the only treatment that can cure the patient
- radioactive iodine and thyroid hormone are not effective treatments for medullary thyroid cancer
- medullary thyroid cancer is more aggressive than differentiated thyroid cancer

The treatment of a patient with medullary thyroid cancer is a total thyroidectomy and removal of the lymph nodes in the nearby "central compartment" of the neck (an area from just below the chin to the upper chest and between the two internal jugular veins). These lymph nodes are removed, even if they appear to be normal, since many patients with medullary thyroid cancer have microscopic lymph node involvement. The surgeon may also perform a modified radical neck dissection (as opposed to a radical neck dissection) if any abnormal lymph nodes are found in the neck outside the central compartment. A patient with residual or recurrent medullary thyroid cancer may receive external-beam radiation, additional surgery, and chemotherapy.

Approximately 95% of patients with MEN 2 have a genetic mutation of the RET proto-oncogene. Therefore, all family members of patients with MEN 2 should have genetic testing for RET proto-oncogene mutations. Family members with mutations should be screened for medullary thyroid cancer and, when indicated, any other associated abnormalities, such as pheochromocytomas and parathyroid tumors. Measurement of calcitonin, either with or without stimulation by an intravenous infusion of calcium, may be useful to determine the timing of surgery in affected family members. Stimulation tests of calcitonin using another hormone, pentagastrin, have also been useful, but pentagastrin is not currently available in the United States. The optimal use of genetic and calcitonin testing and the timing of surgery in family members with RET proto-oncogene mutations have yet to be established.

Evaluation and Treatment of Patients with Undifferentiated (Anaplastic) Thyroid Cancer

An anaplastic thyroid cancer is an undifferentiated tumor arising from thyroid follicular cells. When cells from a thyroid cancer look similar to normal thyroid follicular cells, the cancer is described as differentiated. When the cells from a thyroid cancer appear completely different from normal thyroid follicular cells, the cancer is referred to as undifferentiated (anaplastic). Accounting for approximately 2 to 5% of all thyroid cancers, anaplastic cancers occur primarily among women sixty-five years and older, although 10% of the patients are younger than fifty, and 30 to 40% are men.

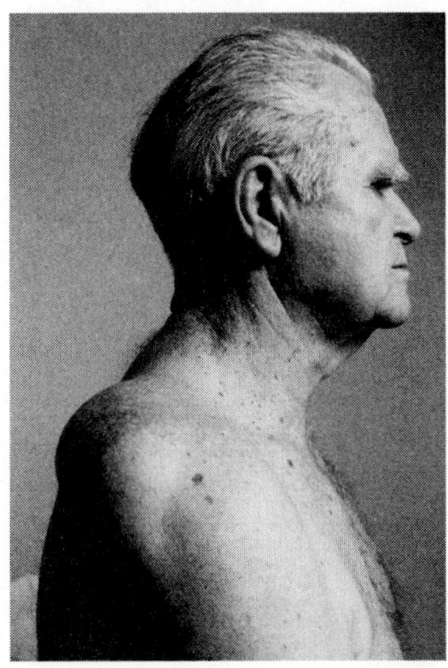

Figure 11.5. Patient with follicular thyroid cancer with metatasis to the right shoulder prior to treatment with external-beam radiation. He died after his follicular cancer transformed into anaplastic cancer.

Many physicians speculate that undifferentiated thyroid cancers arise from pre-existing or co-existing differentiated (papillary or follicular) thyroid cancers. For example, the patient pictured in Figure 11.5 died after anaplastic transformation of his long-standing follicular cancer, which could not be adequately treated because of his severe heart disease. Although small differentiated thyroid cancers are found frequently at autopsy and appear to be of little biological significance, large and aggressive differentiated thyroid cancers have the potential to become undifferentiated thyroid cancers if they are not adequately treated.

Anaplastic thyroid cancer behaves very aggressively. The prognosis is, unfortunately, very poor; most patients do not live for more than one year after they are diagnosed. Ordinarily, physicians do not recommend aggressive surgery, and some patients may not have any surgery at all since most anaplastic thyroid cancers are incurable at the time they are found. When surgery is done, surgeons often do what they can to prevent death caused by airway obstruction. External-beam radiation and chemotherapy are occasionally effective for a short period of time.

Patient Profiles

JERRI LYNN'S STORY

In 1995, Jerri Lynn had trouble losing weight after the birth of her third child and was concerned that her hair was falling out. Jerri Lynn described her symptoms to her grandmother.

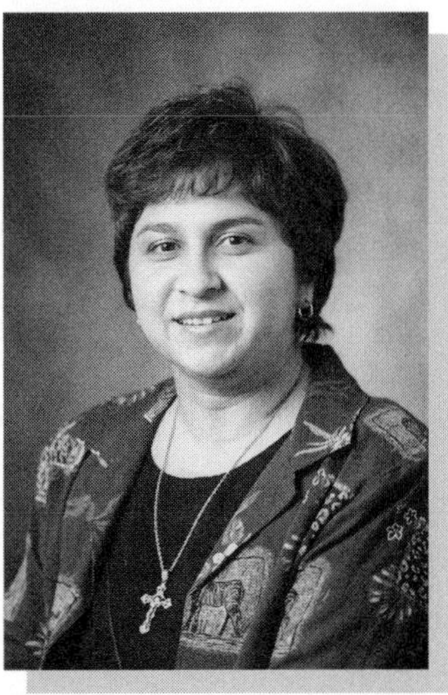

> She was a retired RN [registered nurse] and said, "Let me see your neck. I think it's your thyroid." I had a small lump about the size of a walnut, but I hadn't noticed it until she pointed it out.

Her grandmother was also aware of the family's thyroid history. Jerri Lynn's grandfather, father, and father's sister had had surgery and radioactive iodine treatment for papillary thyroid cancer.

> I went to my GP [general practitioner] right away. He said it was my thyroid and sent me to an ENT [ear, nose, and throat doctor]. [The ENT] had a bad bedside manner. He said men got cancer more and that it was probably just a cyst even though I told him about the thyroid cancer in my family. He said he'd do some tests and sent me for an ultrasound. The ultrasound indicated a tumor, so we skipped the biopsy and did surgery right away. I was twenty-eight years old.
>
> [The ENT] took out all of one lobe and 20% of the other. At first, I cried a lot because my kids were so young. I didn't know how long I had had it. I was worried about the kids, but my ENT told me that it was the

> best kind of cancer; it was slow-growing.
>
> A week or two after surgery, I went to see my ENT, and he gave me [levothyroxine]. He said it would put my thyroid to sleep so it wouldn't develop more tumors. I asked him about radioactive iodine, but he said I didn't need it because he had gotten it all.
>
> About a year later, I still couldn't lose weight, and my hair was still coming out. When I went to my gynecologist for a check-up, I told her about it, and she said that I needed more thyroid medication. But my ENT said it would be too strong, and he would see me again in six months.
>
> I didn't want to wait six months. I had a friend who had seen the same ENT but switched to [an endocrinologist]. So I made an appointment with him. He asked me what type of cancer I had had, but I hadn't been told which kind it was.

The pathologist's report from her surgery indicated that Jerri Lynn had a follicular variant of papillary thyroid cancer. Medical records from her grandfather, father, and aunt revealed that they also had papillary thyroid cancer—a fact too remarkable to be a coincidence.

Her new endocrinologist increased her levothyroxine dosage since Jerri Lynn's thyroid hormone levels were low normal. Slightly high thyroid hormone levels would decrease her chances of cancer recurrence. Jerri Lynn's tumor was larger than 1.5 cm, suggesting that additional surgery followed by radioactive iodine would also improve her prognosis.

> He did an ultrasound in his office and saw something small. He thought it might require surgery and referred me to a different ENT. After [the ENT] examined me, he agreed that I needed another operation.

Thirteen months after her left lobectomy, Jerri Lynn's new ENT removed the remainder of her thyroid gland, which was free of any cancer. Treatment with radioactive iodine would not have been practical without a completion thyroidectomy.

> The surgery was somewhat painful, just like the first time. But compared to the three C-sections I had had, it wasn't bad. My insurance plan wanted me released the same day, but [my surgeon] arranged it so that I could stay overnight.
>
> I remember that they gave me calcium at first, but then I didn't need it. Two days after I went home, my legs felt like they were asleep, then my arms. I had numbness around my mouth. My doctor told me to come to the office right away. I had calcium problems; there was something wrong with my parathyroid glands. [The doctor] said he thought they might be in shock and that this was just temporary, but it's a permanent thing. I take 2,000 milligrams of calcium daily and Rocaltrol [vitamin D].

At the suggestion of both her ENT and endocrinologist, Jerri Lynn was hospitalized for treatment with radioactive iodine six weeks after her completion thyroidectomy.

> Before the uptake and treatment, I had to go off my [levothyroxine]. [My endocrinologist] put me on Cytomel, but I still had a bad drop in energy, and my memory was horrible. I had to count my kids before I drove off to be sure all of them were in the car!
>
> It was really kind of funny in the hospital. They give you this walkway you have to stay on when you walk to the bathroom. Everything is disposable. There's a special box for waste, a warning sign on the door, and even the phone is wrapped. Nurses came in only briefly. And this is supposed to be safe!
>
> I drank lots of water and got out of the hospital the

> next day. I lost my taste for two weeks, but I sucked on hard candies a lot [and the situation improved].

One year after her first radioactive iodine treatment, a withdrawal scan showed residual thyroid tissue. Jerri Lynn returned to the hospital for her second treatment.

> I had to go back off [levothyroxine] for about eight weeks, so I got really forgetful again. After the treatment, it took another six to eight weeks to feel better, so there were three months of feeling bad, dragging, and being forgetful.

Until recently, only medullary thyroid cancer was considered hereditary. However, Jerri Lynn's papillary cancer and those of her family members clearly indicated a strong genetic link. In order to clarify the hereditary nature of the thyroid cancer in her family, researchers asked Jerri Lynn to gather her family for a medical examination.

> They wanted everybody in the family to come to my house, but not everyone came. We had about seventy or eighty people there. [The research endocrinologists] came to my house and did blood work on everybody and checked their necks. They also did a family tree.
>
> The doctors explained that they think something triggers this gene. The gene could have just laid there, but something set it off. No one knows.
>
> They found a lump in another one of my father's sisters, but it turned out to be benign. She had a thyroidectomy two weeks ago.
>
> [My father's third sister] has a lump, but she won't get it checked out because she says if it's there, it's meant to be there. Her blood work was okay, but she's overweight, and her hair's falling out.

> A fourth sister was clear, but her nine-month-old grandson has something wrong with his thyroid. I'm not sure what it is. Of my father's three brothers, one was tested and is okay, but the other two didn't come to be tested.
>
> The [research] doctors checked my children, too. Everything looks clear now, but they said more than likely one of them would get it because it wasn't skipping generations. Now that I know how important it is, when I take my kids to the pediatrician, I always make sure he remembers my history and tests their thyroid. He also examines their neck. He would do it anyway, but I reinforce it, just to be sure.
>
> Grandpa's thyroid cancer came back last year. It had spread to his lungs and trachea. He died, but they said his death wasn't a result of his thyroid. He died because of his bad heart.
>
> The aunt who had two surgeries for her thyroid cancer died of an aneurysm, not cancer. She would go for months without taking her [levothyroxine]. She was always dragging and was so forgetful.

Jerri Lynn has had two consecutive, negative whole body scans since her second treatment, and her prognosis is very good. From not knowing what type of thyroid cancer she had to organizing an entire family for a special research project, Jerri Lynn has made a quantum leap in her understanding of thyroid cancer. Her cooperation and participation have been invaluable to thyroid cancer researchers.■

LISA'S STORY

During a routine physical examination in 1991, a nurse found a small nodule in Lisa's thyroid gland. Her physician referred her to an ENT who performed a fine needle biopsy.

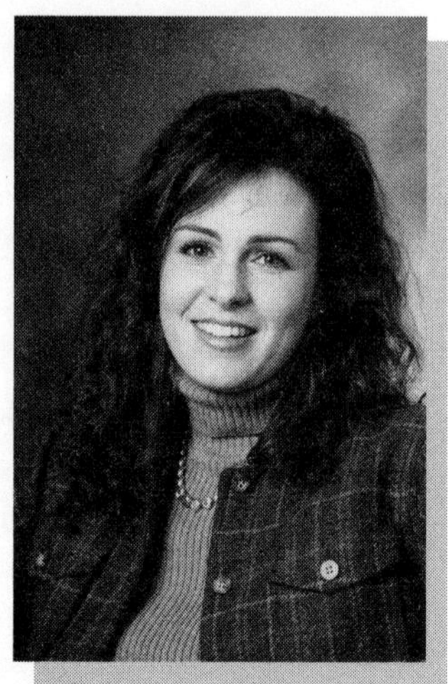

I was a college student at the time. I don't remember exactly what they said except that I should not worry about it—just have it looked at every year. It didn't bother me or cause any problems. As far as any family history of thyroid disease, I think my great-grandfather had thyroid problems, and my great-aunt had something removed from her thyroid that she claimed was the size of a grapefruit.

In 1993, I went to [an endocrinologist], and he did all kinds of tests. He did an ultrasound-guided biopsy that found it was benign. He also said just to watch it.

Afterwards, I had to switch doctors because of my insurance plan. I went to an internist who said the same thing for two years. I just wasn't comfortable with him, so I switched to an endocrinologist. Somewhere in here, [my nodule] grew to about 3 cm. [The new endocrinologist] suggested that I take [levothyroxine] for three months to see if it would shrink, but it got larger. After another biopsy, he said that the results were unsatisfactory and recommended that I have it taken out. He recommended a general surgeon.

I was fairly comfortable with this decision. I was tired of worrying about it for [seven] years. No one could ever really say what it was. I was married by this time, and my husband had heard about another endocrinologist and said, "Let's get a second opinion." We drove through a flood to get to his office! He recommended another biopsy, but I wanted to get it over. So I went ahead and had surgery with a surgeon on our HMO.

He took it out and said there was just one little pea-sized

> cancer. I wasn't really surprised, but I was somewhat alarmed. He said that it was totally encapsulated, so he only took out one lobe. He didn't think I needed radioactive iodine and said he'd just watch it.
>
> After surgery, I felt bad for a few weeks. The muscles in my neck were so sore. But I could sit up and eat the same night I had surgery, and I was surprised that I could swallow pills. I stayed in the hospital for one or two nights.
>
> Then [the second endocrinologist's] office called to see what I had decided to do about the biopsy. I told them I had already had the surgery, and they asked if they could look at the slides.

Lisa's surgeon had removed a nodule measuring 2.5 cm; 90% of it was papillary cancer. After reviewing the slides from the previous negative biopsy and the slides from her surgery, her endocrinologist concluded that Lisa actually had two nodules. The cancerous nodule originated close to the previous nodule and eventually grew into the old nodule—a very unusual situation.

> It was a month or more after surgery, and I thought this was all behind me. But the doctors disagreed. My husband said, "Sit down. You need to see [the endocrinologist] and have a second operation." Now I was upset!

At her husband's insistence, Lisa returned to the endocrinologist they had gone to for a second opinion. He explained that additional surgery was necessary to decrease the chances of recurrence of a papillary cancer larger than 1.5 cm. He referred her to an ENT with years of experience performing thyroidectomies. Lisa returned to the hospital two months after her first surgery to have a completion thyroidectomy, removal of almost all of her remaining thyroid tissue. There was no cancer in the lymph nodes, and she was scheduled for radioactive iodine treatment six weeks later.

> I recovered from the surgery faster; I had a drain this time. I went back to work part-time a week after surgery. The last time it took two weeks.
>
> The end of December [1998], I went into [the hospital] for my radioactive iodine treatment. That was the worst experience I've ever been through psychologically. I felt like such a leper! There was plastic over the phone. They walked in all covered up with this little box of iodine in a concrete container and told me to drink it. Then I drank lots and lots of water and ate lots of lemon candies so that I could get out of there quickly. My biggest concern about radioactive iodine was having kids. Mom thought that I wouldn't be able to have children.

After being reassured that her radioactive iodine treatments would not cause infertility or birth defects, Lisa felt better. She was advised to delay pregnancy until her thyroid function test results were normal. Lisa resumed levothyroxine after her radioactive iodine treatment and, within four months, became euthyroid.

> In April I saw a gynecologist. She said I could get pregnant any time now. My husband and I decided to go ahead and try. I got pregnant immediately. I went to [my endocrinologist] every six weeks until I had the baby. We had to increase and decrease my thyroid medicine several times during the pregnancy. I saw him six weeks after the baby was born, and he made an adjustment to my medicine then, and that's what I've been taking ever since.
>
> I've been breastfeeding, but I'm in the process of stopping now [seven months postpartum] to have a scan to see if all the cancer is gone. I've been off [levothyroxine] for three-and-a-half weeks. I got tired at first, but now I'm on Cytomel. I have to go off of it in a few days to be ready for the scan.

> I'm almost more scared about dying since I had a baby. It's always in the back of my mind. I worry about the chances of getting other cancers like breast cancer. My grandmother died when she was thirty-two, right after having a baby. I'm about that same age now.
>
> I would definitely recommend getting a second opinion to anyone who faces a similar situation. I've learned it's worth the extra money to get better insurance and get the best doctors. I'm going to stay in the medical center for all my medical care now; it's worth it. I no longer think a doctor's a doctor.

Lisa's scan was negative. Shortly thereafter, she became pregnant again and had another healthy baby boy.■

MELANIE'S STORY

Twenty-five-year-old Melanie talked about her thyroid experience as her two-year-old son napped and her four-year-old daughter played on the floor. If it were not for the short new hair growth covering her head like a tight cap, she would have seemed like any other young mother. Melanie's thyroid problem was first detected in 1995, when she was in the Army, stationed in Okinawa.

> I was about two months pregnant when the doctors on the base first noticed that my thyroid was getting larger; it seemed to be swelling. I didn't even know what a thyroid was before all this.

Once she learned about thyroid disease and its tendency to run in families, Melanie discovered that there was some thyroid disease in her family. Her grandmother's sister took thyroid hormone replacement for "a thyroid problem;" her great-grandmother had a swollen thyroid during pregnancy; but nobody in the family could recall more details.

A few months after she learned about her enlarged thyroid, the Army reassigned Melanie to Yuma, Oklahoma.

> A military endocrinologist there saw me when I was five months pregnant. He told me that what I had was called a goiter, and he put me on [levothyroxine] to try to shrink it. He also did a needle biopsy. I don't really remember what he said about the biopsy; I think he said something about it being fast-growing. Anyway, it didn't shrink.
>
> I decided to get out of the military and move back to Texas before having my daughter in December. The goiter was huge by this time. After the baby was born, my medicines ran out. My husband changed jobs, and we got insurance but had to change doctors.
>
> In May, I saw the only endocrinologist on our list, and he just wanted to put me back on medicine to see if he could shrink it. We tried that for about three months, and then he sent me to an ENT. He did another biopsy and told me that it was a tumor that wouldn't shrink. He didn't think it was cancer, but he thought we should remove it since I was having a little trouble breathing and some trouble swallowing. But my endocrinologist said no surgery. I quit going to him and stopped the medicine.
>
> In 1997, my husband changed jobs again, and we got another insurance plan with a new list of doctors. I was pregnant again and went to see a new obstetrician. When he saw how big [the goiter] was, he was afraid it would complicate my pregnancy. He sent me to a new endocrinologist; he did another [fine needle aspiration biopsy]. The tests came back showing rapid-growing cells. The doctor never said the word cancer, but I was afraid it might be. He thought we should remove it, and I agreed, but we had to wait until I was four months pregnant.

Since Melanie was in the first trimester of her pregnancy, she was advised to postpone surgery until her second trimester, when there would be less risk of miscarriage.

> In July 1997, a surgeon removed the right side of my thyroid. I wasn't in the hospital very long, and I was not in much pain. I was out of the hospital when I found out it was cancer. Two weeks later, [the surgeon] removed the left side. They said it was very important to take my thyroid and that they would watch me closely. After the baby was born, they'd give me radioactive iodine.
>
> I was really devastated. "Will I die?" kept going through my mind. But after a month or two, I said I've just got to deal with it, and I put it in God's hands. My husband doesn't show much emotion. He feels he has to be strong. My mother freaked out a little bit. She'd go out of the room and cry, but she tried to hide it.
>
> I didn't really feel bad during the pregnancy; it went smoothly. My son was born in December. I decided not to breastfeed—to go ahead with the radioactive iodine treatment. [My physicians] took me off my thyroid [hormone], and, within eight weeks, a visible lump grew back. They said they couldn't get it all with radioactive iodine, so they did the third surgery in March or April of 1998.
>
> About a month later I did the radioactive iodine. I felt like some kind of freak because of the way they isolated me in the hospital, but I didn't really worry about the safety of treatment. I just wanted it taken care of. I couldn't hold the kids after I got out of the hospital, so I left them with my mother.
>
> The doctors did thyroid scans every six months. The first scan was clear, but the next one showed a little bit of thyroid, so I did another radioactive iodine treatment. I

> had to go off my thyroid medicine before all the scans. They'd put me on T_3 for a few weeks. But I was used to feeling tired, chasing children around all day.

Following her second radioactive iodine treatment, Melanie was encouraged and looked forward to raising her children.

> One day I started feeling sick; I had a headache really bad. My vision was messed up; I was throwing up and had diarrhea. I went to our family doctor, and he said it was just a virus. I went to him two times, but he said the same thing each time. I finally went to the emergency room, and they decided to keep me overnight. When I fell asleep that night, I sort of hallucinated and woke up screaming for the nurses. They did a bunch of tests and found cancer in my head and lungs. They sent me to [a major medical center]; they did more tests.

Melanie had a poorly differentiated follicular thyroid cancer that had spread, or metastasized, to her brain and possibly her lungs. Her surgeons decided to remove the brain metastasis. However, two days before the scheduled surgery, Melanie had difficulty breathing and was rushed into emergency brain surgery.

> I don't remember much after that. I was in [the hospital] almost a whole month before Christmas. I was kind of out of it, not aware of what was going on. I had radiation treatments after the surgery. It made my hair fall out, but I wasn't nauseous.
>
> In January or February, I went back to the hospital, and they started chemotherapy for the lung cancer. It's made me really sick; I've lost forty pounds between December and May. And it's kept my hair from growing back.

More bad news came when Melanie's oncologist discovered that she had a questionable metastasis to her kidney.

> The chemotherapy is working on the kidney, and my tumors in the lung are shrinking. My brain scan is clear; nothing has grown back yet. My vision is still messed up. It's blurred, half vision, so I can't drive.
>
> I get chemotherapy for two days, every three weeks. The first day I get it for three hours and then one hour or so the second day. I take my crochet and get to know the other patients while I'm there. I get nauseous usually two or three days after, then I feel fairly regular.

Taking care of a family with small children is a challenge for anyone who is sick, but it is especially difficult when cancer is involved. During the course of her hospitalization and chemotherapy, Melanie had to determine what was best for her four-year-old daughter and two-year-old son.

> My children went to my husband's family in California when I first got home from the hospital, but I didn't like that; I wanted them back. My parents kept them during the day, and friends from my church helped. I actually feel pretty good now and don't need much help with the kids. They just know that Mommy is sick.

The prognosis for poorly differentiated follicular thyroid cancer with brain metastases is very poor. Melanie faced this grim knowledge with incredible strength and courage, avoiding bitterness.

> Hopefully, God chooses to let me stay a little longer. Having kids and a strong belief in God have kept me going. I try to go to church every Sunday, but sometimes I can only go to Sunday School.
>
> When he first found out I had a growth, I really wish that the first doctor had recommended surgery. Then

> again, I had a second child, and that's a blessing. Things are just working out like they were supposed to. Only God knows why this happened. Faith has really gotten me through this.

When asked what she would tell a person who discovers a thyroid nodule, Melanie had the following advice:

> Go to the doctor and have it checked. It may turn out to be nothing, but it could be worse than you think—it could be cancer.

After Melanie gave this interview, she developed recurrent metastases to the brain and had additional surgery. The masses in her lungs enlarged. Melanie entered a hospice and died shortly thereafter, six years after her thyroid nodule was discovered.■

DICK'S STORY

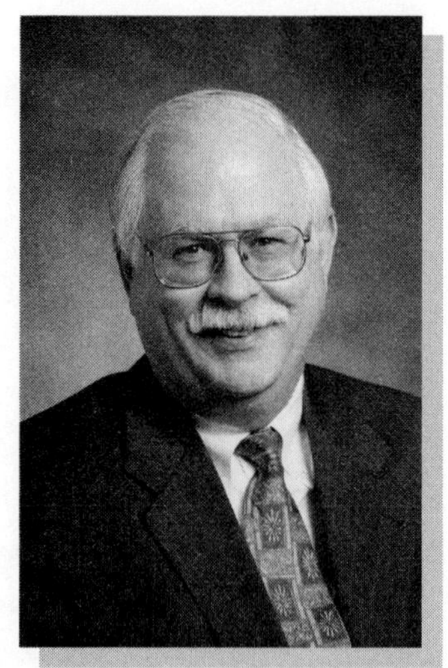

Shortly after Dick was born in the 1940s, his physician prescribed radiation treatments for an enlarged thymus. In 1972, his mother read an article in *Reader's Digest* discussing the increased risk of thyroid cancer in adults who received radiation therapy when they were children.

She attempted to track down his childhood medical records, but there were none. When Dick contacted a cancer treatment center, they advised him to have a thyroid scan. The scan did not show any signs of thyroid cancer, but his physicians recommended that he have a yearly examination of his thyroid gland.

> But I didn't go to the doctor regularly. When I did go

> and mentioned my radiation history, they would just kind of look at me and say that they hadn't felt a thyroid since college. But I followed the literature about thyroid cancer. I read that once you got to fifty, it wouldn't happen. So I decided it was a non-event when I turned fifty.
>
> Then I started seeing a new doctor, and he was very thorough. In October 1998, he did blood tests, and, when they showed some abnormal thyroid results, it set off bells.

Dick's TSH was slightly elevated at 7.16 mU/L, diagnostic of subclinical hypothyroidism.

> When my doctor suggested that I have a thyroid scan, I asked how soon, and he said, "Fairly soon." During the scan, I could see a bump myself, but the [nuclear medicine physician] couldn't feel anything.
>
> Two days later, my doctor called and said that there was a little nodule and that these things were usually benign, but he wanted me to have a biopsy. He referred me to an endocrinologist who felt my neck, drew blood, and said that my neck was too fat for him to be able to do the biopsy in his office. He sent me to [a hospital for an ultrasound-guided biopsy]. They jabbed me eight or nine times and then had to repeat it. A couple of weeks later, the nurse called and said the results were benign, but that my calcitonin was positive. That's when they restained the slides [from the biopsy] and saw cancer cells.

Dick's first calcitonin was 547 pg/mL (picograms per milliliter); normal is less than 8 pg/mL. Since very high calcitonin usually indicates medullary thyroid cancer, a closer look at the specimen from Dick's fine needle aspiration biopsy was crucial. Additional studies confirmed that Dick had medullary thyroid cancer.

> When my doctors recommended surgery, I had no second thoughts; I just wanted to remove it, whatever it took. I didn't care what I looked like, but I wanted it done right. I wanted the best surgeon. I would have gone anywhere.

Dick read everything he could find on the Internet and became quite knowledgeable on the subject of medullary thyroid cancer. He chose a surgeon who specialized in thyroid surgery at a renowned cancer treatment center where he lived.

> The surgeon asked me about my family history, but no one had had medullary thyroid cancer. My mother had a goiter and thyroid surgery to treat it. There was not much history of any cancer in my family. I had a DNA test that didn't show any genetic problem.

In January, three months after the abnormal thyroid function test results, Dick underwent an eight-hour surgery that included a total thyroidectomy, a central compartment dissection, bilateral modified radical neck dissections, and a parathyroid transplant to his left forearm.

> They cleaned house. They removed the entire thyroid and sixty to sixty-four lymph nodes. All the nodes were clear; the cancer was contained in the thyroid. I wanted to go home the next day, but then I started feeling that something was not right; I knew something was wrong. They had just switched my IV bags, and I thought they had hung the wrong stuff.

Dick was experiencing hypocalcemia, or low calcium. His parathyroid glands, the glands that regulate calcium in the body, were injured during his extensive surgery. Furthermore, the parathyroid tissue transplanted into Dick's forearm did not function adequately. Dick became permanently hypoparathyroid, and, as a result, he has hypocalcemia. Therefore, Dick takes 0.25 mcg (micrograms) of Rocaltrol (vitamin D) three times a week and 500 mg (milligrams) of calcium three times a day. Since calcium may block the absorption of levothyroxine, Dick takes his thyroid medication and calcium at different times.

After surgery, Dick tested positively for a very uncommon mutation of the RET proto-oncogene that showed he had a rare hereditary form of medullary thyroid cancer.

> My doctors said I had a very wimpy form of medullary cancer, that it was very slow-growing. The second DNA test showed that I had a gene that was just a little mutant and hereditary. I called my brother in Cincinnati who is four years older and told him about it. His doctors tested him, and he had medullary thyroid cancer, too. His doctors removed his entire thyroid gland, but they did not do a radical [neck dissection]. He doesn't have parathyroid problems.

Ironically, the radiation treatments Dick had as an infant had nothing to do with the development of his medullary thyroid cancer.

> In hindsight, I wouldn't have done it any other way. It's a fluke that it was picked up. If it hadn't been for the radiation treatments I had as a baby, I would have blown it off when the first thyroid tests were abnormal. But I insisted on following up since I was worried about the radiation treatments. The best part is that it didn't take long from discovery to resolution. Everything happened between October and January.

Since his surgery, Dick has been cancer-free, with a calcitonin level less than 1 pg/mL. He takes levothyroxine every day and leads a very productive life.■

CHRISTINE'S STORY

In 1993, Christine had no idea that she had a thyroid problem until an annual physical examination by her gynecologist.

> He noticed a nodule in my throat and asked another doctor to look at it; they both thought the nodule looked suspicious. Two days later, I had a fine needle biopsy. A couple of days later, my doctor told me that the results had come back suspicious. My endocrinologist had me meet with a surgeon, an ENT. He advised a total thyroidectomy if it was cancerous.
>
> You can imagine—I was shocked. It happened so fast! I was thirty-three years old and had two small children. My husband had just started a new company and was frequently out of town. But I didn't think I'd die. My ob-gyn had said that if it was cancer, it would be easy to treat.
>
> When I went in for surgery, I thought it would be something else, not cancer. The surgeon said it would take either one hour or four hours, depending on the results of the pathology report. When I woke up in recovery and realized it had been four-and-a-half hours, I knew I had cancer. That's when I started coming to grips with it.

The pathology report indicated that Christine had a 2.4-cm papillary cancer and two incidental papillary cancers, measuring 0.3 and 0.1 cm. Two of six removed lymph nodes also had evidence of papillary thyroid cancer. Her postoperative whole body scan was positive, indicating either residual thyroid tissue or thyroid cancer.

> It was a week or so before I was up and around. A month later, I had radioactive iodine treatment to make sure the cancer would not spread. The treatment was painless. It wasn't any fun, but it wasn't bad. I have five siblings and a mother and father who helped my husband and me with the children.

Christine began levothyroxine therapy, but she was not feeling well.

> I was on the synthetic hormone, but I didn't feel like myself yet. I didn't have enough energy, but my endocrinologist kind of shunned me. He made me think I was wasting his time. A friend gave me [another endocrinologist's] name, and I started seeing him. He did much more comprehensive blood work and increased my medicine. Within a month, I was feeling like I had felt prior to my operation.

A second scan was negative. Like so many other thyroid cancer patients, Christine did not look forward to the preparation necessary for another whole body scan.

> Going off the hormone was no fun. You lose all your energy. One year ago, I did Thyrogen and got to stay on my thyroid hormone. I had moved to [another city], but I wanted to remain with [my endocrinologist]; he's great. He talked to my internist here who ordered the Thyrogen. I went to [my endocrinologist] for the scan. Thyrogen is a dramatic improvement!

Christine wanted to have another child, and there was no reason she could not do so. As instructed, she visited her endocrinologist periodically during her pregnancy. Pregnant women often need additional thyroid hormone, but in Christine's case, she needed to make an adjustment for quite a different reason.

> When I was two months pregnant, I went on vacation in New Orleans. I was so cold that I called my endocrinologist, and he said to come in to see him when I got back. He did tests and found out that my thyroid hormone level was low.
>
> When I got home, I looked at the milligrams on the bottle [of levothyroxine] and realized that the pharmacy had made a mistake. They had filled it with half the dose I was supposed to have. They didn't apologize;

> they didn't do anything. I switched to another pharmacy. I always look at the milligrams now. It took several weeks for me to feel better.

Since her treatment for thyroid cancer, Christine has continued to lead a busy life, raising her three children and operating a business with her husband. She says she would like for fellow patients to know, "...that thyroid cancer is usually treatable. You can live your life as if you never had cancer at all."■

JOAN'S STORY

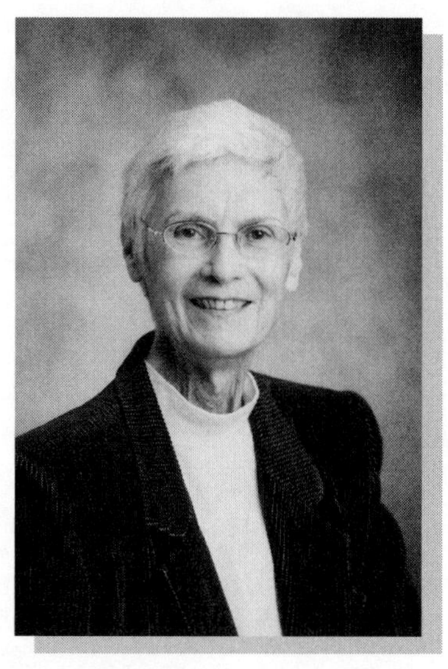

As one of the first thyroid cancer patients treated with radioactive iodine, sixty-eight-year-old Joan offers a fascinating insight into the treatment of patients with thyroid cancer fifty years ago. Her story also underscores a very important lesson for current thyroid cancer patients.

> In 1948, when I was sixteen years old, I became extremely tired. I was so tired, I couldn't ride my bicycle. I was living in South Jersey at the time, and, when the local doctors could not find out what was wrong with me, they told my mother to take me to Philadelphia. The doctors there put me in the hospital for three months solid without letting me go home. The hospital got to be my home! My family was afraid I was going to die.
>
> I had thyroid cancer, but you couldn't see or feel it. It didn't show up in any blood work. [My thyroid gland] was almost completely removed during surgery.

In 1949, Joan's surgeon performed a thyroidectomy and bilateral radical neck dissections to remove as much of her thyroid gland and as many lymph nodes in her neck as possible. Today, patients rarely have radical neck dissections.

> They probably cut more out than needed to be. After the surgery, the doctor told my mother that I would never talk again because half of my voice box was paralyzed from the surgery. My mother responded, "But, Doctor, she was just talking to me!" I haven't had any trouble with my voice. The doctors also said that I would never be able to work. That's how they thought in those days. I worked for forty-five years—from the time I was seventeen until I retired a few years ago. For seventeen years, I worked two jobs a day!
>
> I had [external-beam] radiation to my neck daily for a while. In 1957, I also drank some clear liquid like water that came from Oakridge; I called it an iodine cocktail in the journal I kept. I remember that they said it was only good for twenty-four hours, so I had to get to the hospital right away when they got it from Tennessee.
>
> Remember how in the movies they'd show a patient sitting in an amphitheater surrounded by doctors in white coats? Well, I was one of those patients. I was kind of a guinea pig then. They were still learning about thyroid cancer and radioactive iodine. The machines they used to treat me had big dials. I remember being in a lab where they were experimenting on white mice. It was like science fiction compared to today.
>
> They didn't put me on thyroid medication right away because they wanted to see what I did on my own without the stuff. At some point, they put me on natural animal thyroid, but my body rejected it, so they put me on [synthetic levothyroxine].

> I would go to the thyroid clinic and see so many patients who looked horrible because they wouldn't take their medicine like they were told. You know, as a teenager, you're so weight-conscious. I weighed myself all the time, and, if I gained even a couple of pounds, I would lose it right away instead of letting it add up on me. I followed what the doctor ordered right to the letter.
>
> Back then, they put me on a high dose of [levothyroxine]. They thought that would prevent the cancer from coming back. Eventually, they discovered I was developing osteoporosis as a result of taking so much thyroid medication. They put me on several medications; one was a prescription vitamin D. Now I take half of [the levothyroxine] I used to take. I continued to see an endocrinologist once or twice a year.

After her thyroidectomy in 1949, Joan continued to lead a very productive life despite mastectomies in 1986 and 1996 for breast cancer. In 1999, fifty years after the initial treatment of her thyroid cancer, a chest x-ray revealed a growth the size of a quarter in her lung.

> I didn't worry about cancer. I had no idea it could return. I thought they got it all out and that was that. When I was sixteen, they told me that a piece of my thyroid fell in my lung. It didn't cause any trouble, so they left it alone. So one-and-a-half years ago, it decided to grow. I was really scared this time. Maybe it was because I was older and lived by myself.
>
> I went to [a hospital], and [my surgeon] took out a fourth of a lobe in my lung; it was cancer. When tests showed that it was thyroid tissue, they were glad that it was [metastatic] thyroid cancer, not lung cancer and not from my breast cancer. I didn't have to have chemotherapy. I never, never had chemotherapy for any of my cancers.

> After my lung operation, I had a thyroid scan—my first since 1957. Some thyroid tissue showed up in my neck, so I drank radioactive iodine, and that got rid of it. Back then in 1957, they used to take you off thyroid [medication before performing a thyroid scan] and didn't give you anything to help you through it. It was awful; I got so tired. I kept working, but I couldn't even remember how to get home one day. That didn't happen this time. They gave me something to get through this period. Technology is so much better these days.

Joan received 200 millicuries of radioactive iodine in December of 1999. Sixteen months later, her thyroglobulin was elevated to 16.7 ng/ml while taking enough levothyroxine to suppress her TSH. Elevated thyroglobulin in patients with a suppressed TSH suggests the presence of residual thyroid tissue or recurrent thyroid cancer. Joan's repeat withdrawal scan in May of 2001 was negative, but her thyroglobulin was elevated to 126 ng/ml off of levothyroxine, very suggestive of either residual or recurrent cancer. In November of 2001, her thyroglobulin remained elevated at 15.7 ng/ml while her TSH was suppressed on levothyroxine. She is awaiting a repeat withdrawal scan, a PET scan, and, possibly, another radioactive iodine treatment.

Treating patients with an elevated thyroglobulin and a negative scan presents a challenge—there is no consensus among physicians concerning the best treatment for patients like Joan.

> I never knew all this would happen. I just took one day at a time. I just lived. My advice to other thyroid cancer patients is to do exactly what the doctor tells you. Follow his instructions, take your medicine, and keep your appointments.

Joan's story highlights the fact that thyroid cancer generally grows very slowly. Most importantly, her story makes it clear that long-term follow-up of patients with thyroid cancer is necessary. Recurrences can occur long after apparently successful initial treatment, although the overwhelming majority of patients with thyroid cancer do well and are usually cured.■

Thyroid Newsmakers

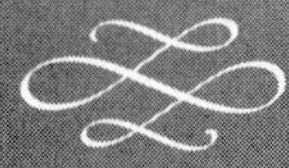

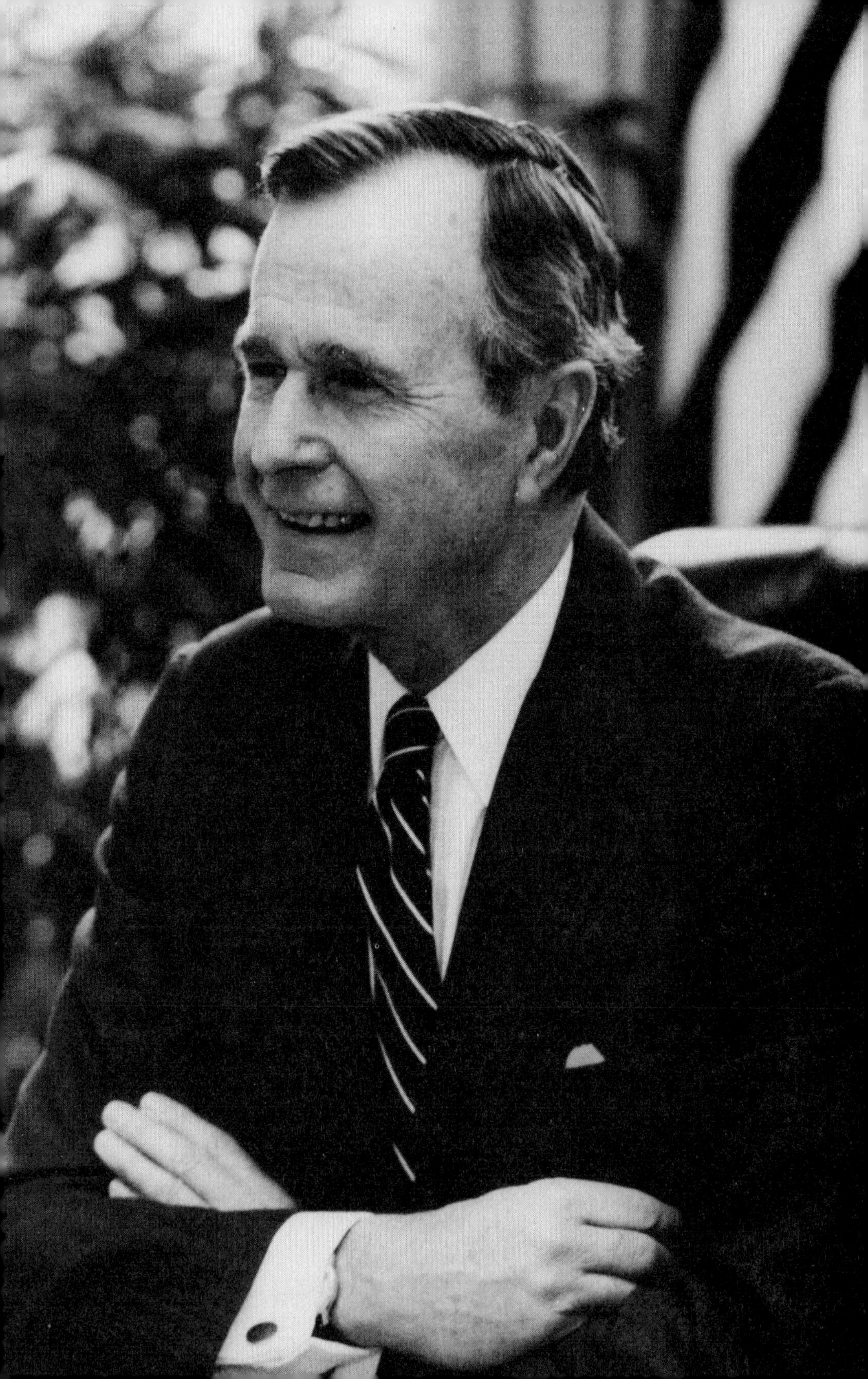

GEORGE H. W. BUSH

When the forty-first President of the United States developed a heart rhythm disturbance while jogging, it stunned America. Tests revealed that the President was suffering from atrial fibrillation caused by Graves' disease. Against improbable odds of more than 10,000 to one, both President and Mrs. Bush had developed Graves' disease within two years of each other. President Bush was treated with drugs to control his heart rhythm, blood thinners to prevent blood clots, and radioactive iodine to control his hyperthyroidism. He is now euthyroid on levothyroxine and continues to lead a very active and productive life.

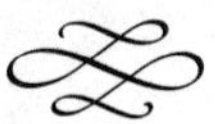

"Take it from someone whose thyroid gland has been the subject of national media scrutiny: having my problem diagnosed and treated has helped me to continue to lead a full and productive life. To anyone who may be facing a similar situation, I highly recommend that you take action and consult a doctor. You owe it to yourself and your loved ones."

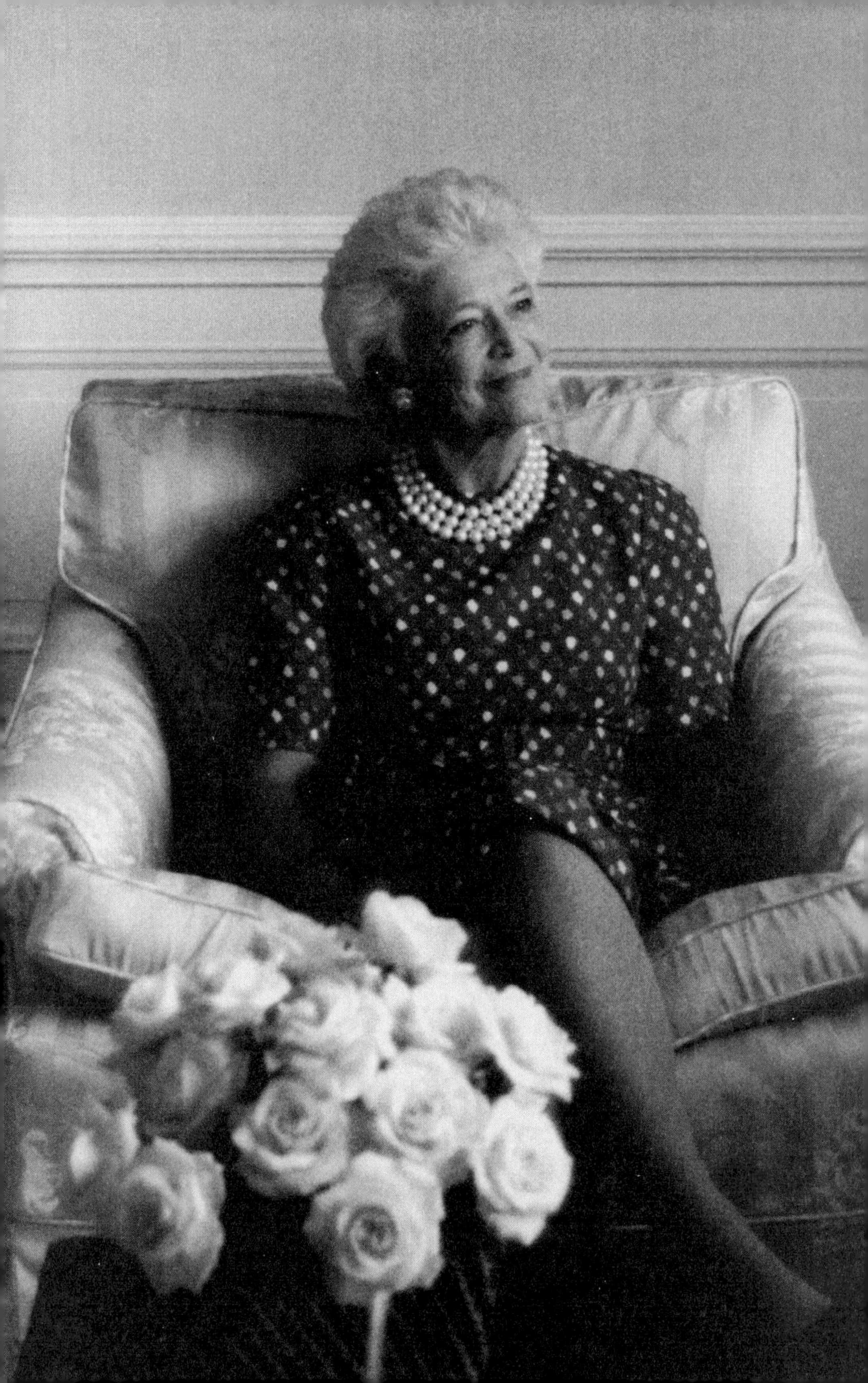

BARBARA BUSH

In the last few months leading up to her husband's Presidential Inauguration in 1989, Barbara Bush had never felt better and was very pleased that she was losing weight. The week before the ceremony, however, her eyes began to bother her. Tests revealed that the First Lady was suffering from Graves' disease, which affected her thyroid gland and her eyes. Her hyperthyroidism was successfully treated with radioactive iodine, and she received both steroids and radiation for her Graves' eye disease. Throughout her ordeal, Mrs. Bush maintained a busy schedule; she is now euthyroid on levothyroxine and is enjoying life to the fullest.

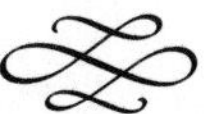

"There are several physical signs in advanced cases of Graves' disease. I encountered puffy, tearing, swollen eyes, eyelids that didn't close, and double vision, while George experienced heart fibrillations. Luckily, I was blessed with wonderful doctors and an early diagnosis, so treatment was relatively easy and very successful."

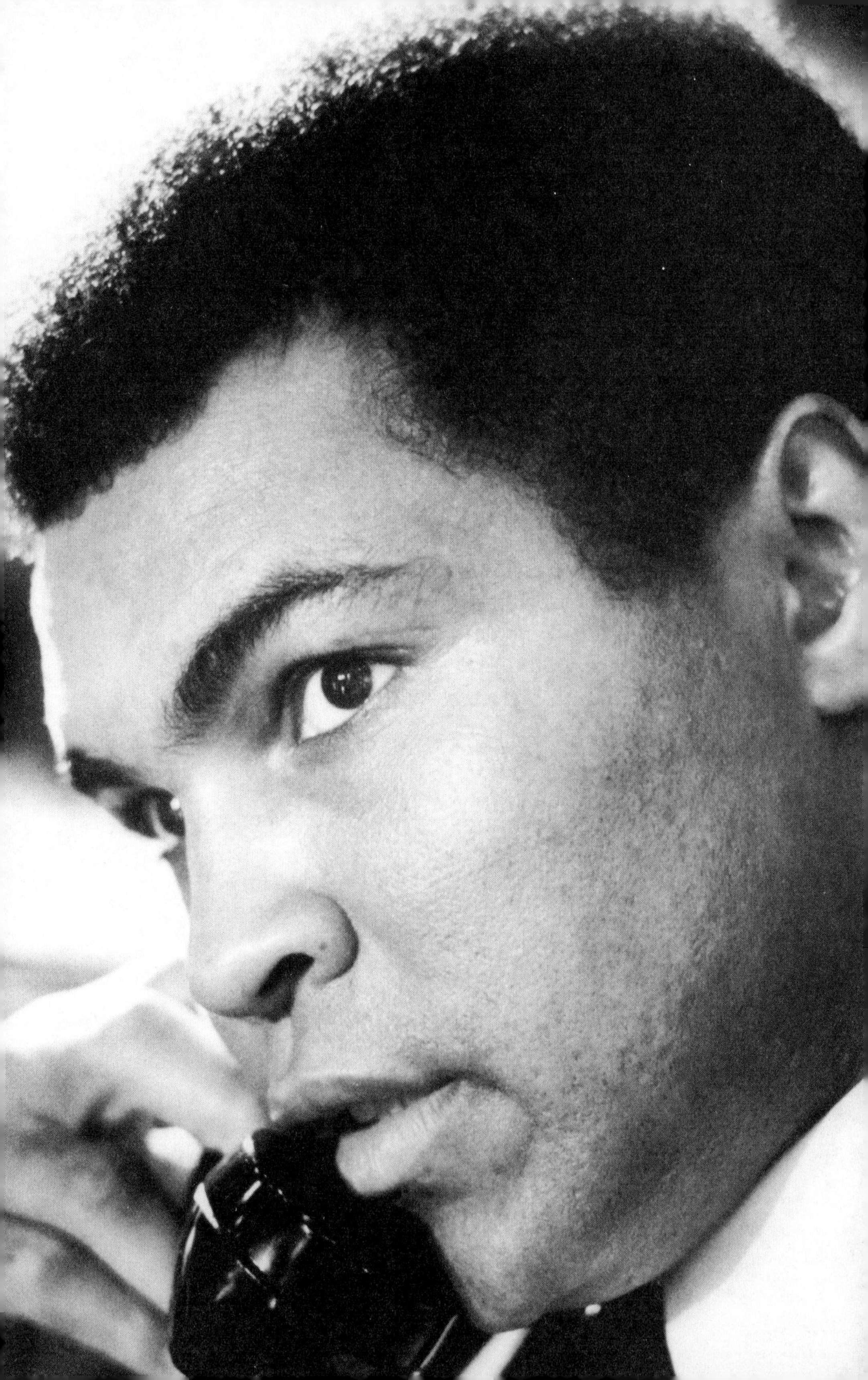

MUHAMMAD ALI

Considered one of the greatest heavy-weight boxing champions of all time, Muhammad Ali entertained and thrilled his fans, not only with his powerful, lightning-quick punches but also with his poetic gift of gab. While preparing to fight Larry Holmes in what was to be Ali's last boxing match, Ali was incorrectly diagnosed with hypothyroidism and given thyroid hormones. Unfortunately, excessive thyroid hormones contributed to his muscle weakness and loss of strength, which led to the match being stopped in the tenth round when it was obvious that it was only Ali's iron will that kept him standing.

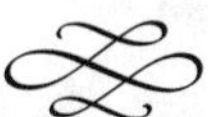

"In September of 1980, I was misdiagnosed with a thyroid disorder and given prescription medication to correct the condition. Several weeks later, after a complete physical, tests showed my thyroid was functioning normally, and I did not have a thyroid disorder. Immediately, I was taken off the medication. While being tested, I learned of the possible side effects the misdiagnosis could have caused, including heart failure. I was one of the lucky ones—I survived the misdiagnosis and intake of thyroid medication without incurring any long-term damage to my thyroid or my overall health.

"Please don't let this happen to you. If you suspect you have a thyroid disorder or you have been diagnosed with a thyroid disorder, make sure you get a complete diagnosis from a qualified physician—hopefully, an endocrinologist. I was lucky, but I could have easily been a statistic."

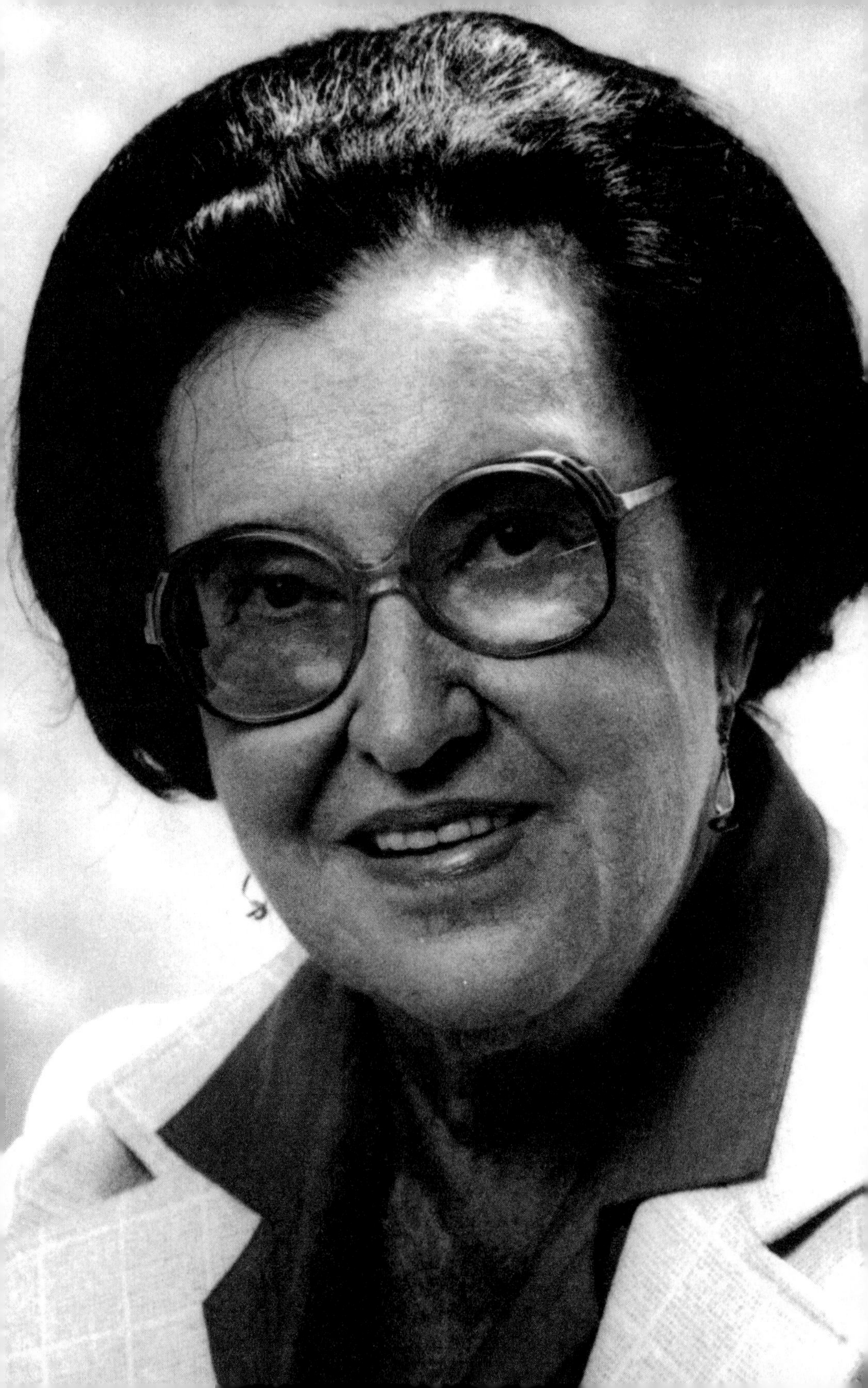

ROSALYN YALOW

In 1977, Dr. Rosalyn Yalow was awarded the Nobel Prize in Physiology and Medicine for her invention of the radioimmunoassay (RIA). Because of her invention, hundreds of substances in the blood can be accurately measured and patients' conditions more definitively assessed. Thyroid patients, in particular, have benefited from Dr. Yalow's research; thyroid hormones and TSH can be precisely measured and appropriate treatment prescribed.

"There has always been concern about the safety of radioactive materials for both diagnostic and therapeutic purposes. However, years of research and study have confirmed the safety of radioactive iodine for diagnostic and therapeutic use in thyroidology. Nothing says this more clearly than the treatment of both President and Mrs. Bush with radioactive iodine for their Graves' disease.

"Radioimmunoassay and subsequent assay methods have improved both the measurement of thyroid hormones and TSH and the physician's ability to accurately diagnose thyroid disorders. As research efforts continue, there will be future advances and refinements in the diagnosis and treatment of thyroid diseases. Support of these research efforts will enable thyroid patients to get the full benefit of new techniques and procedures as they become available."

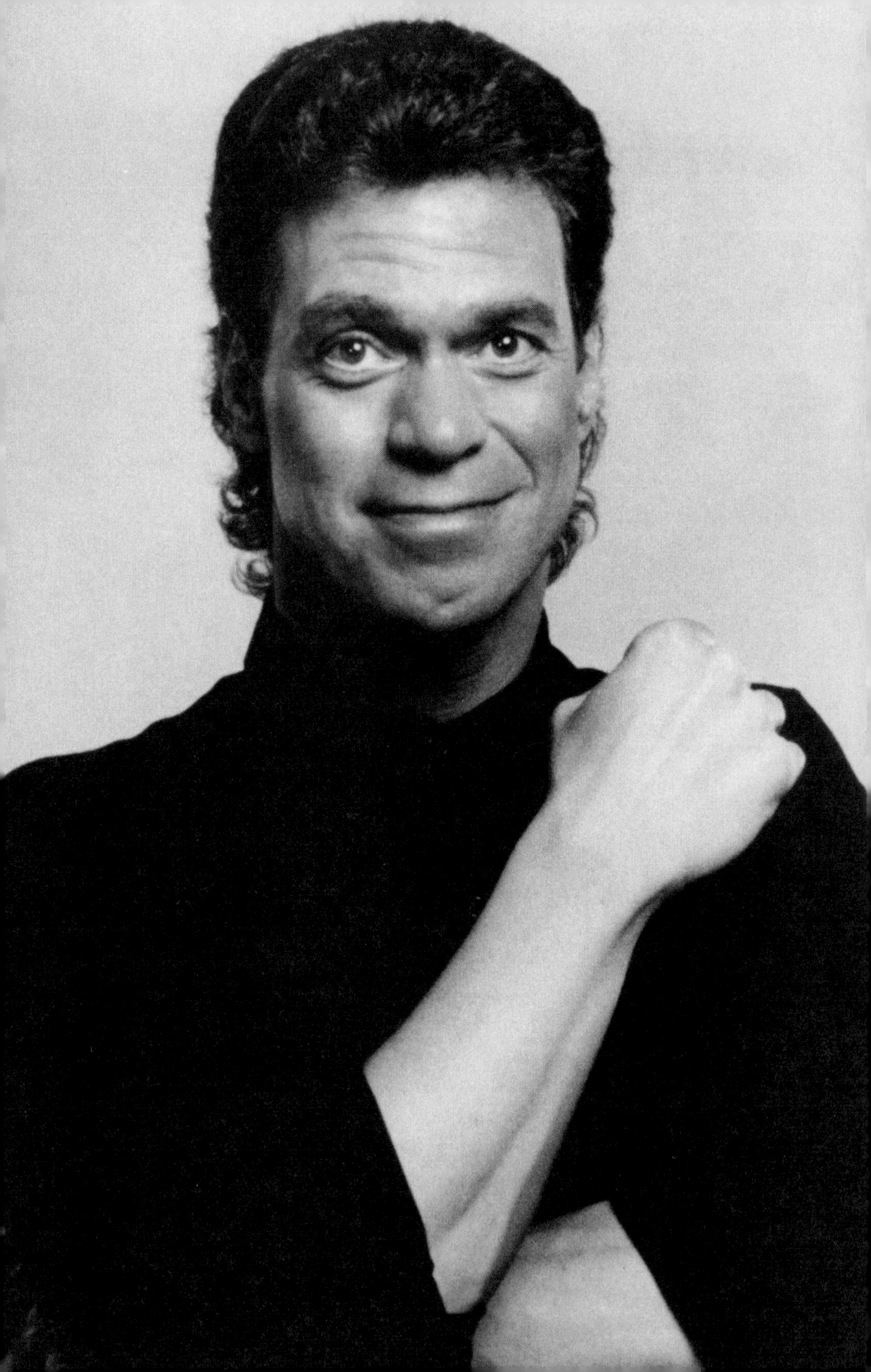

JOE PISCOPO

Star of television and movies, Joe Piscopo is probably best known to millions of people for his comedy sketches and impersonations on *Saturday Night Live!* Imagine his surprise when, over ten years ago, his doctor found a cancerous tumor the size of an egg in his thyroid. Thanks to successful surgical and medical treatment, Mr. Piscopo has not missed a beat and continues to bring laughter and entertainment into everyone's life.

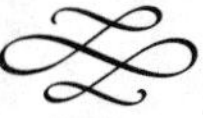

"Hey—I had no idea where my thyroid even was! Fortunately, I was diagnosed early enough to catch it. As I take my thyroid medicine everyday, I realize how lucky I am.

"I wish you all the best in your quest to educate people about thyroid disease and in helping those who might not have been as fortunate as me."

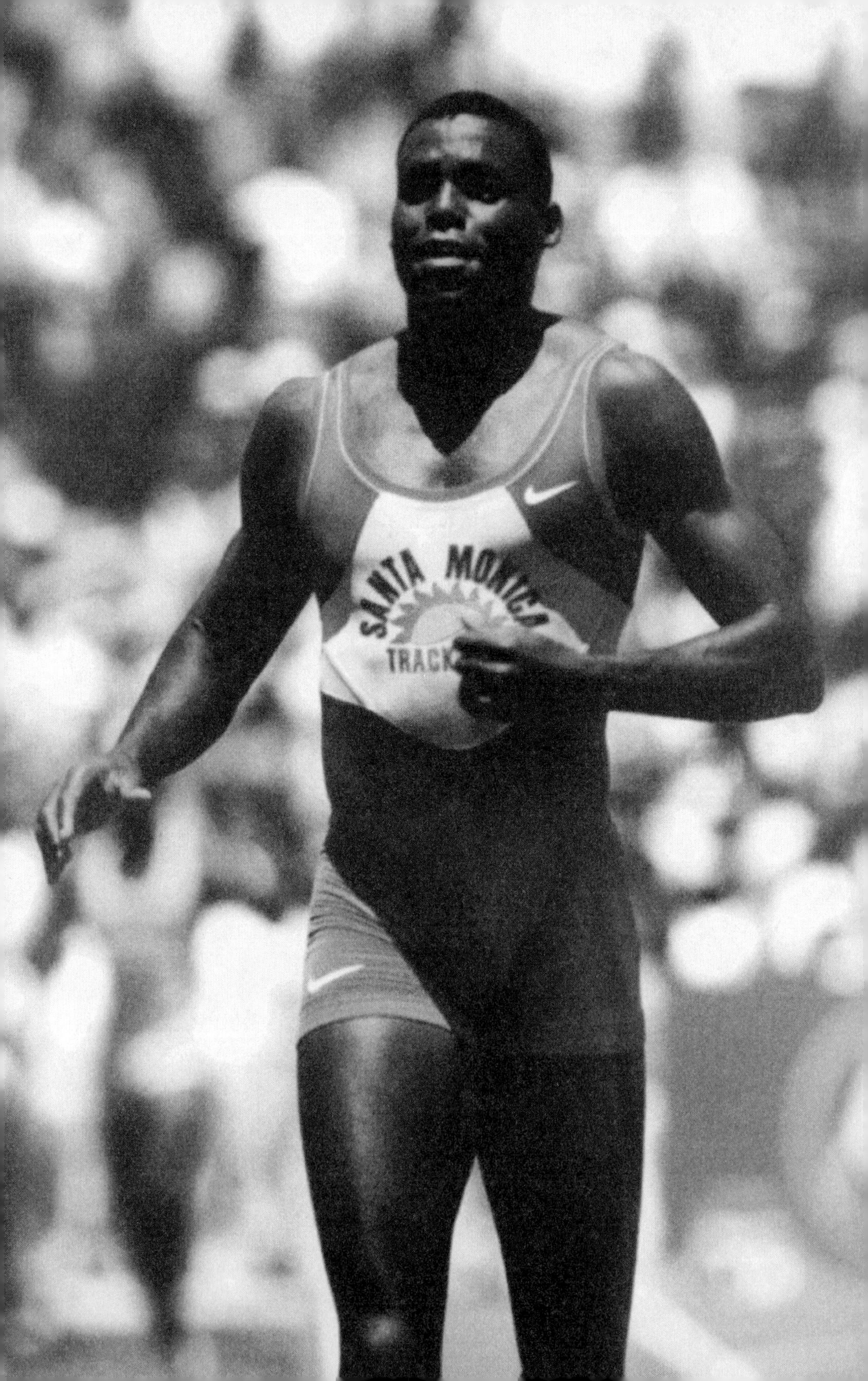
SANTA MONICA
TRACK

CARL LEWIS

Carl Lewis is an Olympic and World Championship medalist in the long jump, the 100 and 200 meter races, and the 4 x 100 relay. Five months before participating in his fifth and final Olympic competition, he learned that he had Hashimoto's thyroiditis and hypothyroidism. Being a true champion, he started taking levothyroxine while continuing his strenuous schedule of training, track meets, and promotional activities. Lewis, however, questioned whether he could rebound sufficiently to compete in the Olympics. On July 29, 1996, soaring through the air in the long jump, he answered that question and became one of only two people in the history of the Olympic Games to win nine gold medals during an Olympic career. Today he remains euthyroid on levothyroxine and continues to lead a very active, healthy life.

"As is the case with most people with thyroid conditions, I had no clue that I had the condition at all. The fact that I was checked was a fortunate accident. I can't emphasize enough the importance of being checked by a doctor for thyroid problems, especially if there is a family history of problems.

"I knew nothing about thyroid problems before discovering that I had one myself. Educate yourself, and follow prescribed treatment. As I showed in the Olympics, you can go back to being 100%. I feel even better now than I did in Atlanta, now that my stress level is on a more even keel and my medication levels are just right."

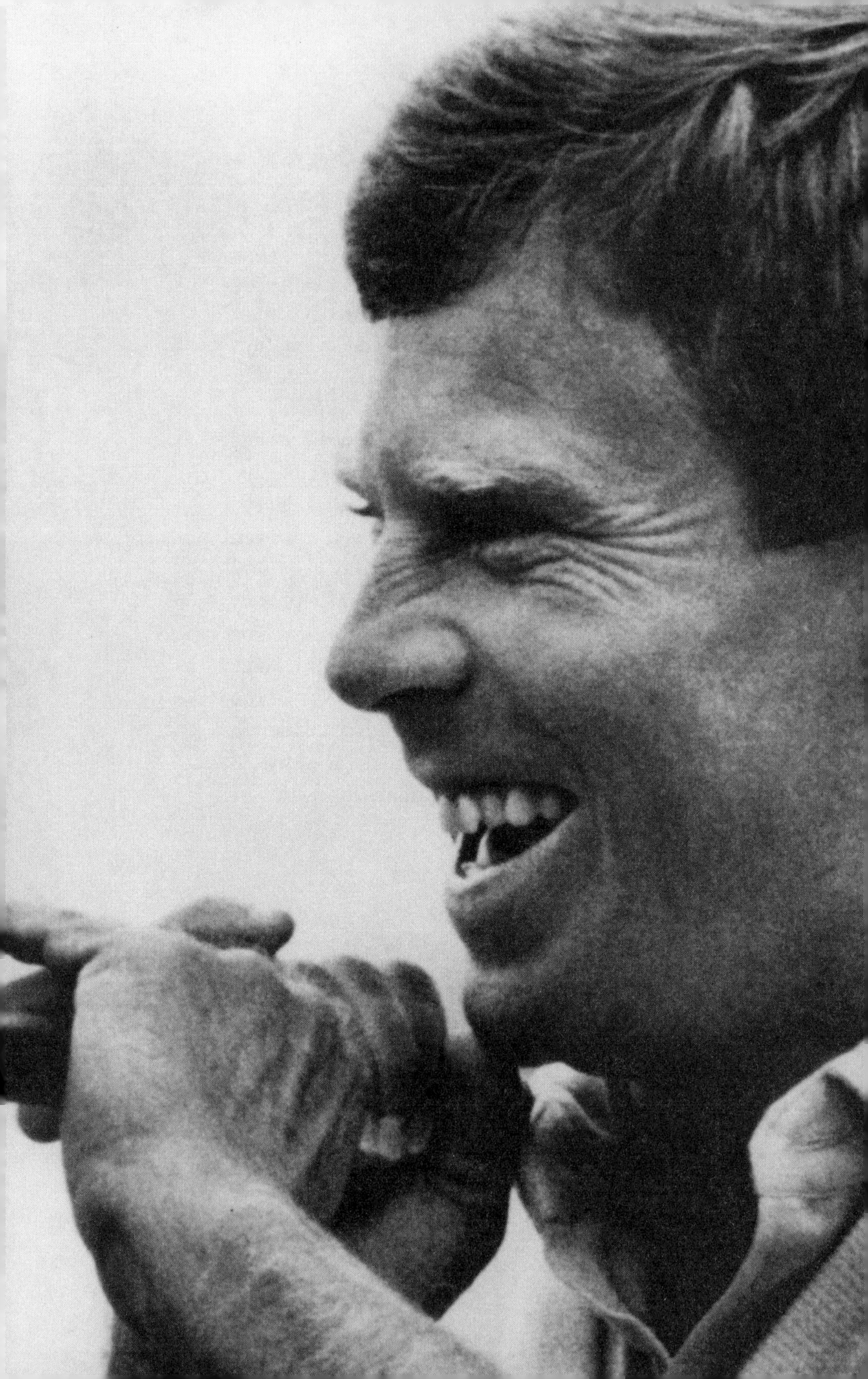

BEN CRENSHAW

In 1985, Ben Crenshaw, a professional golf veteran, was mystified about why his golf game was not "up to par," why his swing didn't have that zing. The explanation for his difficulties became apparent when he sought the advice of his physician; Ben Crenshaw had Graves' disease. Shortly after receiving radioactive iodine, Mr. Crenshaw was once again on the PGA Tour, and no one was more pleased than he when, in the summer of 1995, he won his second Master's Golf Tournament Championship in Augusta, Georgia.

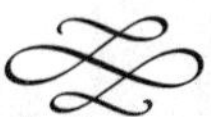

"Since contracting Graves' disease in 1985, and with subsequent treatment (radioactive iodine and supplemental [levothyroxine] daily), I was able to enjoy my former health status as a professional golfer. I continue to test my blood every 3 to 5 months. Stabilizing my thyroid was obviously vitally important to me."

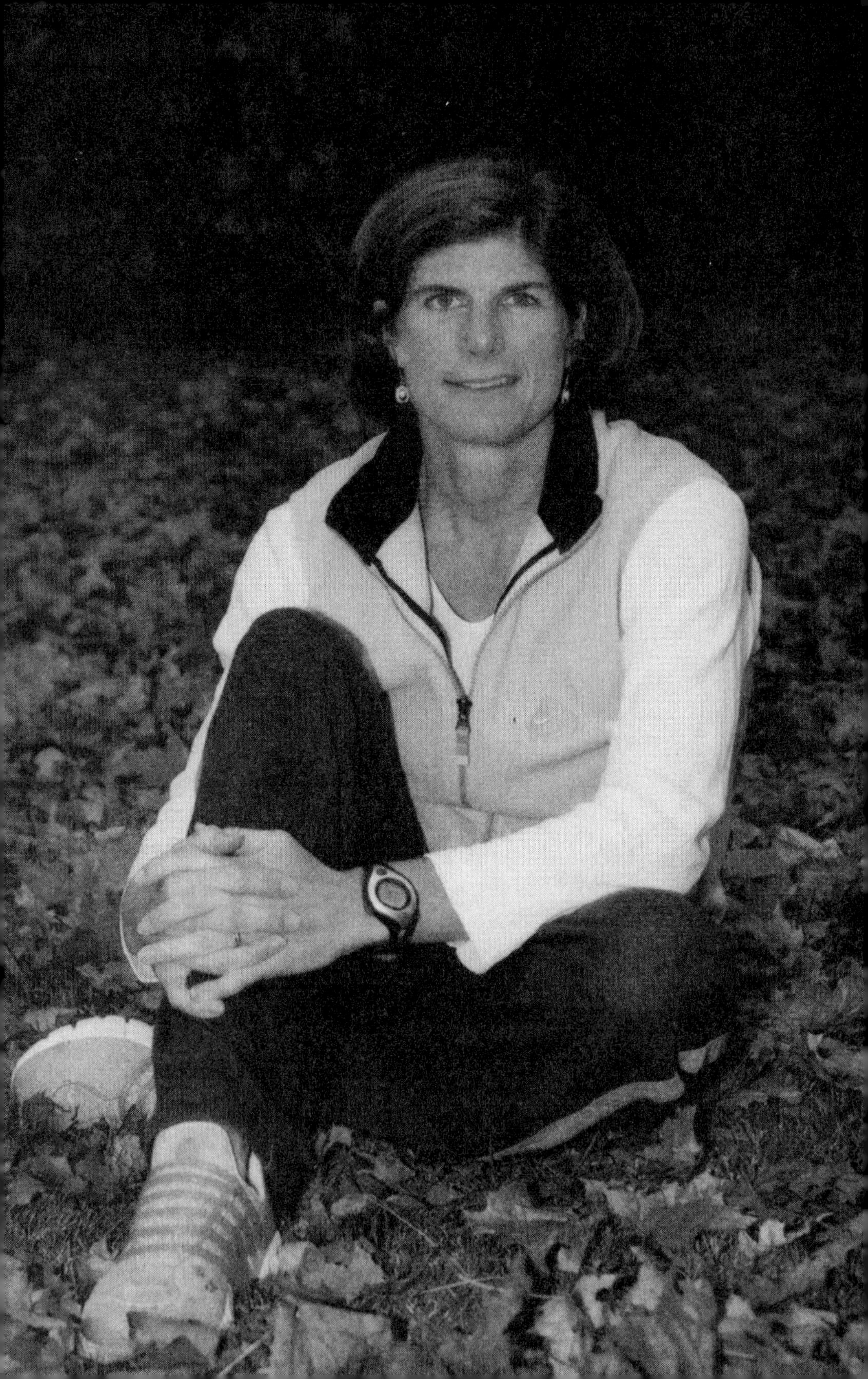

KAREN SMYERS

Karen Smyers won both the Hawaiian Ironman World and the short-course Triathlon World Championships in 1995, becoming the only woman ever to win these two races in the same year. During her seventeen-year career as a professional triathlete, Karen faced many challenges, including the diagnosis of thyroid cancer. Nonetheless, within a year of successful thyroid cancer treatment, she won the USA Triathlon Elite National Championship, her seventh national championship title.

"As a professional triathlete who makes a living from having my body fit and healthy, I was shocked beyond belief when the ultrasound indicated a high possibility of thyroid cancer. I thought that cancer was something that happened to other people—certainly not someone who trained twenty hours a week and was capable of doing nine-hour races in the heat of the Hawaiian Ironman.

"When the biopsy confirmed the cancer, I was forced to confront my worst fears. But I found that knowledge is power, and I learned all I could about the best treatment, support groups, and possible side effects. And, to my great relief, I read about other athletes with thyroid cancer who not only survived, but thrived.

"These role models provided me with the positive attitude and determination I needed to get through two surgeries and radioactive iodine treatment while continuing to pursue my athletic goals. And, as long as I take my daily dose of [levothyroxine], my body doesn't even know that my thyroid is missing!"

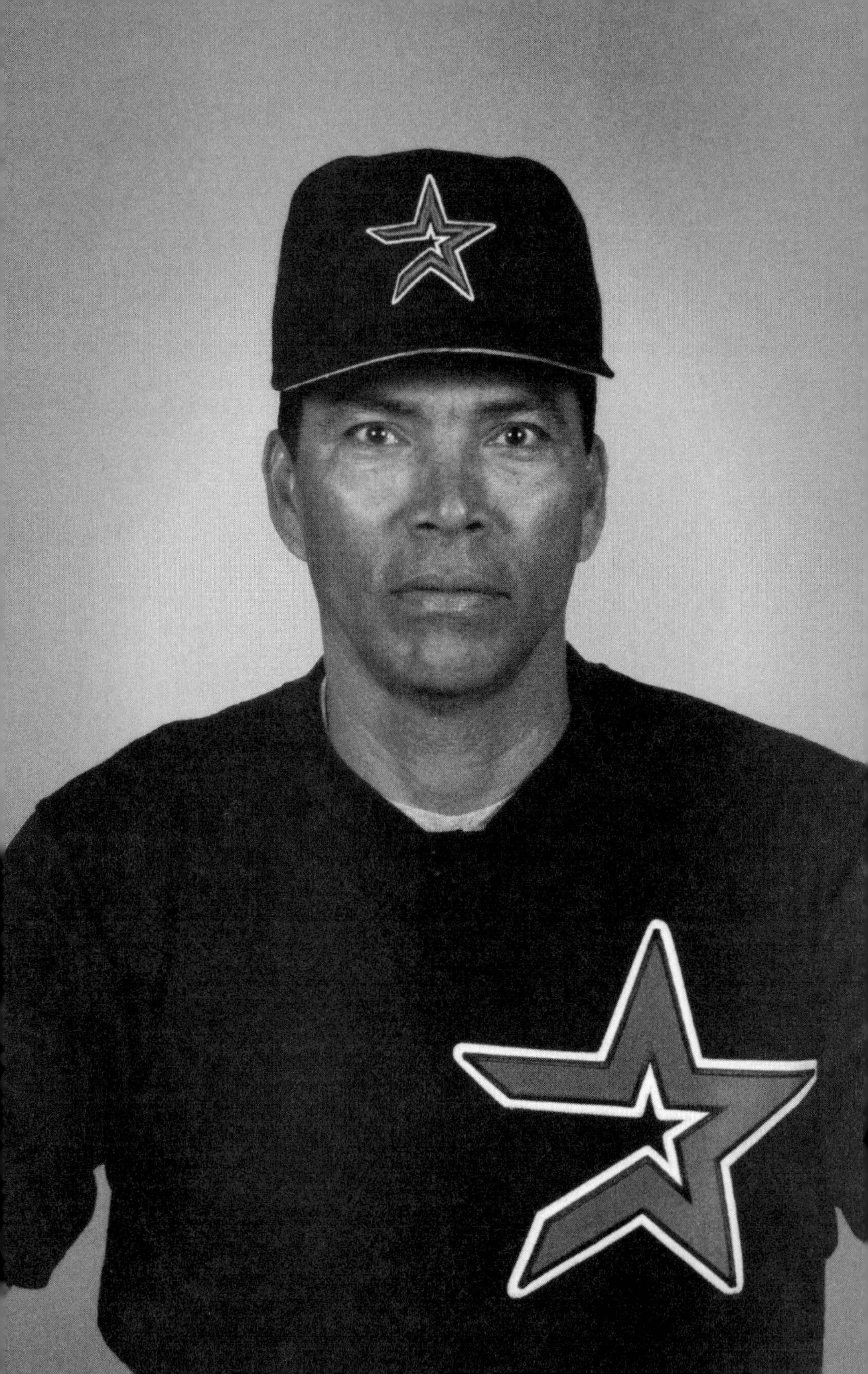

JOSÉ CRUZ

José Cruz's major league baseball career spanned nineteen years, most of which he spent as a record-setting batter and outfielder for the Houston Astros. Prior to becoming the Astros' first base coach, he played in more games (1,870) than any other player in the history of the franchise. In 1999, however, he was sidelined when an EKG demonstrated a rapid heart beat. Cruz had developed atrial fibrillation from Graves' hyperthyroidism. After treatment with radioactive iodine, Cruz became hypothyroid and began taking levothyroxine daily. He returned to the baseball field after missing thirty-four games. Today he is euthyroid, and his heart rate is normal.

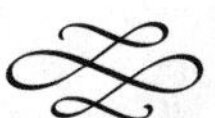

"I don't know for sure how long I had Graves' disease—maybe one or two years before I was treated. I lost about twenty pounds in three or four months. I was sweating, anxious, and not sleeping at night. I was also losing muscle, and my legs hurt when I touched them. I would overreact to everything. I would walk away when I got angry, to be alone, so I wouldn't explode. Everybody told me to 'calm down.' Then my heart started beating very fast, and everybody thought I had a heart problem. One doctor even put me to sleep and shocked my heart to get the heart rhythm normal. But one guy knew right away what was wrong. He was an endocrinologist.

"People should check with a specialist if they have these symptoms. Graves' disease can happen to anybody."

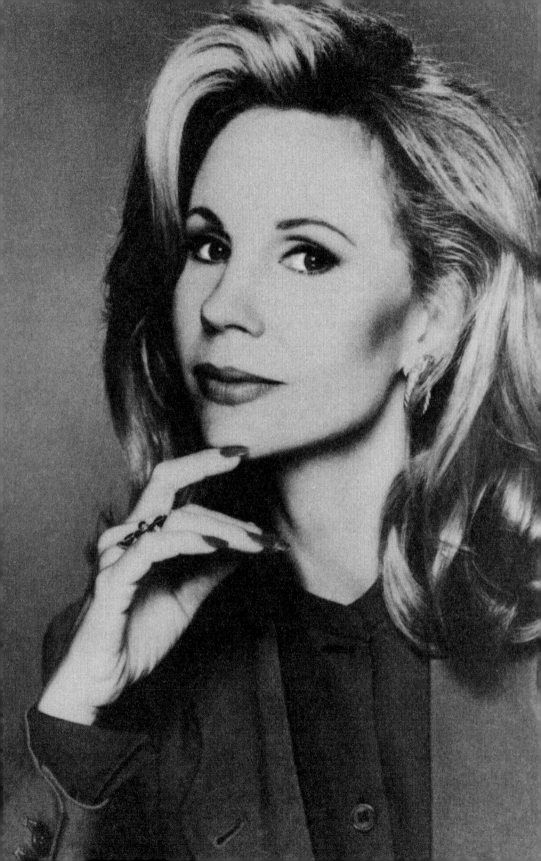

CAROLYN FARB

Carolyn Farb is a well-known Houstonian who devotes most of her time to helping other people. A familiar face and motivating dynamo behind many charitable organizations, her advice and expertise in organizing special fund raising events is highly sought after. Fortunately, Ms. Farb has shared her fund raising knowledge in her book, *How to Raise Millions Helping Others, Having a Ball!*

"Your symptoms may not be obvious, but I can remember putting on a couple of pounds when I had always been slim and not being able to lose that weight and feeling tired when I had always been 'high energy.' During a routine checkup, the doctor examined my thyroid, and a nodule was discovered. Sometimes we are so involved in the act of living that we forget to see how we are really feeling and take our health for granted.

"Once the nodule was determined to be the 'good kind,' I was given medication to suppress it. I now take daily medication and have my thyroid hormone and TSH levels checked on a regular basis. I feel very fortunate that my hypothyroid condition was identified early and has not interfered with my living life to the fullest. Remember, that butterfly-shaped thyroid gland touches all of our organs."

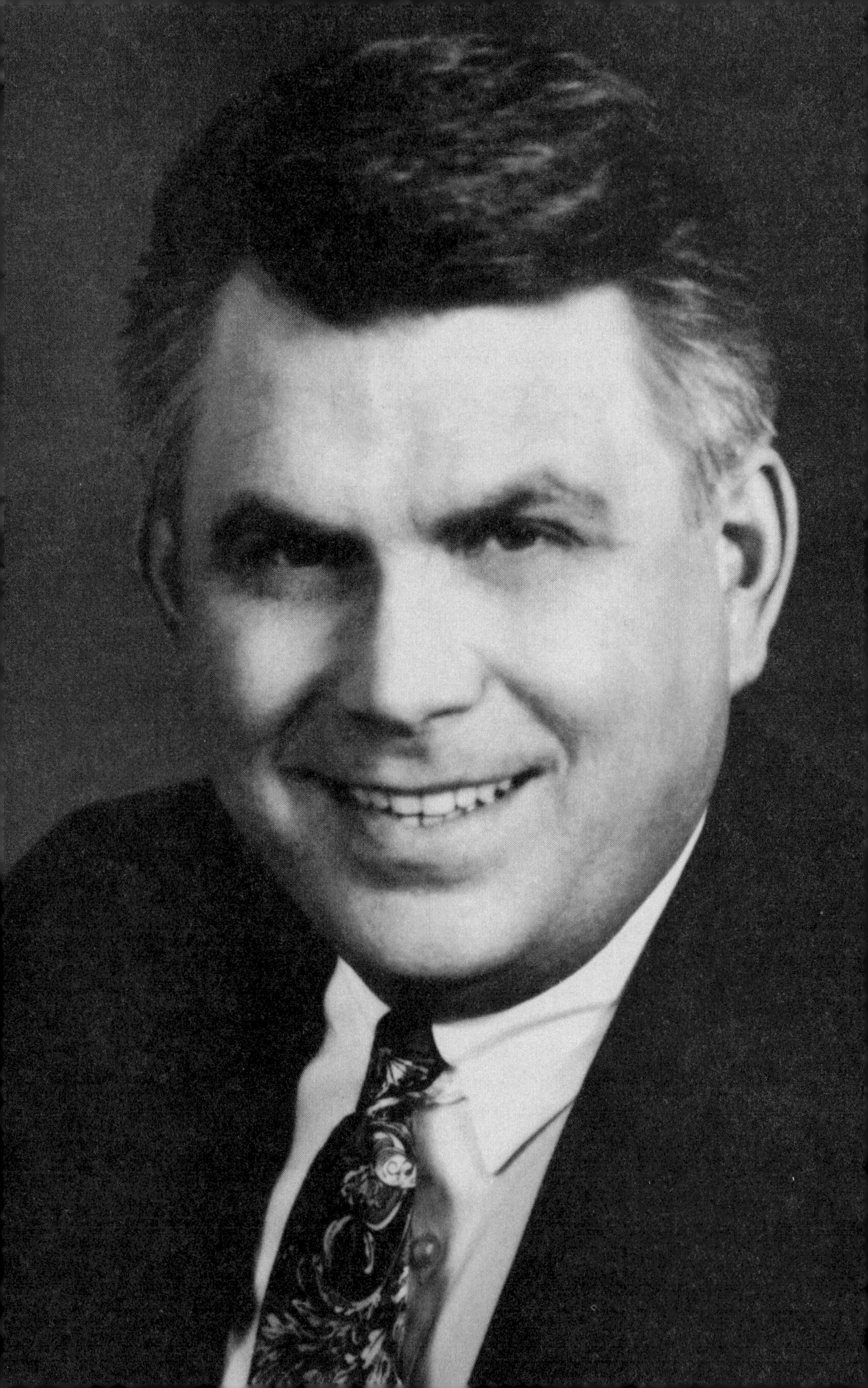

DON NELSON

Don Nelson has been working for more than twenty years at KTRK-TV in Houston, Texas; for sixteen of those years, he served as co-host of a weekday morning show, *Good Morning Houston*. One day Don began to feel very strange—his heart was racing; he was hot and sweaty; he thought he was having a heart attack. After being rushed to the hospital, he was diagnosed with Graves' disease. Following his doctor's advice, Don took radioactive iodine and started taking levothyroxine as soon as he became hypothyroid. Today Don is busier than ever, reporting on traffic, community events, and entertainment news on three newscasts a day.

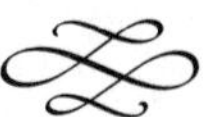

"When I look back on this whole episode, I realize how willingly I accepted my horrible mood swings and how easy it was to attribute them to the crazy type of business I'm in. After treatment, it was quite a revelation for me when I realized what 'normal' behavior really is. My experience has been that thyroid disease either exhilarates you or depresses you; there is no in-between.

"Now that I have a handle on what happened to me, I realize the incredible influence thyroid disease has on a person's psychological well-being. I worry about other people out there who might be second guessing their behavior, and not seeking help. My advice is not to dismiss changes in behavior too easily; have your thyroid checked."

Appendix A

SOURCES OF THYROID INFORMATION

Your physician is the best person to answer additional questions you may have about thyroid disease; however, if you would like more information, there are other resources available.

Lay Organizations for Thyroid Patients

Thyroid Foundation of America
410 Stuart Street
Boston, MA 02116
www.allthyroid.org
info@allthyroid.org
Phone: 1-800-832-8321
Fax: 617-726-4136

The Thyroid Foundation of Canada
P. O. Box/CP 1919 STN MAIN
Kingston, Ontario K7L 5J7
Canada
www.thyroid.ca
Phone: 613-544-8364 or 1-800-267-8822 (in Canada)
Fax: 613-544-9731

National Graves' Disease Foundation
P. O. Box 1969
Brevard, NC 28712
www.ngdf.org
ngdf@citcom.net
Phone: 1-828-877-5251
Fax: 1-828-877-5250

ThyCa: Thyroid Cancer Survivors' Association
P. O. Box 1545
New York, NY 10159-1545
www.thyca.org
thyca@thyca.org
Phone: 1-877-588-7904
Fax: 503-905-9725

The Hormone Foundation
4350 East West Highway, Suite 500
Bethesda, MD 20814-4426
www.hormone.org
Phone: 1-800-HORMONE (1-800-467-6663)

Professional Thyroid Organizations

The American Thyroid Association
6066 Leesburg Pike
P. O. Box 1836
Falls Church, VA 22041
www.thyroid.org
admin@thyroid.org
Phone: 703-998-8890 or 1-800-THYROID (1-800-849-7643)
Fax: 703-998-8893

American Association of Clinical Endocrinologists (AACE)
1000 Riverside Avenue, Suite 205
Jacksonville, FL 32204
www.aace.com
Phone: 904-353-7878
Fax: 904-353-8185

The Endocrine Society
4350 East West Highway, Suite 500
Bethesda, MD 20814
www.endo-society.org
Phone: 1-888-ENDOCRINE (1-888-363-6274)
Fax: 301-941-0259

Thyroid Books for Patients

The Thyroid Book: What Goes Wrong and How to Treat It by Martin I. Surks, M.D.

The Thyroid Source Book by M. Sara Rosenthal

Your Thyroid: A Home Reference by Lawrence C. Wood, M.D., David S. Cooper, M.D., and Chester Ridgway, M.D.

Thyroid Disease: The Facts by R. I. S. Bayliss, M.D., and W. M. G. Turnbridge, M.D.

Thyroid for Dummies by Alan L. Rubin, M.D.

The Thyroid Guide by Beth Ann Ditkoff, M.D., and Paul Lo Gerfo, M.D.

Sources of Physician Referral Lists

Your physician is usually the best source of physician referral. If you wish to locate a specialist on your own, the most important fact that you should bear in mind is that *experience counts.*

Patient Organizations Providing Physician Referral Lists

Thyroid Foundation of America
410 Stuart Street
Boston, MA 02116
www.allthyroid.org
info@allthyroid.org
Phone: 1-800-832-8321
Fax: 617-726-4136

The Hormone Foundation
4350 East West Highway, Suite 500
Bethesda, MD 20814-4426
www.hormone.org
referrals@endocrinologist-society.org
Phone: 1-800-HORMONE (1-800-467-6663)

Professional Associations Providing Physician Referral Lists

The American Thyroid Association
6066 Leesburg Pike
P. O. Box 1836
Falls Church, VA 22041
www.thyroid.org
Phone: 703-998-8890 or 1-800-THYROID (1-800-849-7643)
Fax: 703-998-8893

The Endocrine Society
4350 East West Highway, Suite 500
Bethesda, MD 20814
www.endo-society.org
Phone: 1-888-ENDOCRINE (1-888-363-6274)
Fax: 301-941-0259

American Association of Clinical Endocrinologists (AACE)
1000 Riverside Avenue, Suite 205
Jacksonville, FL 32204
www.aace.com
Phone: 904-353-7878
Fax: 904-353-8185

American Society of Ophthalmic, Plastic and Reconstructive Surgery
1133 West Morse Blvd., #201
Winter Park, FL 32789
www.asoprs.org
Phone: 407-647-8839

National Directories

You may also find several national medical directories in medical libraries or public libraries that have lists of physicians in your area. Below are the names of three directories that could be helpful.

American Medical Association Directory of Physicians in the United States, 33rd Edition published by the American Medical Association

Directory of Medical Specialists published by Marquis' *Who's Who*

Directory of Board Certified Medical Specialists published by the American Board of Medical Specialties

Bookstores

Guide to Top Doctors, published by the Center for the Study of Service

Websites

www.abms.org
1-866-ASK-ABMS (1-866-275-2267)
maintained by the American Board of Medical Specialties
to confirm whether a particular physician is board certified

www.bestdoctors.com
provided by Best Doctors®
to obtain a list of doctors ranked by other physicians

www.EndocrineWeb.com/docsearch
provided by YourDoctor™
to find medical and surgical specialists

www.medem.com
provided by Medem™
to locate physicians by specialty in certain geographic areas

Other Sources

local medical societies

endocrinology and surgery departments of hospitals associated with medical schools

Some websites, street addresses, and phone numbers may have changed since the printing of this book.

APPENDIX B

ONE LAST "TAIL"

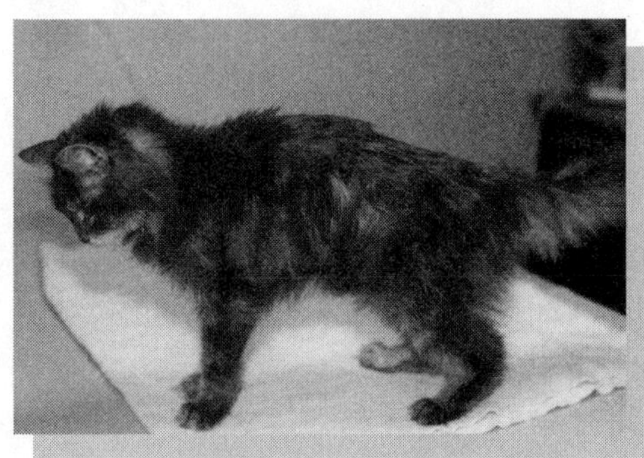

Hyperthyroid cat

Thyroid disease in humans is the primary focus of this book. However, some readers, especially pet owners, might find it interesting that animals, particularly cats and dogs, develop thyroid disease, too. Cats are more likely to develop hyperthyroidism, and dogs (like mine, described on page 126) are more prone to develop hypothyroidism.

According to Dr. Brian Poteet, a veterinary radiologist, the cause of hyperthyroidism in cats is unknown. However, the typical hyperthyroid cat is an older cat (fourteen years or older) with a toxic multinodular goiter. Symptoms include weight loss of up to half their body weight in two to three months, ravenous appetite, intermittent vomiting and diarrhea, increased urination, restlessness, dull coat, increased shedding, and patchy loss of hair. Approximately 30% of hyperthyroid cats become apathetic and do not want to eat.

Owners sometimes do not notice any changes in their cats, and, if they do, they may attribute the cat's symptoms to advancing age. Therefore, many cats are diagnosed only when they have a geriatric feline profile, routine blood work that is done annually in cats twelve years and older. Although measurement of T_4 is part of this profile, there is no TSH for cats.

To confirm a diagnosis of feline hyperthyroidism, a veterinarian will usually order a thyroid scan. Thyroid images with radioactive materials for cats are the same as thyroid scans for humans with one exception. Since cats are unlikely to lie still while the gamma camera scans them, they are put under general anesthesia for about ten minutes.

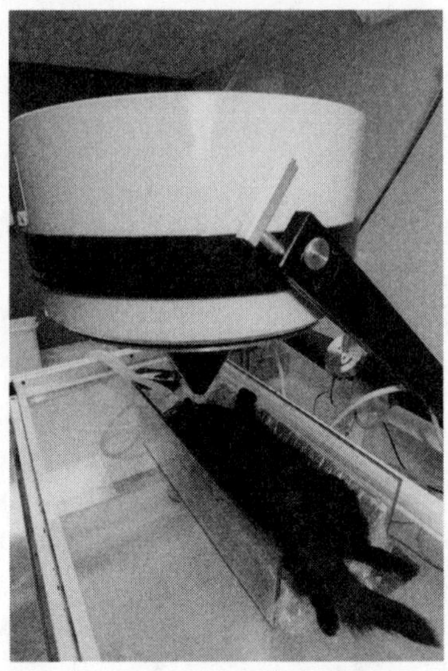

Cat having a thyroid scan (a real cat scan?).

The treatment options for feline hyperthyroidism are the same as for humans—radioactive iodine, anti-thyroid drugs, and surgery. Treating cats for hyperthyroidism can be costly, but it can be done effectively, especially when radioactive iodine treatment is chosen. According to Dr. Poteet, "the success rate of radiaoctive iodine treatment is close to 100%." He also pointed out that unlike humans, "Cats almost never become hypothyroid after treatment."

GLOSSARY

aberrant thyroid – thyroid tissue that migrates from its usual path and appears in other places in the neck

ablative dose – the amount of radioactive iodine required to destroy residual thyroid tissue after surgical treatment of thyroid cancer

acropachy – a rare disorder in patients with Graves' disease that may include elevation of the nail beds, soft-tissue swelling of the hands and feet, and new bone formation

acute suppurative thyroiditis – an inflammation of the thyroid gland due to bacterial infection

AFTN – *see* autonomously functioning thyroid nodule

agenesis – the complete absence of the thyroid gland at birth

agranulocytosis – a very low white blood cell count

AIH – *see* amiodarone-induced hypothyroidism

AIT – *see* amiodarone-induced thyrotoxicosis

albumin – one of three proteins in the bloodstream to which thyroid hormones attach themselves

alopecia – hair loss

amiodarone – a medication for the control of dangerous heart rhythm disturbances (arrhythmias)

amiodarone-induced hypothyroidism (AIH) – hypothyroidism caused by amiodarone

amiodarone-induced thyrotoxicosis (AIT) – hyperthyroidism caused by amiodarone; two different types, I and II, have been identified

anaplastic thyroid cancer – *see* undifferentiated thyroid cancer

anemia – reduced number of red blood cells

angina pectoris – chest pain from coronary artery disease

antibodies – proteins formed by the immune system to protect the body against chemicals, bacteria, or viruses

antithyroid antibodies – antibodies against the thyroid gland; also called antithyroid autoantibodies

antithyroid autoantibodies – *see* antithyroid antibodies

antithyroid drugs – drugs that block the production of thyroid hormones by the thyroid gland

apathetic hyperthyroidism – a form of hyperthyroidism seen primarily in older patients whose major symptom is a lack of interest in life

aplasia cutis – a birth defect that may be caused by a pregnant woman's ingestion of antithyroid drugs

assays – laboratory tests

atrial fibrillation – a dangerous heart rhythm disturbance seen in some hyperthyroid patients

atrophic – smaller than normal

autoantibodies – antibodies formed against the body's own tissues

autoimmune disease – a disease characterized by the presence of autoantibodies

autoimmunity – the development of antibodies against one's own tissues

autonomously functioning thyroid nodule (AFTN) – a thyroid nodule that functions independently of the usual control mechanisms

basal metabolic rate (BMR) – the rate at which energy is expended for cellular and tissue processes that maintain life

benign – noncancerous

beta-blockers – medications that slow down the heart rate and reduce the tremor of hyperthyroid patients

block-replace method – a method of treating hyperthyroid patients using antithyroid drugs (block) and then adding levothyroxine (replace)

C cells – thyroid cells that produce calcitonin; also called parafollicular cells

calcitonin – a hormone, whose function is not known, secreted by the C cells; a tumor marker for medullary thyroid cancer

calcium – an essential element whose level in the blood is maintained by the parathyroid glands

calcium infusion test – calcium given intravenously to stimulate calcitonin

carcinoembryonic antigen (CEA) – a tumor marker for medullary thyroid cancer and other nonthyroidal cancers such as colon cancer

carotidynia – pain in the carotid artery

CAT scan – a computerized axial tomographic scan; an x-ray procedure

CEA – *see* carcinoembryonic antigen

central compartment – the area in the front of the neck, from the hyoid bone to the innominate veins and in between the jugular veins

central hypothyroidism – hypothyroidism caused by failure of either the pituitary gland (secondary hypothyroidism) or the hypothalamus (tertiary hypothyroidism)

cholesterol – a fatty substance present in the blood and tissues of the body as well as many foods

choriocarcinoma – a cancer causing excessive secretion of hCG

cold nodule – a nodule that takes up less radioactive material than the surrounding thyroid tissue on a thyroid image or scan

colloid – a jelly-like material in the center of a thyroid follicle that stores thyroid hormone

completion thyroidectomy – additional surgery on a thyroid cancer patient, designed to remove all or nearly all of the remaining thyroid tissue

congenital abnormality – a defect that exists at birth

congenital hypothyroidism – hypothyroidism that exists at birth

congestive heart failure – a condition resulting from failure of the heart to pump blood effectively, resulting in the accumulation of fluid in the lungs and legs

coronary artery disease – disease of the arteries supplying blood to the heart that leads to chest pain, heart attacks, angioplasty, and bypass ("open heart") surgery

creatine kinase (CK) – a muscle enzyme

cretin – a hypothyroid patient with mental retardation and short stature

cutting needle biopsy (CNB) – a biopsy using a needle with a tip for cutting tissue

cyst – a fluid-filled structure

cystic thyroid nodule – a fluid-filled thyroid nodule

Cytomel® – the brand-name of triiodothyronine (T_3)

Cytomel® suppression test – *see* T_3 suppression test

de Quervain's thyroiditis – *see* subacute thyroiditis

differentiated thyroid cancer – papillary or follicular thyroid cancer

diffuse goiter – a generalized, relatively symmetrical enlargement of the thyroid gland

diplopia – double vision

dominant nodule – a nodule much larger than others present in a multinodular goiter

dosimetry – the determination, based upon a calculation of the radiation delivered to cancer cells, of the radioactive iodine dosage to treat a patient with thyroid cancer

dysphagia – difficulty in swallowing

dyspnea – difficulty in breathing

endemic goiter – a goiter that occurs among large segments of a population living in areas of the world with widespread iodine deficiency

endocrine glands – glands that secrete hormones internally

endocrinologist – a doctor who cares for patients with disorders of the endocrine glands

ENT – an ear, nose, and throat doctor; also called an otorhinolaryngologist

enzyme – a protein that speeds chemical reactions

estrogens – female hormones

ethanol injection – a direct injection of alcohol into a thyroid nodule to destroy it

euthyroid Graves' disease – Graves' eye disease in a patient with normal thyroid function

euthyroid sick syndrome (ESS) – *see* nonthyroidal illness syndrome

euthyroidism – the state of having the proper amount of thyroid hormone in the body

exophthalmometer – an instrument for measuring the protrusion of an eyeball from its orbit

exophthalmos – protrusion of an eyeball from its orbit

external-beam radiation – radiation therapy originating from a source outside of the patient's body

factitious thyrotoxicosis – condition resulting from excessive ingestion of thyroid hormone in a covert fashion

familial – hereditary

familial dysalbuminemic hyperthyroxinemia – an elevated T_4 caused by a hereditary abnormality of albumin, a thyroid hormone-binding protein

FDA – *see* Food and Drug Administration

fine needle aspiration biopsy (FNAB) – a biopsy obtained by inserting a thin needle into a thyroid nodule and extracting cells for analysis

FNAB – *see* fine needle aspiration biopsy

follicles – microscopic spherical units that make up the thyroid gland

follicular adenoma – a noncancerous growth composed of thyroid follicular cells

follicular thyroid cancer – a type of cancerous growth derived from thyroid follicular cells; also called follicular carcinoma

follicular thyroid carcinoma – *see* follicular cancer

Food and Drug Administration (FDA) – United States governmental agency that regulates the manufacturing of drugs

free T_3 – unbound triiodothyronine in the bloodstream

free T_3 assay – measurement of unbound triiodothyronine in the bloodstream

free T_4 – unbound thyroxine in the bloodstream

free T_4 assay – measurement of unbound thyroxine in the bloodstream

free thyroxine index (FTI) – a calculation using T_3 resin uptake and total T_4 to estimate free T_4 in the bloodstream

frozen section – rapid freezing and then slicing (sectioning) of a tissue specimen for immediate viewing under the microscope

FTI – *see* free thyroxine index

galactorrhea – a milky discharge from the breast

gamma camera – a stationary instrument that produces images of the thyroid gland after administration of radioactive materials

ganglioneuromatoses – tumors arising from nerves

gestational transient hyperthyroidism – hyperthyroidism that occurs in some women during the eighth through fourteenth week of an otherwise normal pregnancy; also called gestational thyrotoxicosis

glaucoma – increased pressure in the eye

globus hystericus – an anxiety-related tightening of throat muscles that causes a sensation of something stuck in the throat

goiter – an enlargement of the thyroid gland

Graves' dermatopathy – a disease of the skin associated with Graves' disease

Graves' disease – an autoimmune disease of the thyroid, eyes, and skin

Graves' eye disease – an eye disease associated with Graves' disease; also called Graves' orbitopathy or Graves' ophthalmopathy

Graves' ophthalmopathy – *see* Graves' eye disease

Graves' orbitopathy – *see* Graves' eye disease

gynecomastia – an abnormal growth of breast tissue in a male

Hashimoto's thyroiditis – a chronic destructive autoimmune inflammation of the thyroid gland

hCG – *see* human chorionic gonadotropin

HDL – *see* high-density lipoprotein

hemiagenesis – the absence of one lobe of the thyroid gland at birth

high-density lipoprotein (HDL) – the "good" cholesterol

homocysteine – an amino acid; elevated levels of homocysteine in the blood may be a risk factor for heart disease

hot nodule – a nodule that takes up more radioactive material than the surrounding thyroid tissue on a thyroid image or scan

human chorionic gonadotropin (hCG) – a hormone produced during pregnancy that can stimulate the thyroid gland

Hürthle cell cancer – a distinctive type of follicular cancer

hydatidiform mole – an abnormal growth in pregnant women that can cause excessive secretion of hCG

hypercalcemia – too much calcium in the blood

hypercholesterolemia – too much cholesterol in the blood

hyperemesis gravidarum – excessive vomiting during pregnancy

hyperparathyroidism – production of too much parathyroid hormone by the parathyroid glands

hyperthyroidism – production of too much thyroid hormone by the thyroid gland

hypocalcemia – a low calcium level in the blood

hypoparathyroidism – low parathyroid hormone production by the parathyroid glands

hypothalamus – the part of the brain that controls the pituitary gland

hypothyroidism – a condition resulting from insufficient production of thyroid hormone by the thyroid gland

I^{123} – a radioactive isotope of iodine used for diagnostic purposes

I^{131} – a radioactive isotope of iodine used in the diagnosis and treatment of some thyroid disorders

iatrogenic thyrotoxicosis – too much thyroid hormone in the blood caused by a physician prescribing too much thyroid hormone medication

ICCIDD – *see* International Council for the Control of Iodine Deficiency Disorders

IDD – *see* iodine deficiency disorders

idiopathic hypothyroidism – hypothyroidism from an unknown cause

IFNa – *see* interferon alpha

IL-6 – *see* interleukin-6

incidentalomas – thyroid nodules found during diagnostic procedures examining other parts of the neck

interferon alpha (IFNa) – a drug used to treat patients with hepatitis B or C and certain types of cancer

interleukin-6 (IL-6) – one of many cytokines, or hormone-like proteins, that play an important part in the body's immune response

International Council for the Control of Iodine Deficiency Disorders (ICCIDD) – a multinational network of experts who help develop, implement, and monitor national programs to eliminate iodine deficiency

internship – the first year of a medical school graduate's hospital training program

iodine – an essential element in thyroid hormones

iodine deficiency disorders (IDD) – disorders, such as goiter, hypothyroidism, and mental retardation, caused by insufficient iodine intake

isotopes – radioactive materials used in the diagnosis and treatment of some thyroid disorders

isthmus – the thyroid tissue that connects the two lobes of the thyroid gland

isthmusectomy – the surgical removal of the isthmus of the thyroid gland

Jod-Basedow's disease – hyperthyroidism caused by taking excessive amounts of iodine

LDL – *see* low-density lipoprotein

Levothroid® – a brand-name levothyroxine preparation

levothyroxine – a thyroid hormone containing four atoms of iodine; also called T_4 or thyroxine

Levoxyl®– a brand-name levothyroxine preparation

libido – interest in sex

lingual thyroid – thyroid tissue located at the back of the tongue

lobectomy – *see* thyroid lobectomy

low-density lipoprotein (LDL) – the "bad" cholesterol

lymph node – a collection of protective white blood cells

lymphatic system – an interconnected system of channels and lymph nodes through which fluid (lymph) containing protective lymphocytes travels

lymphatics – channels through which fluid (lymph) containing protective lymphocytes travels

lymphocyte – a white blood cell

lymphocytic thyroiditis – *see* painless thyroiditis

lymphoma – a cancer of lymphocytes

malignant – cancerous

medullary thyroid cancer (MTC) – thyroid cancer arising from C cells

MEN 2 – *see* multiple endocrine neoplasia type 2

MEN 2A – *see* multiple endocrine neoplasia type 2A

MEN 2B – *see* multiple endocrine neoplasia type 2B

menopause – the time when a woman's ovaries stop functioning or are surgically removed

metastasis – the spread of cancer beyond its site of origin

methimazole – an antithyroid medication; also called Tapazole®

microcarcinoma – *see* occult thyroid cancer

mild thyroid failure – *see* subclinical hypothyroidism

millicurie (mCi) – a unit of measurement of radioactive materials

modified radical neck dissection – the surgical removal of selected lymph nodes from one side of the neck

MRI – magnetic resonance imaging; an x-ray procedure

multifocal papillary cancer – a papillary cancer arising from more than one site within a thyroid gland

multinodular goiter – an enlarged thyroid gland with multiple growths or lumps

multiple endocrine neoplasia type 2 (MEN 2) – a hereditary syndrome that includes tumors in multiple endocrine glands

multiple endocrine neoplasia type 2A (MEN 2A) – a hereditary syndrome that includes medullary thyroid cancer and tumors of the adrenal and parathyroid glands

multiple endocrine neoplasia type 2B (MEN 2B) – a hereditary syndrome that includes medullary thyroid cancer, tumors of the adrenal glands, and ganglioneuromatoses

myxedema – 1. a severe form of hypothyroidism; 2. thickening of the skin in Graves' disease

myxedema coma – a coma resulting from severe, untreated hypothyroidism

NDA – *see* New Drug Application

neonatal hyperthyroidism – temporary hyperthyroidism seen in some babies born to mothers with Graves' disease

New Drug Application (NDA) – a process pharmaceutical manufacturers follow to meet FDA standards of safety, effectiveness, consistency, and reliability of a brand-name drug

nodule – *see* thyroid nodule

nonsteroidal anti-inflammatory drugs (NSAIDs) – certain drugs containing no steroids used to treat inflammation

nonthyroidal illness syndrome (NTIS) – abnormal thyroid function tests in a patient with a severe nonthyroidal illness; also called euthyroid sick syndrome

ob-gyn – *see* obstetrician-gynecologist

obstetrician-gynecologist (ob-gyn) – a doctor who specializes in women's diseases and in the delivery of babies

occult thyroid cancer – a papillary thyroid cancer less than 1.0 centimeter in diameter

oncologist – a physician who specializes in the treatment of cancer

onycholysis – the separation of fingernails from the nail beds

ophthalmologist – a physician specializing in eye diseases

orbital decompression – the surgical removal of inflamed and swollen tissue from the orbit

orbital expansion – the surgical removal of some of the bone around the orbit to provide more space for the eye

orbital rim augmentation – the surgical procedure to move facial bones forward to make more room for the eye

osteopenia – a milder form of osteoporosis

osteoporosis – thinning of the bones

otorhinolaryngologist – *see* ENT

painless thyroiditis – a painless inflammation of the thyroid gland; also called subacute lymphocytic thyroiditis, silent thyroiditis, or lymphocytic thyroiditis

palpation-induced thyroiditis – thyroiditis caused by vigorous physical examination of the thyroid gland by the physician or by the patient

papillary-follicular thyroid cancer – a form of thyroid cancer with elements that look like both papillary and follicular cancers; also called follicular variant of papillary cancer

papillary thyroid cancer – a type of cancerous growth composed of thyroid follicular cells; also called papillary carcinoma

papillary thyroid carcinoma – *see* papillary thyroid cancer

parafollicular cells – *see* C cells

parathyroid glands – glands that produce parathyroid hormone

parathyroid hormone – a hormone produced by the parathyroid glands that is responsible for maintaining a normal calcium level in the blood

pathologist – a doctor who examines cells and tissue for disease and supervises laboratories where blood tests are performed

Pemberton's sign – a redness of the face that appears after fully extending the arms upright along the side of the head

pentagastrin – a hormone used to stimulate calcitonin

permanent section – the meticulous preparation of a tissue sample for viewing under the microscope by a pathologist

PET scan – a positron emission tomography scan

pheochromocytoma – a type of tumor of the adrenal glands

pituitary gland – the "master gland," located in the brain, that makes TSH (thyroid-stimulating hormone) and other hormones

postpartum period – the year following the birth of a child

postpartum thyroiditis – an inflammation of a woman's thyroid gland that begins during the first few months after delivery of a child

post-treatment scan – a whole body scan performed two to seven days after radioactive iodine treatment for thyroid cancer

prematurely gray hair – gray hair before the age of thirty

premature menopause – a failure of the ovaries before the age of forty

pretibial myxedema – a thickening of the skin on the shins seen in patients with Graves' disease

primary hypothyroidism – hypothyroidism caused by failure of the thyroid gland

prognosis – a prediction of the outcome of an illness

prolactin – a pituitary hormone required for lactation and breastfeeding

proptosis – the protrusion of an eyeball from the orbit

propylthiouracil (PTU) – an antithyroid medication

pruritus – itching

PTU – *see* propylthiouracil

pyramidal lobe – a small lobe of the thyroid gland rising upward from the isthmus

radiation-induced thyroiditis – an inflammation of the thyroid gland due to radiation

radical neck dissection – the surgical removal of all lymph nodes, certain muscles and veins, and a nerve from one side of the neck

radioactive iodine – a radioactive isotope of iodine used in the diagnosis and treatment of some thyroid disorders

radioactive iodine uptake (RAIU) – the amount of orally administered radioactive iodine taken up by the thyroid gland

RAIU – *see* radioactive iodine uptake

receptor – a specific site on a cell that selectively captures its corresponding hormone

recombinant human TSH – *see* Thyrogen®

rectilinear scanner – an instrument that scans back and forth to provide life-size images of the thyroid gland after oral administration of radioactive materials

recurrent laryngeal nerves – nerves that control the vocal cords

remission – the disappearance of the signs and symptoms of a disease

residency – a medical school graduate's hospital training program in a specialized area of medicine

resistance to thyroid hormone (RTH) – the failure of the pituitary gland or other organs to properly sense the amount of thyroid hormone in the blood

RET proto-oncogene – a gene in which a mutation can identify patients with familial medullary thyroid cancer

rhTSH – *see* Thyrogen®

Riedel's struma – a form of thyroiditis, characterized by scarring of the thyroid gland and, sometimes, the tissue surrounding the thyroid gland

Rocaltrol® – a man-made vitamin D

screening – a process for detecting a disease among people who do not have, or are unaware that they have, the disease

secondary hypothyroidism – hypothyroidism caused by the pituitary gland's failure to produce sufficient TSH (thyroid-stimulating hormone)

secrete – to release into the bloodstream

sedimentation rate – the rate at which proteins in the blood settle to the bottom of a small tube in a laboratory

sign – physical evidence of an illness

silent thyroiditis – *see* painless thyroiditis

simple euthyroid goiter – a diffusely enlarged thyroid gland in a patient with normal thyroid function and without Hashimoto's thyroiditis

sleep apnea – intermittently not breathing during sleep

solitary thyroid nodule – a single lump or growth in the thyroid gland

spontaneous remission – disappearance of the signs and symptoms of an illness without treatment

steroids – powerful anti-inflammatory drugs, such as prednisone and Decadron®

struma ovarii – thyroid tissue in an ovary

subacute lymphocytic thyroiditis – *see* painless thyroiditis

subacute thyroiditis (SAT) – a painful inflammation of the thyroid gland; also called subacute granulomatous thyroiditis, giant cell thyroiditis, subacute nonsuppurative thyroiditis, and de Quervain's thyroiditis

subclinical hyperthyroidism – a condition characterized by low TSH (thyroid-stimulating hormone) with normal thyroid hormone levels in a patient without signs or symptoms of hyperthyroidism

subclinical hypothyroidism – a condition characterized by an elevated TSH (thyroid-stimulating hormone), or an elevated TSH response to thyrotropin-releasing hormone (TRH), with normal thyroid hormone levels in a patient without signs or symptoms of hypothyroidism; also called mild thyroid failure

substernal goiter – thyroid tissue located in the chest behind the breast bone (sternum)

subtotal thyroidectomy – the surgical removal of one lobe, the isthmus, and almost all of the other lobe of the thyroid gland

synthetic TSH – *see* Thyrogen®

Synthroid® – a brand-name levothyroxine preparation

T_3 – *see* triiodothyronine

T_3 resin uptake (T_3RU) – an indirect measurement of thyroid hormone-binding proteins in the bloodstream

T_3 suppression test – radioactive iodine uptakes performed before and after oral administration of T_3 for ten days; also called Cytomel® suppression test

T_3RU – *see* T_3 resin uptake

T_4 – *see* thyroxine and levothyroxine

TAFTN – *see* toxic autonomously functioning thyroid nodule

Tapazole® – a brand name of methimazole, an antithyroid medication

TBG – *see* thyroxine-binding globulin

TBII – *see* TSH-binding-inhibitory immunoglobulins

TBPA – *see* thyroxine-binding prealbumin

technetium – a radioactive isotope used to obtain a thyroid image

tertiary hypothyroidism – hypothyroidism caused by the hypothalamus' failure to produce enough TRH (thyrotropin-releasing hormone)

testosterone – a male hormone

Tg – *see* thyroglobulin

TgAb – *see* thyroglobulin antibody

thymus – an organ in the chest that works with the immune system to protect the body against disease

Thyrogen® – brand-name, man-made human TSH (thyroid-stimulating hormone); also called synthetic TSH, thyrotropin alfa, or recombinant human TSH (rhTSH)

Thyrogen® scan – a whole body scan after thyroid cancer patients have been injected with Thyrogen®

thyroglobulin (Tg) – a protein in which thyroid hormones are made and stored

thyroglobulin antibody (TgAb) – an autoantibody against thyroglobulin, often seen in patients with Hashimoto's thyroiditis

thyroglossal duct – a channel connecting the fetal thyroid gland and tongue; the pyramidal lobe, present in about one-third of people, may be a remnant of this channel

thyroglossal duct cyst – a cystic structure formed from a thyroglossal duct that did not disappear by birth

thyroid bed – the location of the thyroid gland before surgery

thyroid carcinoma – a cancer of the thyroid gland

thyroid gland – an endocrine gland that produces, stores, and secretes thyroid hormones

thyroid hormone-binding proteins – proteins to which thyroid hormones attach themselves and circulate in the blood

thyroid image – a picture of the thyroid gland obtained with radioactive materials and a gamma camera or a rectilinear scanner; also called a thyroid scan

thyroid lobectomy – the surgical removal of one lobe of the thyroid gland

thyroid nodule – a lump in the thyroid gland

thyroid remnant – the thyroid tissue remaining after a subtotal thyroidectomy

thyroid scan – a picture of the thyroid gland obtained with radioactive materials and a rectilinear scanner

thyroid storm – a life-threatening hyperthyroid crisis

thyroidectomy – partial or complete surgical removal of the thyroid gland

thyroiditis – inflammation of the thyroid gland

thyroidologist – a doctor specializing in diseases of the thyroid gland

thyroid-stimulating antibodies (TSAb) – antibodies to the thyrotropin (TSH) receptor that stimulate production of thyroid hormone from the thyroid gland; also called thyroid-stimulating immunoglobulins (TSI)

thyroid-stimulating hormone (TSH) – a hormone produced by the pituitary gland that stimulates production of thyroid hormones by the thyroid gland; also called thyrotropin

thyroid-stimulating immunoglobulins (TSI) – *see* thyroid-stimulating antibodies

thyroperoxidase – a chemical or enzyme facilitating chemical reactions in the thyroid gland

thyroperoxidase antibody (TPOAb) – an autoantibody against thyroperoxidase, often seen in patients with Hashimoto's thyroiditis

thyrotoxicosis – a condition resulting from too much thyroid hormone in the bloodstream

thyrotropin – *see* thyroid-stimulating hormone (TSH)

thyrotropin alfa – *see* Thyrogen®

thyrotropin (TSH) receptor – the site on a thyroid cell that selectively captures TSH (thyroid-stimulating hormone)

thyrotropin receptor antibodies (TRAb) – antibodies against the thyrotropin (TSH) receptor; also called TSH receptor antibodies

thyrotropin-releasing hormone (TRH) – a hormone secreted by the hypothalamus that stimulates the pituitary gland to produce TSH (thyroid-stimulating hormone)

thyroxine (T_4) – a thyroid hormone containing four atoms of iodine; also called levothyroxine

thyroxine-binding globulin (TBG) – the main protein to which thyroid hormones attach themselves and circulate in the blood

thyroxine-binding prealbumin (TBPA) – one of three proteins to which thyroid hormones attach themselves and circulate in the blood

TMNG – *see* toxic multinodular goiter

total body scan – *see* whole body scan

total T_4 – the total of bound and unbound T_4 in the bloodstream

total thyroidectomy – the surgical removal of the entire thyroid gland

toxic autonomously functioning thyroid nodule (TAFTN) – a thyroid nodule that functions independently of the usual control mechanisms and produces sufficient thyroid hormone to cause hyperthyroidism

toxic multinodular goiter (TMNG) – a thyroid gland with multiple nodules that function independently of the usual control mechanisms and produce sufficient thyroid hormone to cause hyperthyroidism

TPOAb – *see* thyroperoxidase antibody

TRAb – *see* thyrotropin receptor antibodies

trachea – the windpipe

tracheostomy – a surgical opening in the trachea (windpipe)

trauma-induced thyroiditis – a form of thyroiditis that may occur after fine needle aspiration biopsy, manipulation of the thyroid gland during surgery, and repetitive trauma to the thyroid gland from a seat belt

TRH – *see* thyrotropin-releasing hormone

TRH test – a test performed by injecting thyrotropin-releasing hormone intravenously and then drawing blood several times to measure TSH

triiodothyronine (T_3) – a thyroid hormone containing three atoms of iodine

TSAb – *see* thyroid-stimulating antibodies

TSBAb – *see* TSH-stimulation-blocking antibodies

TSH – *see* thyroid-stimulating hormone

TSH-binding-inhibitory immunoglobulins (TBII) – antibodies that inhibit the binding of TSH to its receptors on thyroid cells

TSH receptor antibodies – *see* thyrotropin receptor antibodies

TSH-stimulation-blocking antibodies (TSBAb) – antibodies that inhibit the binding of TSH to its receptor

TSI – *see* thyroid-stimulating immunoglobulins

tumor – a collection of abnormally growing cells that can be either benign or malignant

tumor marker – a chemical made by cancer cells that can be measured and used to follow the course of the cancer

ultrasound – a technique used to obtain pictures by bouncing sound waves off an object

ultrasound-guided thyroid biopsy – a technique using ultrasound to guide the placement of the needle in a thyroid nodule during a biopsy

undifferentiated thyroid cancer – a thyroid cancer whose cells look entirely different from normal cells; also called anaplastic cancer

Unithroid® – a brand-name levothyroxine preparation

vital signs – a patient's blood pressure, pulse rate, respiratory rate, and temperature

vitiligo – the patchy loss of skin pigmentation

warm nodule – a nodule that appears to take up the same amount of radioactive iodine as the surrounding thyroid tissue on a thyroid image or scan

whole body scan – images of the entire body taken after ingestion of radioactive iodine; also called total body scan

withdrawal scan – a whole body scan performed after a thyroid cancer patient discontinues levothyroxine approximately six weeks before the scan

INDEX

A

B

C

D

G

M

N

O

R

S

U

Notes

Notes

SHELDON RUBENFELD, M.D.

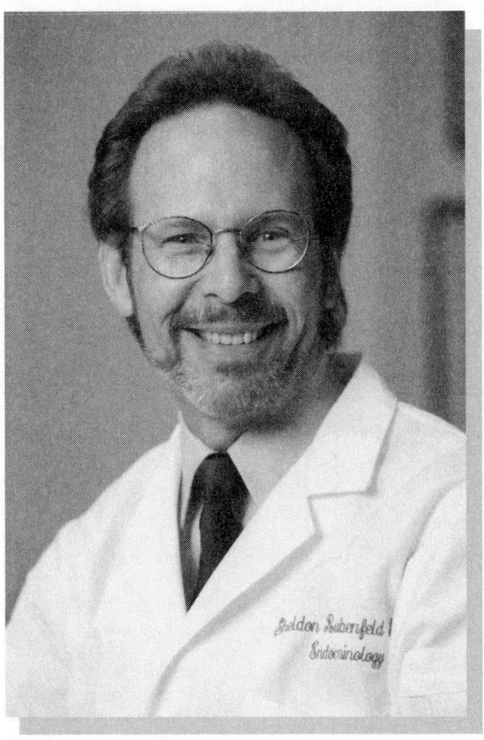

Sheldon Rubenfeld is a practicing thyroidologist who pioneered the use of fine needle aspiration biopsy of the thyroid in Texas. He is a Professor of Medicine at Baylor College of Medicine and a Fellow in both the American College of Endocrinology and in the American College of Physicians. His scientific articles have been published in many medical journals, and he is a member of numerous professional medical societies.

In a survey of nurses conducted by *Houston Metropolitan* magazine in 1992, Dr. Rubenfeld was voted the Best Endocrinologist in Houston. His peers selected Dr. Rubenfeld as the Top Endocrinologist in Houston in the first two editions of *Guide to Top Doctors* published by The Center for the Study of Services in 2000 and 2002. In addition, Dr. Rubenfeld is one of approximately 4% of the outstanding physicians in the United States listed by Best Doctors, an Internet medical service referral system. He, his wife, two children, and two hypothyroid dogs live in Houston.